The Electrocardiogram in Emergency and Acute Care

The Electrocardiogram in Emergency and Acute Care

Edited by

Korin B. Hudson, | MD, FAAEM, FACEP, CAQ-SM
Amita Sudhir, | MD, FACEP
George Glass, | MD, FACEP
William J. Brady, | MD, EMT-B, FACEP, FAAEM

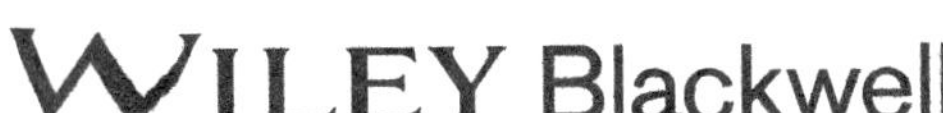

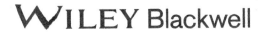

This edition first published 2023

Registered Offices
John Wiley & Sons, Inc., 111 River Street, Hoboken, NJ 07030, USA
John Wiley & Sons Ltd, The Atrium, Southern Gate, Chichester, West Sussex, PO19 8SQ, UK

For details of our global editorial offices, customer services, and more information about Wiley products visit us at www.wiley.com. Wiley also publishes its books in a variety of electronic formats and by print-on-demand. Some content that appears in standard print versions of this book may not be available in other formats.

Library of Congress Cataloging-in-Publication Data
Names: Hudson, Korin B., editor. | Sudhir, Amita, editor. | Glass, George (George F.), editor. | Brady, William, 1960- editor.
Title: The electrocardiogram in emergency and acute care / edited by Korin B. Hudson, Amita Sudhir, George Glass, William J. Brady.
Description: Hoboken, NJ : Wiley-Blackwell, 2023. | Includes index.
Identifiers: LCCN 2022037475 (print) | LCCN 2022037476 (ebook) | ISBN 9781119266891 (paperback) | ISBN 9781119266860 (Adobe PDF) | ISBN 9781119266792 (epub) | ISBN 9781119266938 (obook)
Subjects: MESH: Electrocardiography–methods | Emergencies | Critical Care | Heart Diseases–diagnosis
Classification: LCC RC683.5.E5 (print) | LCC RC683.5.E5 (ebook) | NLM WG 140 | DDC 616.1/207547–dc23/eng/20221110
LC record available at https://lccn.loc.gov/2022037475
LC ebook record available at https://lccn.loc.gov/2022037476

Cover Design: Wiley
Cover Image: © JY FotoStock/Shutterstock

Set in 9.5/12.5pt STIXTwoText by Straive, Pondicherry, India

SKY10048233_052323

Korin B. Hudson – I would like to thank my husband, Christopher for his unwavering support and patience; our children, Andrew and Alexander, for encouraging me and making me laugh; my parents, Kathy and David, for supporting and inspiring a career in academics; and to all my mentors and colleagues who demonstrate excellence in clinical medicine, education, and patient care every day. A special thanks to Bill Brady who has been a friend and mentor for 25 years and to our co-editors and authors who have helped to bring this project to life.

Amita Sudhir – Thank you to my husband, Aaron, my children, Anisha and Anand, and my parents, Romila and Sudhir for their support. Thank you also to Bill Brady for his educating me about ECGs during residency, and for his continued mentorship ever since.

George Glass – I'd like to thank my wife, Heather, for her constant support and my six kids who inspire me every day to be a little bit better. To my parents, for teaching the meaning of love and service. Finally, to my patients: thank you for teaching me every shift and trusting me to care for you. It's truly an honor.

William J. Brady – To my wife, King Brady, my partner and a truly amazing person, thank you for everything; to my children, Lauren (and husband Robert), Anne, Chip, and Katherine, and to my new grandson Eli, all my inspiration; to Amal Mattu, MD, my friend, fellow ECG nerd, and mentor in many ways, thank you for years of collaboration (past, present, and future); and finally to emergency healthcare providers across the globe, both prehospital- and hospital-based, for the your dedication to patient care and your expertise in emergency medicine . . . and for always "being there" when needed. And, of course, I want to thank my co-editors and authors for their hard work and expertise in the creation of this work.

Contents

[†] Deceased.

Editors and Contributors

Editors

Korin B. Hudson, MD, FACEP, FAAEM, CAQ-SM
Professor of Clinical Emergency Medicine
Department of Emergency Medicine
Georgetown University School of Medicine
MedStar Health
Team Physician: Georgetown Athletics, Washington Wizards, Washington Mystics
Consulting Physician: Washington Capitals, Maryland Jockey Club EMS
Washington, D.C. USA

Amita Sudhir, MD, FACEP
Associate Professor and Program Director of Emergency Medicine
University of Virginia Health System
Charlottesville, USA

George Glass, MD
Assistant Professor of Emergency Medicine
University of Virginia Health System
Charlottesville, USA

William J. Brady, MD, FACEP, FAAEM
Professor of Emergency Medicine, Medicine (Cardiovascular), and Nursing
Vice Chair for Faculty Affairs
The David A. Harrison Distinguished Educator
University of Virginia Health System
Charlottesville, USA
EMS Physician and Operational Medical Director
Albemarle County Fire Rescue
Charlottesville, USA

The editors would like to acknowledge and thank the following physician colleagues who served as editors on a prior text which served as the foundation for this volume. Their support is greatly appreciated and highly valued.

Dr. Robin Naples
Dr. Steven Mitchell
Dr. Jeffrey Ferguson
Dr. Robert Reiser

Contributors

J. Aidan Boswick, BA, EMT-B
Senior Director, Crossix Analytics Services, Veeva Systems Inc, New York, NY, USA

David Carlberg, MD
Associate Program Director, Georgetown Emergency Medicine Residency, Assistant Professor of Emergency Medicine, Georgetown University School of Medicine, Washington, DC, USA

Jeffrey D. Ferguson, MD, FACEP, FAEMS, NRP
Associate Professor, Department of Emergency Medicine, Virginia Commonwealth University, Richmond, VA, USA

Christopher P. Holstege, MD
Professor of Emergency Medicine and Paediatrics, Director, Division of Medical Toxicology, University of Virginia School of Medicine, Charlottesville, VA, USA

Erik Iszkula, MD
Clinical Assistant Professor of Emergency Medicine, University of Pittsburgh, Pittsburgh, PA, USA

Michael Levy, MD, FAEMS, FACEP, FACP
Chief Medical Director Anchorage Areawide EMS, Medical Director State of Alaska Emergency Programs, Anchorage, AK, USA

Steven H. Mitchell, MD, FACEP
Associate Professor, Department of Emergency Medicine, Medical Director, Harborview Medical Center, University of Washington, Seattle, WA, USA

Peter Monteleone, MD
Assistant Professor, Department of Internal Medicine, University of Texas at Austin Dell School of Medicine, Austin, TX, USA

Robin Naples, MD
Clinical Professor of Emergency Medicine, Sidney Kimmel Medical College at Thomas Jefferson University, Philadelphia, PA, USA

Francis X. Nolan Jr, BS, MICP[†]
Chief Medical Officer (Ret.), Anchorage Fire Department, Anchorage, AK, USA

Peter Pollak, MD
Consultant and Chair, Division of Interventional Coma Ischemia & Structural Heart Disease, Interventional Cardiology Specialist, Mayo Clinic Specialist, Jacksonville, FL, USA

Robert C. Reiser, MD
Associate Professor, Department of Emergency Medicine, University of Virginia, Charlottesville, VA, USA

Robert Rutherford, MD
Attending Physician, Swedish Medical Centre-Edmonds Campus, Edmonds, WA, USA

Courtney B. Saunders, MD
Department of Cardiology, Vidant Health, Greenville, NC, USA

Robert C. Schutt, MD
Department of Cardiology, Ascension Medical Group, Austin, TX, USA

Megan Starling, MD
Assistant Professor of Emergency Medicine, University of Virginia School of Medicine, Charlottesville, VA, USA; Attending Physician, Culpeper Memorial Hospital, Culpeper, USA

Richard B. Utarnachitt, MD, MS
Clinical Associate Professor, Medical Director, Airlift Northwest, Department of Emergency Medicine, University of Washington, Seattle, WA, USA

Alvin Wang, DO, NREMT-P
Emergency Medicine Specialist, Jefferson Health System, Philadelphia, PA; Chief, Emergency Medical Services, Jefferson Health System Northeast

Kelly Williamson, MD
Associate Professor and Assistant Program Director, Residency Program of Emergency Medicine, Northwestern University, Chicago, IL, USA

[†] Deceased.

Foreword

The electrocardiogram (ECG) is an essential instrument in the evaluation of a broad array of clinical conditions related to cardiac and non-cardiac disorders. The ECG is commonly used to evaluate the electrical and mechanical function of the heart, but the tracing can also be used to detect systemic disorders such as electrolyte disarray or toxic and metabolic abnormalities. The indications for an ECG encompass all aspects of medical care. In fact, the only contraindication to obtaining an ECG tracing is patient refusal. Acquisition of an ECG tracing is an easily learned skill, but the interpretation can be difficult and nuanced, thus requiring significant effort on the part of the learner to develop competence and confidence in the skill. Reading an ECG can be a high-stakes endeavor as incorrect interpretation can have profound consequences. Because the stakes are so high, it is incumbent on any health care providers responsible for ECG interpretation to study the full spectrum of clinical conditions that may be evident on the tracing.

The history of the ECG is a relatively recent one. An understanding that electrical impulses were produced by the heart was not known until the 1850s, but it took four more decades to develop instruments to measure the myocardial action potential. Willem Einthoven, a Dutch physiologist devoted the 1890s to gain an understanding the heart's electrical activity and how to best measure it. By 1902, he had devised the first ECG machine consisting of a fine (less than 3 μm in diameter) filament made of silver and quartz suspended in a powerful magnetic field. The electrical activity of the heart caused the string to resonate within the field and these vibrations were recorded photographically. The photographic plate was set to move at 25 mm per second, a convention that is used on paper tracings to this day. An obscure 1902 paper by Einthoven was the first known writing to describe the device. Einthoven was awarded the 1924 Nobel Prize for his invention.

The first machines commercially available were built between 1905 and 1907, were expensive, weighed 300 kg, and required a team of highly trained personnel to operate. Refinements of the machines brought down the size and weight, but doctors needed to transmit electrical impulses from the patient at the hospital to the machine in the laboratory off-site. Early clinical applications refined the understanding of, what was termed at the time as delirium cordis; which became known as atrial fibrillation. These early machines grew in popularity to aid clinicians in diagnosing cardiac arrhythmias, but information was limited owing to the fact that the machine had only the three leads.

By the 1920s, hypertrophy and infarction had been identified and described as the ECG became an essential medical device. In the 1930, angina pectoris was being identified by ECG, which led to an understanding of the ailment's vascular etiology. Precordial leads were developed, initially as a single lead, but later as multiple leads. In the 1940s, our contemporary precordial leads, V1 through V6 were standardized, and a refinement of the limb leads led to use of leads AVR, AVL, and AVF. During the 1950s and 1960s, acquisition of the ECG became widespread, and training in tracing interpretation became standard for medical students. The 1970s saw the introduction of computer interpretation to assist clinicians in identifying rate, rhythm, axis, hypertrophy, intervals, ischemia and infarction, but reading by a trained eye was (and is) still required.

By 1990, 50 million ECGs were performed annually in the United States, and time from first medical contact to ECG image acquisition became a measured performance standard for emergency medicine and EMS. By

2010, ECG acquisition an essential skill for EMS Basic Life Support personnel and ECG interpretation of STEMI was an essential skill for Paramedics. By 2020, the 300 kg behemoth from 1903 had been miniaturized to something that can be worn on a wrist.

The Electrocardiogram in Emergency and Acute Care is a text where readers are guided through a systematic approach to understanding the physics behind the ECG and are given clinical examples where the tracing can be interpreted to make a diagnosis. This approach places ECG interpretation within the reach of learners at every level making the text valuable to students learning about the ECG for the first time to experienced clinicians. Enjoy!

Robert E. O'Connor, M.D., MPH
Marcus L. Martin Distinguished Professor
and Chair of Emergency Medicine
University of Virginia
Daniel A. Griffith, DHA, MBA
Assistant Administrator for Operations
Department of Emergency Medicine
University of Virginia

Preface

Electrocardiographic monitoring is one of the most widely applied diagnostic tests in clinical medicine today; its first application to the patient occurs in the prehospital setting, in the clinician's office or by emergency medical services (EMS) . . . its use continues on into the hospital. The electrocardiogram, whether in monitor mode using single or multichannel rhythm monitoring or in diagnostic mode using the 12-lead ECG, is an amazing tool; it assists in establishing a diagnosis, ruling-out various ailments, guiding the diagnostic and management strategies in the evaluation, providing indication for certain therapies, offering risk assessment, and assessing end-organ impact of a syndrome. As noted in this impressive list of applications, the ECG provides significant insight regarding the patient's condition in a range of presentations, whether it be the chest pain patient with ST segment elevation myocardial infarction (STEMI), the patient in cardiac arrest with ventricular tachycardia, the poisoned patient with bradycardia, or the renal failure patient with rhythm and morphologic findings consistent with hyperkalemia, among many, many other presentations. This extremely useful tool is non-invasive, portable, inexpensive, quickly obtained, and easily performed. Yet, ECG interpretation is not easily performed and, in fact, requires considerable skill and experience as well as an awareness of the limitation surrounding its use.

This textbook has been prepared to assist clinicians who wish to learn, review, and refine the skills required to interpret the electrocardiogram and develop a deeper understanding of its use across the range of presentations and applications. This textbook is arranged into five sections. Section 1 is a brief introduction and review of the ECG in the clinical setting. Section 2 focuses on the electrocardiographic rhythm diagnosis, considering the electrocardiographic findings from an in-depth differential diagnostic perspective – in other words, rhythms with normal rates as well as bradycardia and tachycardia, allowing for the QRS complex width and regularity. Section 3 reviews the 12-lead ECG in patients suspected of acute coronary syndrome, including ST segment elevation myocardial infarction. Section 4 discusses the range of special presentations, patient populations, and uses of the electrocardiogram. Section 5 is a listing of various electrocardiographic findings, again from the differential diagnostic perspective; in this section, various rhythm and morphologic presentations are discussed, such as the narrow and wide complex tachycardias and ST segment elevation syndromes.

This textbook addresses the use of the ECG in its many forms by clinicians in a wide range of clinical settings. The novice electrocardiographer can use this text as his or her primary ECG reference; additionally, the experienced interpreter can use this textbook to expand his or her knowledge base. This work stresses the value of the ECG in the range of clinical situations encountered daily by health care providers – it illustrates the appropriate applications of the electrocardiogram in emergency and acute care scenarios.

Most importantly, this textbook is written by clinicians for clinicians, with an emphasis on the reality of the patient care. I and my co-editors and authors have enjoyed its creation – we hope that you, the clinician, will not only enjoy its content but also find it of value in the care of your patients. We thank you for what you do every day.

William J. Brady, MD
Charlottesville, USA

Section I

The ECG in Clinical Care

1

Clinical Applications of the Electrocardiogram

George Glass

Department of Emergency Medicine, University of Virginia School of Medicine, Charlottesville, VA, USA

The electrocardiogram (ECG) is a useful tool for identifying and evaluating abnormal heart rhythms, underlying heart disease, current or past myocardial infarction, and various other metabolic conditions. It is used ubiquitously by clinicians and has proven to be one of the most valuable diagnostic tools in modern medicine. The ECG is a safe, non-invasive, and relatively inexpensive to obtain. It is particularly useful in identifying patients with acute ischemia and in identifying abnormal heart rhythms in patients with known risk factors for heart disease. The ECG may also provide timely information that can aid in early diagnostic or therapeutic decision making; for example, detection of peaked T waves in a critically ill patient with end stage renal disease may prompt timely and life-saving treatment for hyperkalemia prior to the availability of laboratory results.

ECG interpretation is an important and useful skill for any clinician, and skillful ECG interpretation requires appropriate attention and training. Section 1 of this book will cover the basics of such ECG interpretation.

Standard ECG Formatting and the Normal Electrocardiogram

In order to identify abnormal, we must first recognize "normal." A normal ECG in the standard 12-lead ECG format is shown in Figure 1.1. In simple terms, the ECG tracing represents a time vs. intensity graph of the electrical signal (in mV) as measured by surface electrodes placed on the patient, though technically, the values for augmented leads – avR, avL, and avF – are calculated, not measured. At standard recording speed, each small box on the x-axis (1 mm of ECG paper) represents 0.04 seconds (40 msec) and each large box represents 0.2 seconds (200 ms). Each small box on the y-axis represents 1 mV.

As cardiac myocytes depolarize, the subsequent summation of electrical current is detected by electrodes placed on a patient's body. A positive deflection in any given lead represents that the current detected is traveling in the direction of the positive terminal of that lead. Conversely, a negative deflection represents that the dominant electrical current is traveling away from the positive terminal of that lead.

ECG Components, Durations, and Intervals

The ECG recording of a standard cardiac cycle largely consists of several distinct phases: namely, the p-wave, QRS-complex, and T-wave. The p-wave represents atrial depolarization. This is followed by the QRS complex, representing ventricular depolarization. Finally, the T-wave represents ventricular repolarization. ECG "segments" comprise the portions of the ECG between these components. The PR segment consists of the portion of the ECG from the end of the P wave to the initiation of the QRS complex. The ST segment comprises the portion of the ECG from the end of the QRS to the beginning of the T-wave. The TP segment includes the portion of the ECG signal from the end of the T-wave to the beginning of the P-wave.

The time (or distance along the y-axis) comprising the individual ECG components are known as "durations" or "intervals" (Figure 1.2). A table of normal intervals is seen in Table 1.1.

The Electrocardiogram in Emergency and Acute Care, First Edition.
Edited by Korin B. Hudson, Amita Sudhir, George Glass, and William J. Brady.

Systematic Interpretation of the ECG

It is helpful to approach reading the ECG in a systematic fashion as to assure a comprehensive evaluation. Failure to do so may result in missed findings. For example, an ECG with findings obviously and dramatically consistent with ST-elevation myocardial infarction might also demonstrate a high degree heart block. This finding may be more subtle and easily missed, especially if one is otherwise occupied with the care of a clinically ill

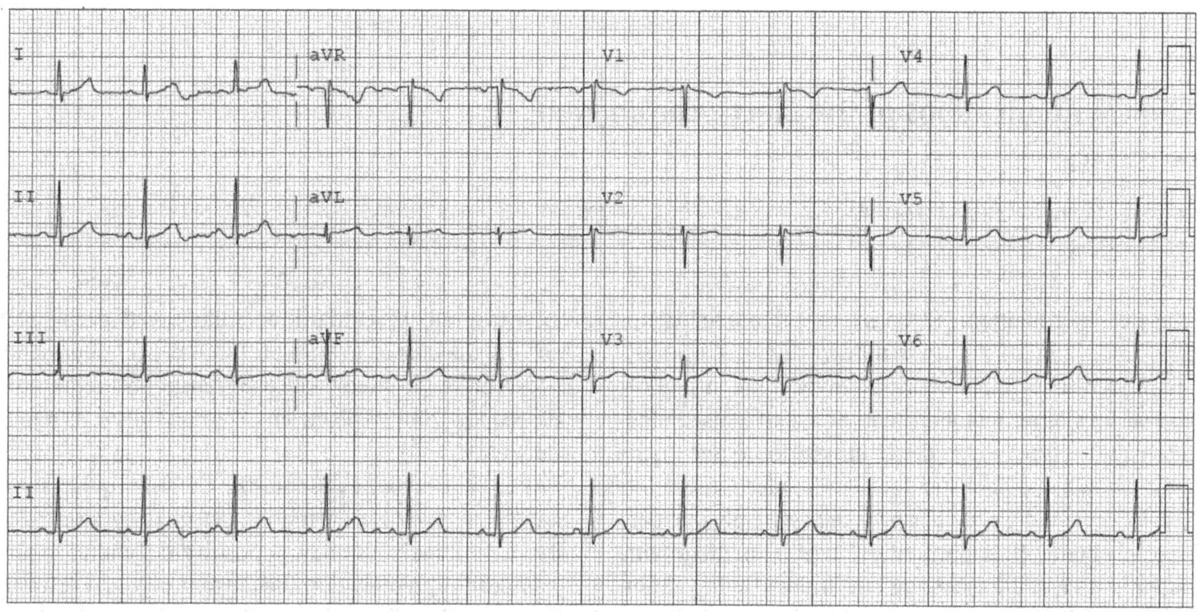

Figure 1.1 A normal 12-lead electrocardiogram.

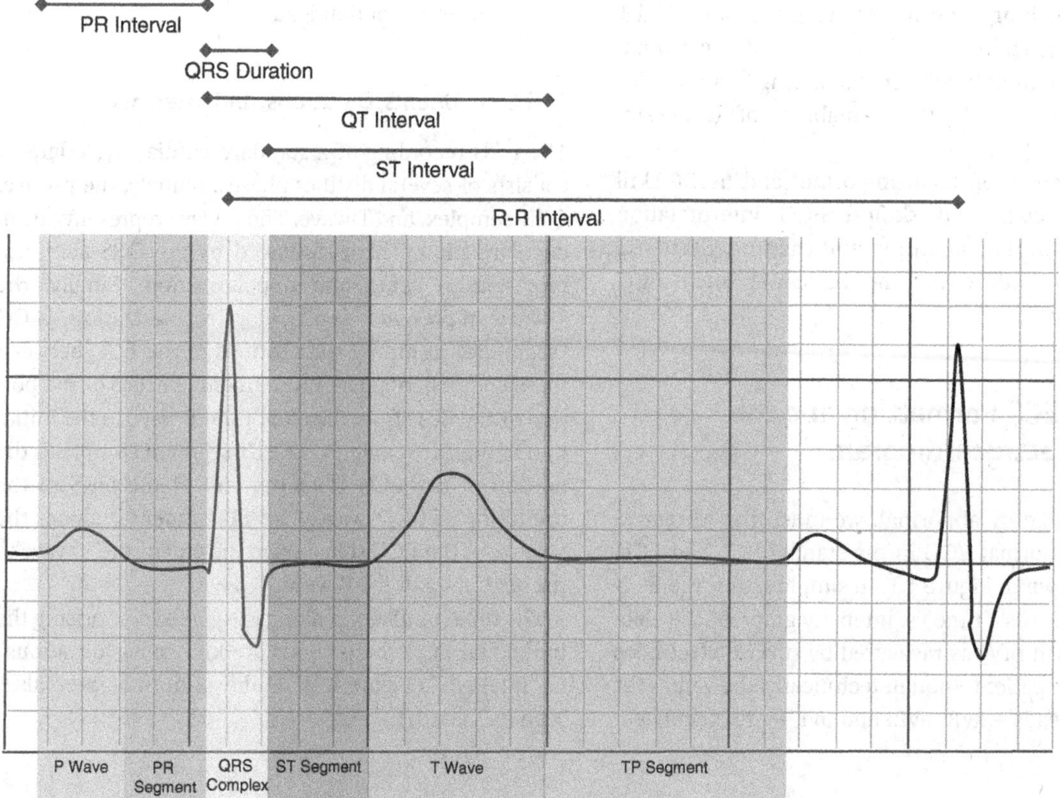

Figure 1.2 Normal cardiac cycle segments and intervals.

Table 1.1 Normal ECG Intervals.

ECG component	Normal duration
P-wave	≤120 msec
PR interval	≥120 and ≤200 msec
QRS duration	Usually ≤100 msec ≥120 msec in bundle branch block
QT interval	Prolonged QT is normally defined by a corrected QT (QTc) >440 msec $QTc = \frac{QT}{\sqrt{RR\ Interval}}$

patient. Appropriate identification of an abnormal rhythm may profoundly influence clinical decision making, however, and is key to optimal patient care.

Rate

A normal heart rate in the adult patient is generally between 60 and 100 beats per minute. Rates faster than this represents tachycardia, whereas slower rates represent bradycardia. A simple method for calculating the rate is to count the number of large squares between two QRS complexes and then divide 300 by this number. For example, if two QRS complexes are four large squares apart, then the calculated rate is 300/4, or about 75 beats per minutes. Note that this method is only effective for regularly spaced QRS complexes – in the case of irregular spacing (atrial fibrillation, or frequent premature contractions, for example), it is more appropriate to average the rate over a longer time period. One way to do this is to count the number of QRS complexes on a 10-second rhythm strip, then multiply this by six to determine the average rate over that 10-second interval.

Rhythm

Sinus rhythm is present if there is a p-wave preceding every QRS complex, as well as a QRS complex following every p-wave. A normal rate, combined with sinus rhythm, is aptly called "normal sinus rhythm." Deviations from a normal rate are termed either sinus tachycardia or sinus bradycardia. P waves should generally be upright in leads I, II, and III. A deviation from this may indicate an ectopic atrial rhythm or another atrial dysrhythmia (atrial flutter, for example).

The appropriate identification of the underlying ECG rhythm is essential for appropriate care. Sinus bradycardia, for example, is seldom pathologic and usually does not require emergency intervention. Bradycardia associated with a Mobitz II second-degree or third-degree heart block, however, represents a patient at high risk for decompensation. Atrial fibrillation and supraventricular tachycardia (SVT) can both present with rapid, narrow complex tachycardia, but acute management and follow-up needs may differ (Figure 1.3).

ECG Orientation and Axis

Utilizing standard ECG lead placement, the 12-lead ECG will provide information in six leads in a vertical or coronal plane (frontal or limb leads – I, II, III, aVL, aVR, aVF), as well as six in the axial plane (precordial leads – V1 through V6). The major direction of QRS vector in the frontal plane is commonly referred to as the ECG "axis." This can be calculated via several methods. The simplest method is to look at leads I and aVF. A positive deflection in the QRS complex in a given lead indicates an axis in the same direction as that lead. A positive deflection in leads I and avF would therefore indicate an axis between 0 and 90°. The relative magnitude of the deflection can help indicate the amplitude of the true ECG "vector" in the direction of that lead. For example, a large, positive deflection in lead I and a near isoelectric deflection in lead aVF would indicate a true EKG vector of about 0°. A normal ECG will have an axis of −30° to 90°. Axis deviation of −30° to −90° is considered "left axis deviation," whereas deviation of 90°–180° is considered "right axis deviation." An axis of −90° to 180° is indeterminate (could be due to severe right or left axis deviation) and is termed extreme axis deviation (Figure 1.4).

Axis deviation is helpful in diagnosing left fascicular blocks, right and left ventricular hypertrophy, or certain toxicologic and metabolic pathologies. A list of common causes of axis deviation are seen in Table 1.2.

Intervals

Abnormal ECG intervals may not be immediately obvious on a cursory look at the ECG. As such, they are easily overlooked, and skilled clinicians should make a concerted effort to look for such abnormalities. Deviations from normal intervals can be indicative of pathologies of the conduction system (e.g. heart block, long or short QT syndromes, or Wolf-Parkinson-White syndrome).

Morphology

Deviations in morphology can occur in any segment of the ECG and may indicate a wide array of pathologies. The ST-segment, for example, should be closely

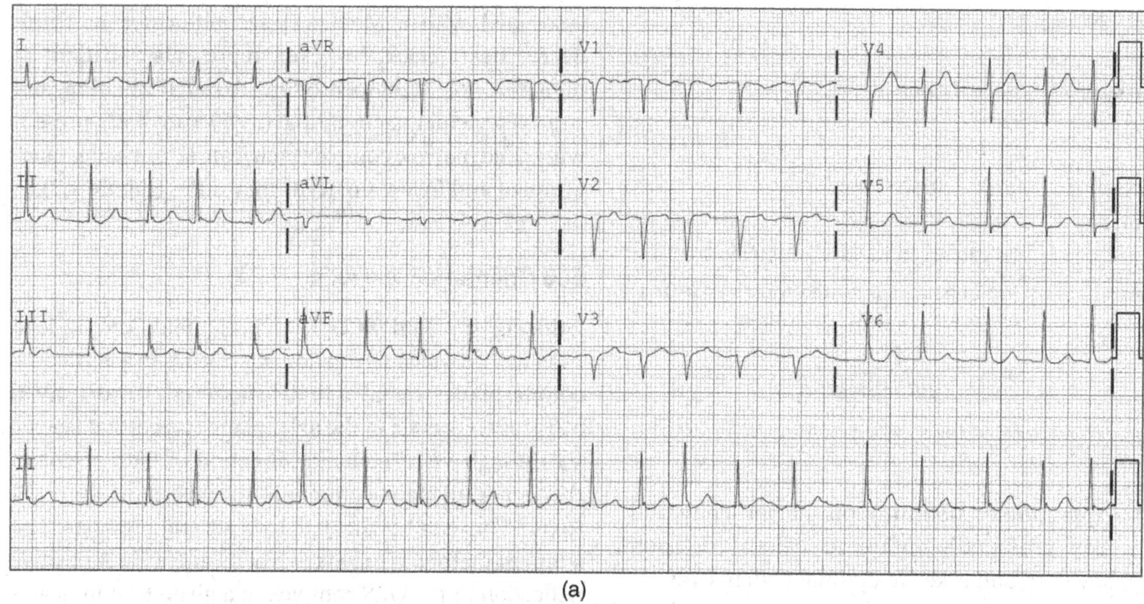

(a)

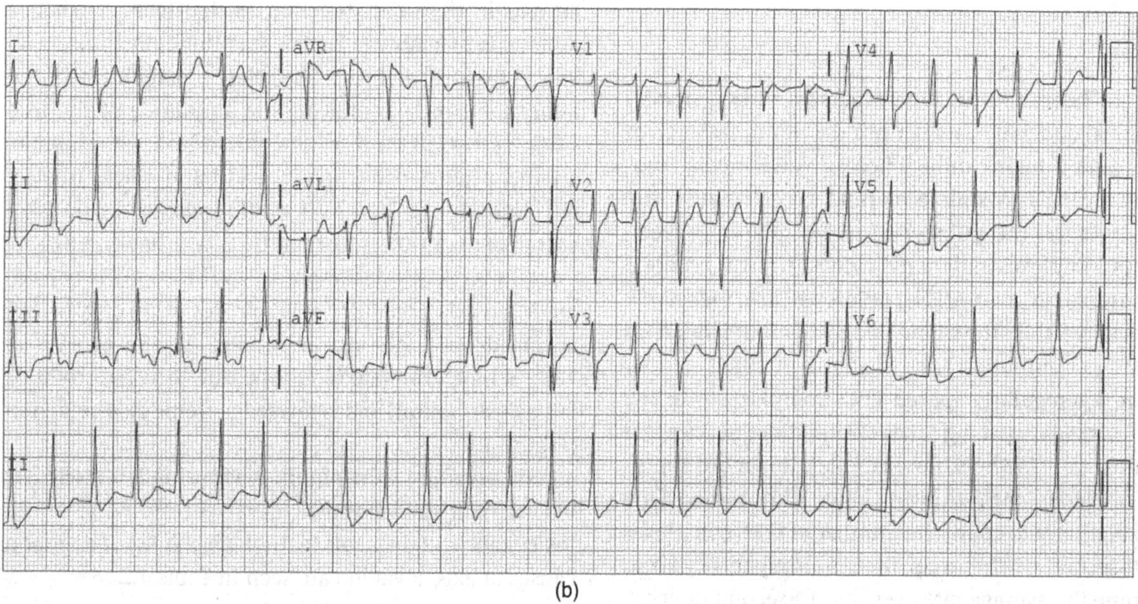

(b)

Figure 1.3 Rapid, narrow complex tachycardia. (a) Demonstrates an irregular rhythm with rapid rate and no discernable p waves, most consistent with atrial fibrillation. (b) Demonstrates a regular, narrow complex tachycardia. Note the p-waves in leads II and III that follow the QRS complex, most consistent with SVT with retrograde p-waves.

scrutinized in patients with suspected acute coronary syndrome (ACS), as ST-elevation and ST-depression may both be indicative of acute myocardial ischemia. ST-elevation myocardial infarction (STEMI), for example, is specifically defined as the presence of ST-elevation of a specific magnitude in two anatomically contiguous leads.

Another key morphologic change, "peaked T-waves," may be the first indicator a clinician may have of life-threatening hyperkalemia. Specific morphologic changes and their corresponding clinical findings will be discussed in later chapters.

Common Indications and Clinical Applications

Syncope

The ECG represents critical data in the evaluation of syncope. In fact, in addition to a thoughtful history and physical exam, the ECG may be the most important diagnostic test in this setting. Many causes of sudden cardiac death may present with an initial episode of syncope and the ECG may be diagnostic. Careful interpretation of the ECG can assist in risk stratification.

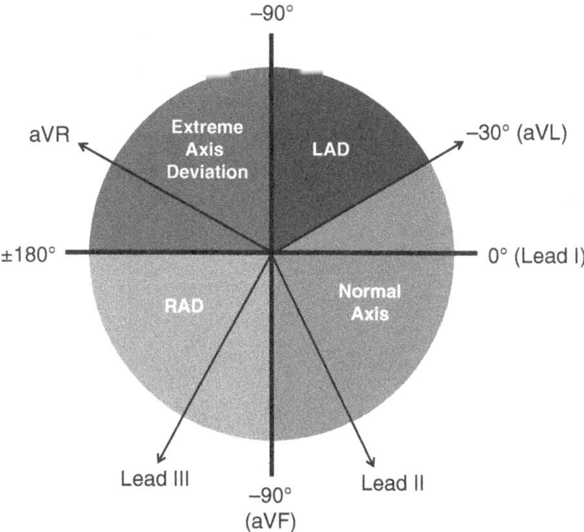

Figure 1.4 ECG axis determination.

Table 1.2 Causes of axis deviation.

Potential causes of ECG axis deviation	
Right axis deviation	• Right ventricular hypertrophy • RV strain • Left posterior fascicular block • Wolff–Parkinson–White syndrome • Lateral wall ischemia/infarcation • Congenital heart defects (ASD, dextrocardia)
Left axis deviation	• Left ventricular hypertrophy • Left bundle branch block • Left anterior fascicular block • Wolff–Parkinson–White syndrome • Inferior wall ischemia/infarcation • Hyperkalemia • Congenital heart defects (double outlet right ventricle, tricuspid atresia, corrected transposition of the great arteries)

Conditions such as prolonged QT syndrome, Brugada syndrome, and hypertrophic cardiomyopathy may not provide many symptoms or additional clinical clues prior to the development of a fatal arrythmia. As such, the ECG is crucial in the diagnosis of these entities and a screening ECG should be obtained in all patients with unexplained syncope. Prolonged monitoring of the ECG tracing, through a rhythm strip, telemetry, or ambulatory monitoring (Holter monitor) may provide additional information, especially if paroxysmal rhythm abnormalities are suspected. Section 2 of this book will cover specific cardiac rhythms and dysrhythmias with their corresponding ECG and clinical findings.

Chest Pain

The ECG is used ubiquitously in the evaluation of patients with chest pain and most patients with chest pain should have a 12-lead ECG performed. Anatomically oriented ST-elevation is diagnostic for STEMI and an indication for acute reperfusion therapy (O'Gara and Kushner 2013). Additionally, other ECG changes, such as ST segment depression, left ventricular hypertrophy (LVH), or other repolarization changes can be indicative of heart disease and are useful for risk stratification in patients with suspected ischemic cardiac disease. As such, the ECG is vital component of the HEART score, a validated clinical decision tool useful in risk stratification of such patients (Six and Backus 2008). Dynamic ECG changes – that is, variability in ST segment deviation – can also be indicative of an evolving process, such as ongoing ischemia or changes associated with ischemia and subsequent reperfusion. Such changes may prompt further diagnostic testing or consideration of early intervention, potentially reducing the impact of ongoing ischemia and associated morbidity. The ECG may also be diagnostic of other causes such of chest pain, such as pericarditis, usually characterized by diffuse ST-segment elevation with associated PR-segment depression. Section 3 of the book will cover the use of the ECG in the diagnosis of ACS.

Shortness of Breath

Shortness of breath, or dyspnea, is common patient complaint. Initial evaluation may include an ECG, which may reveal signs of lung disease or underlying cardiac disease which may be contributing to the patient's symptoms. For example, patients with pulmonary embolism will often present with sinus tachycardia and may have other, more specific findings, including the "S1Q3T3 pattern" – that is, the presence of S-waves in lead I, and Q waves with associated T-wave inversion in lead III – an indicator of associated heart strain (Digby 2015). Other findings, such as right axis deviation, may be indicative of right ventricular hypertrophy, which could be due to chronic lung conditions (cor pulmonale) or valvular disease (mitral stenosis). Shortness of breath may also be associated with certain dysrhythmias or ACS.

Other Indications

Specific ECG findings may also be noted in certain clinical contexts, including certain electrolyte disorders (e.g. hyper- and hypokalemia, hyper- and hypocalcemia), use of therapeutic agents (e.g. digoxin), or ingestion or overdose on toxins or medications (e.g. tricyclic antidepressant overdose). The findings of the "normal" ECG may also be altered in patients with certain conditions such as Wolff–Parkinson–White Syndrome or in patients with an implanted pacemaker. These special situations will be covered in Section 4. The ECG may also be significantly altered in hypothermia, intracranial hemorrhage or stroke, and trauma. A list of selected examples of non-coronary pathology that may be seen on ECG is listed in Table 1.3. Patients presenting with stable wide complex tachycardia (Figure 1.5) or bradyarrythmias may also benefit from ECG in order to elucidate the nature of the presenting dysrhythmia (Section 5).

Table 1.3 Abnormal ECG findings not related to coronary pathology.

Pericarditis
- Diffuse non-anatomical ST segment elevation without reciprocal changes
- Diffuse PR segment depression
- Isolated ST segment depression and PR elevation in aVR

Pericardial tamponade
- Electrical alternans
- Low QRS complex voltage
- Diffuse PR segment depression hypothermia
- Osborn "J" waves
- Bradycardias and AV blocks
- Prolongation/widening of PR interval, QRS complex, and QT interval
- Atrial fibrillation with slow ventricular response

Hyperkalemia
- Diffuse non-anatomical peaked T waves
- Widening of PR interval and QRS complex widths

Central nervous system (CNS) events
- Diffuse, deep T wave inversions
- Minor ST segment elevations in leads with T wave inversions overdose and intoxication
- Rhythm disturbances
- Widened QRS complex
- Prolonged QT interval

Source: Reproduced from Brady et al., 2013/John Wiley & Sons.

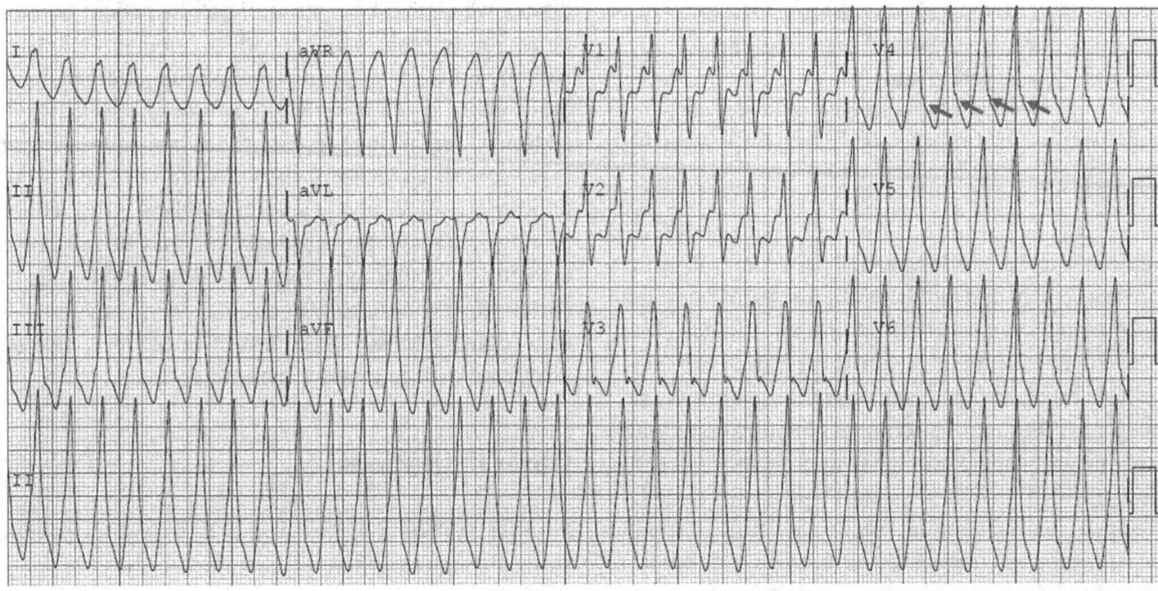

Figure 1.5 Wide complex tachycardia. The presence of retrograde P-waves (arrows) and positive concordance (similar, upright QRS axis) throughout the precordial leads is highly suggestive of ventricular tachycardia.

Clinical Context

The ECG does not exist in a vacuum; each ECG belongs to a patient with a corresponding clinical history. Appropriate ECG interpretation must occur within this context. For example, ST-elevation discovered incidentally on the ECG of an asymptomatic 18-year-old male undergoing a sports physical is clinically vastly different than a similar finding on the ECG of an elderly, obese patient with ongoing chest pain and diaphoresis. While one might split hairs about the inflection point of the ST segment and concavity or convexity of the ST segment, clinically it is highly likely that the finding in the first case represents benign early repolarization (BER), whereas the second scenario represents ACS. Clinicians who fail to interpret the ECG within the clinical context in which they were obtained do so at their own peril. The ECG contains an enormous amount of information pertaining to cardiac function. When used appropriately, the ECG is an invaluable tool, and expertise in its interpretation will undoubtedly enhance clinical care.

References

Digby, G.C. (2015). The value of electrocardiographic abnormalities in the prognosis of pulmonary embolism: a consensus paper. *Ann. Noninvasive Electrocardiol.* 20 (3): 207–223.

O'Gara, P.T. and Kushner, F.-G. (2013). ACCF/AHA guideline for the management of ST-elevation mycoardial infarction: a report of the American College of Cardiology Foundation/American Heart Association Task Force. *J. Am. Coll. Cardiol.* 61 (4): e78–e140.

Six, A.J. and Backus, B. (2008). Chest pain in the emergency room: value of the HEART score. *Neth. Heart J.* 16 (6): 191–196.

2

Clinical Impact of the Electrocardiogram (ECG)

Robert C. Schutt[1], William J. Brady[2], Korin B. Hudson[3], and Steven H. Mitchell[4]

[1] *Department of Cardiology, Ascension Medical Group, Austin, TX, USA*
[2] *Departments of Emergency Medicine and Medicine, University of Virginia School of Medicine, Charlottesville, VA, USA*
[3] *Department of Emergency Medicine, Georgetown University School of Medicine, Medstar Health, Washington, DC, USA*
[4] *Department of Emergency Medicine, University of Washington School of Medicine, Seattle, WA, USA*

The impact of the electrocardiogram (ECG) on clinical care is wide ranging and significant. The ECG is a primary tool for evaluating the unstable patient and a useful tool in the assessment of the stable patient. The ECG aids in clinical decision making for patients experiencing primary cardiac pathology. This includes conduction disturbances, acute coronary syndrome (ACS), and also such non-cardiac pathology as pulmonary embolism (PE), metabolic disarray, and poisoning or overdose. The use of the ECG is widespread and requires every clinician to work toward competence in the efficient and accurate use and evaluation of the ECG.

Management of the Patient with Dysrhythmia

From its inception, rudimentary ECGs have been used to diagnose and treat rhythm disturbances. There are now well-established treatment algorithms for both prehospital and in hospital treatment of life-threatening cardiac dysrhythmias, and the ECG findings are paramount in these algorithms. The rapid diagnosis and management of life-threatening dysrhythmias is often based on the interpretation of the single-lead ECG (also called a rhythm strip).

A significant impact of the ECG and an area of continued research is in the treatment of sudden cardiac death. Symptomatic dysrhythmias may occur both outside the hospital and in patients who are under inpatient care. Sudden cardiac death is a commonly encountered extreme example of symptomatic dysrhythmia in which the ECG plays a pivotal role in assessment and management. Non-cardiac arrest rhythms are also frequently identified, especially in hospitalized patients. These rhythm possibilities range from bradycardia to tachycardia, with and without conduction block. Clearly, the single-lead ECG enables the clinician to diagnose the rhythm and initiate the most appropriate care based on the ECG information as well as the patient's clinical situation.

Management of the Patient with Acute Coronary Syndrome

Beyond the recognition and treatment of cardiac rhythm disturbances, the ECG has impacted the care of patients with ACS with both the single- and the 12-lead ECG. The 12-lead ECG (as opposed to laboratory evaluation with a cardiac enzyme assay such as troponin) is the primary tool for identifying patients with ST segment elevation myocardial infarction (STEMI). In STEMI, the ECG rapidly identifies patients who are in emergent need of revascularization. The ECG is used in both the prehospital and in hospital environments to detect STEMI and has been shown to favorably impact the time to revascularization. Also, when used in the out of hospital setting, including clinics, urgent cares and Emergency Medical Services (EMS), the ECG may detect ischemic changes that resolve before the patient arrives at the emergency department and provides a valuable snapshot of an ischemic event. The benefits of out of hospital ECG are realized with little increase in time to transport, even in the emergency setting. Furthermore, many EMS systems have the capability to transmit the 12-lead ECG for

The Electrocardiogram in Emergency and Acute Care, First Edition.
Edited by Korin B. Hudson, Amita Sudhir, George Glass, and William J. Brady.

"real-time" interpretation by a physician. This allows for rapid consultation with an EP and/or cardiologist who can make transport and treatment decisions including planning for reperfusion strategies even before the patient arrives to the hospital.

The interpretation of the 12-lead ECG, however, is a skill that requires advanced training and practice in order to assure proficiency. Inaccurate interpretation of the ECG has been shown to impact the care of patients with ACS. In particular, clinicians must be particularly aware of ominous changes of the ST segment and the T wave. Inaccurate interpretation of the ECG, including the lack of recognition of ST segment and T wave abnormalities can have grave consequences for the patients and potentially expose them to inappropriate and dangerous therapies. A significant limitation of the 12-lead ECG in the evaluation of the ACS patient is that it has rather poor sensitivity (i.e. often falsely negative) for the diagnosis of myocardial infarction. The ECG initially suggests acute infarction in only 50% of patients ultimately found to have an acute myocardial infarction.

Single-lead ECG monitoring is also of significant importance in the ACS patient – not aimed at the detection of ST segment and T wave abnormalities associated with ACS but rather for the detection of complicating rhythm disturbances, such as sinus bradycardia, complete heart block, and ventricular fibrillation.

Management of non-ACS Presentations

The impact of the ECG has been extended beyond the diagnosis and treatment of primary cardiac pathologies. In the patient with chest pain or dyspnea, the ECG can suggest alternative diagnoses to ACS; for instance, the ECG can suggest PE. Historically, the "S1Q3T3 pattern" (S wave in lead I, Q wave in lead III, and T wave inversion in lead III) is classically associated with PE (Figure 2.1). It is important to note that these changes suggest right ventricular "strain" directly, rather than

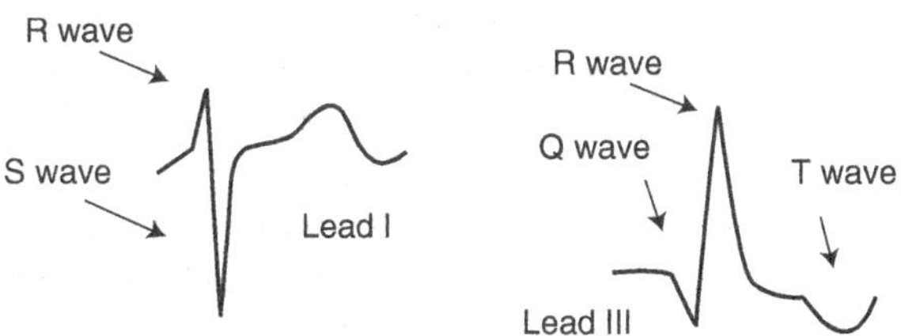

Figure 2.1 Findings of right heart strain in pulmonary embolism. The "S1Q3T3 pattern."

PE. S1-Q3-T3 is typically present only in large PE and the absence cannot be used to exclude the diagnosis.

In the setting of poisoning or overdose, the ECG is used not only as a diagnostic study to rule in the condition but also as an indicator of risk to guide the intensity of therapy. For instance, cardiac sodium channel and potassium efflux blockade will produce worrisome ECG findings, such as widening of the QRS complex and prolongation of the QT interval, respectively. These findings can occur in patients taking prescribed medications as well as in the patient who has overdosed. In the setting of tricyclic antidepressant (TCA) overdose (a potent sodium channel blocking agent), an R wave (positive deflection of the QRS complex) that is 3 mm above the isoelectric line in lead aVR has been shown to be predictive of significant cardiotoxicity including the development of seizures and ventricular arrhythmias (Figure 2.2).

The ECG also impacts the care of patients with underlying metabolic or electrolyte disorders such as hyperkalemia. In hyperkalemia, T waves become peaked as the serum potassium level increases (Figure 2.3). Left

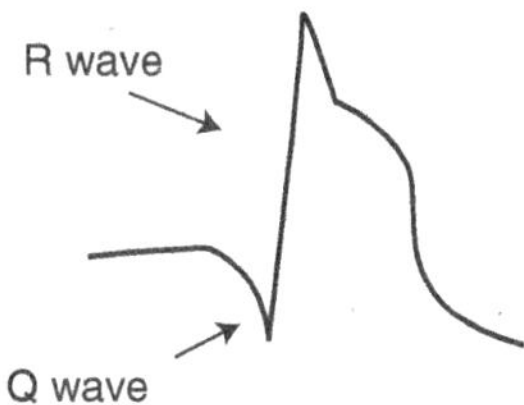

Figure 2.2 Lead aVR with terminal rightward axis; R wave is ≥3 mm above isoelectric line in a patient with significant TCA toxicity.

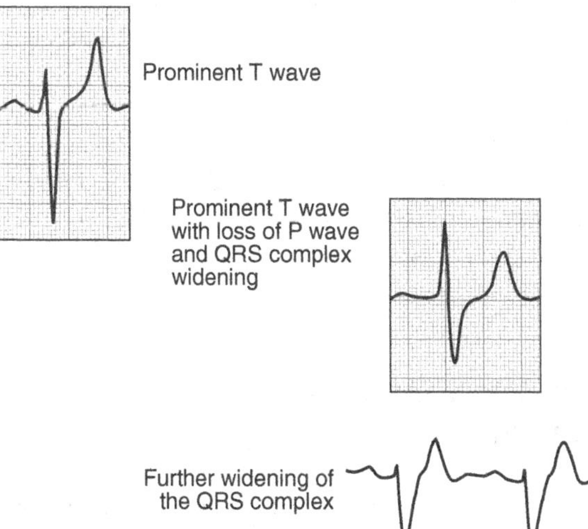

Figure 2.3 Prominent T waves and widened QRS complex of hyperkalemia.

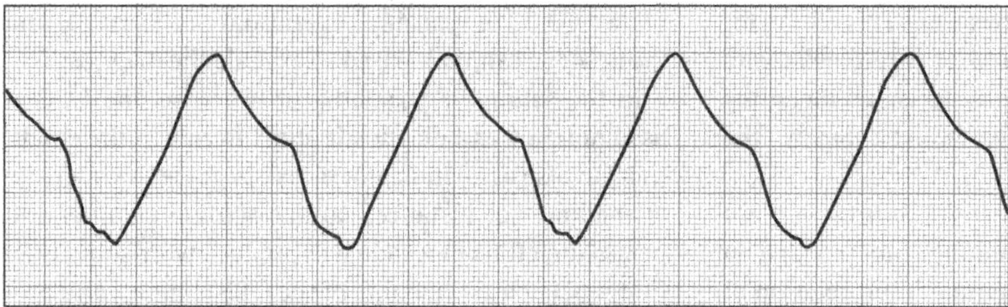

Figure 2.4 Sine wave pattern in untreated hyperkalemia – this rhythm is termed the *sinoventricular rhythm*. Most often, this rhythm has a slow ventricular response.

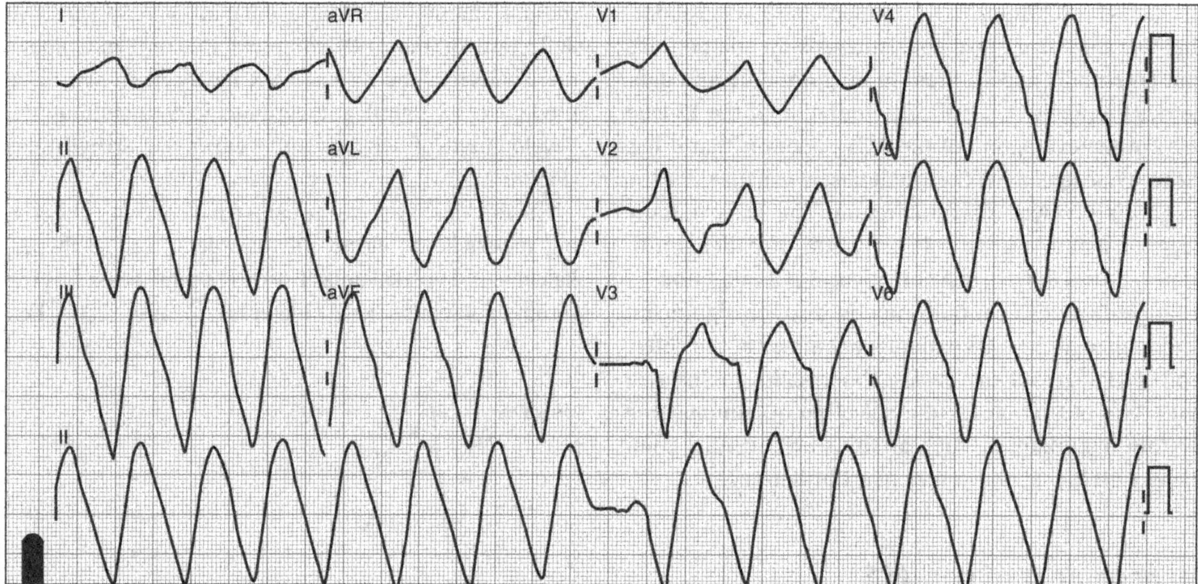

Figure 2.5 ECG of a patient with an elevated potassium level of 7.5 mEq/dl; this is another example of the sinoventricular rhythm of severe hyperkalemia – in this case, the ventricular response is more rapid.

untreated, rising serum potassium level leads to changes in the P wave and QRS complex (Figure 2.3). The PR interval will lengthen and the QRS complex progressively widens (Figure 2.3); ultimately, the ECG continues to change, terminating as a sine wave when the P wave (Figures 2.4 and 2.5), the QRS complex, and the T wave fuse, forming a sine wave – this finding is called the *sinoventricular rhythm of severe hyperkalemia* (Figures 2.4 and 2.5). The ECG provides important information to guide therapy.

Ambulatory Electrocardiogram Monitoring

One significant problem for evaluating patients with suspected dysrhythmia is that frequently dysrhythmias are transient. It is not uncommon for a patient to no longer have evidence of a rhythm abnormality when the patient is evaluated at the emergency department or the physician's office. It is often exceptionally difficult to determine if symptoms such as chest pain or syncope are related to a cardiac dysrhythmia unless there is electrocardiographic evidence of a rhythm abnormality at the time the patient is symptomatic. With this in mind, it is extremely important that any evidence of a dysrhythmia or electrocardiographic abnormality be included in the medical record for review by all treating clinicians. Simply recording/printing an abnormal ECG in certain circumstances may avoid unnecessary, expensive, and potentially invasive diagnostic testing.

To solve the problem of evaluating intermittent dysrhythmias, devices to record both continuous and intermittent ECG readings were developed, which allow the patient to continue with day-to-day activities at home with ECG monitoring available. This technology is referred to as *ambulatory ECG monitoring*.

Computer Interpretation of the Electrocardiogram

Significant advances in detecting and managing abnormal ECG findings occurred in conjunction with the development of the microprocessor. As computer algorithms were developed that could reliably detect and identify cardiac dysrhythmias, the ability to treat abnormal rhythms was expanded significantly. One significant advance is that a layperson with little to no medical training can now provide definitive treatment for patients in cardiac arrest with ventricular tachycardia (VT) or ventricular fibrillation using an automated external defibrillator (commonly referred to as an AED). Locations with widespread AED availability have seen a significant survival benefit associated with the use of this device. However, the computer algorithms are not infallible and in particular when considering the evaluation of the 12-lead ECG, the clinician should follow the steps outlined here to arrive at their own interpretation of the rhythm and its significance rather than relying solely on the printed computer interpretation.

With advancement in technology, artificial cardiac pacemakers and implantable cardioverter-defibrillators (ICDs) were developed that could both identify and treat a wide variety of dysrhythmias. Although the initial cardiac pacemakers did not detect or interpret the ECG rhythm, devices now interpret and respond to ECG changes. Pacemakers have evolved from single-chamber devices that only produced a repeated asynchronous discharge from the right ventricle to newer devices with leads in three chambers that can monitor and respond to the sensed cardiac rhythm, equipped with adjustable timing to synchronize ventricular contraction and mechanisms to sense metabolic needs and increase heart rate with activity. Pacemakers are used to treat heart rates that are too slow (Figure 2.6), and may also be used to synchronize ventricular contraction in patients with both heart failure and ventricular conduction delay, which results in improved cardiac function and reduced mortality in select patient groups.

An ICD is a device similar to a pacemaker that has the ability to cardiovert and defibrillate a patient who has VT or ventricular fibrillation (Figure 2.7). Although devices that have a combination of an advanced pacemaker with an ICD exist, the use of the term pacemaker does not imply the presence of an ICD, but all ICDs usually have at least a rudimentary pacemaker function to treat unexpected bradydysrhythmias. One significant feature of an ICD is that it can painlessly terminate VT with antitachycardia pacing (also called ATP), thereby avoiding cardioversion/defibrillation. In ATP, a short burst (e.g. 8 s) of pacing at a rate slightly faster than the underlying VT is delivered by the ICD, which frequently (~75–90% of the time) will terminate the episode of VT without defibrillation. As repeated defibrillations can be traumatic for the patient, typically the cardiologist will program the ICD to deliver a few rounds of ATP before the device delivers a shock. An ICD is most beneficial in patients with heart failure or for patients with reduced cardiac function after a myocardial infarction.

Although ICDs clearly save lives, significant anxiety is common following repeated defibrillations, and many patients with a poor prognosis would rather not experience repeated painful shocks at the time of their death. In patients experiencing repeated shocks (e.g. a patient in VT storm), it is certainly reasonable and humane to administer an amnestic agent (such as midazolam) if no medical contraindications exist. It is also important to know that placing a magnet over a pacemaker or ICD will typically alter the function of the device but will not completely turn off the device. Although device response to inhibition with a magnet may vary between devices and can be individually

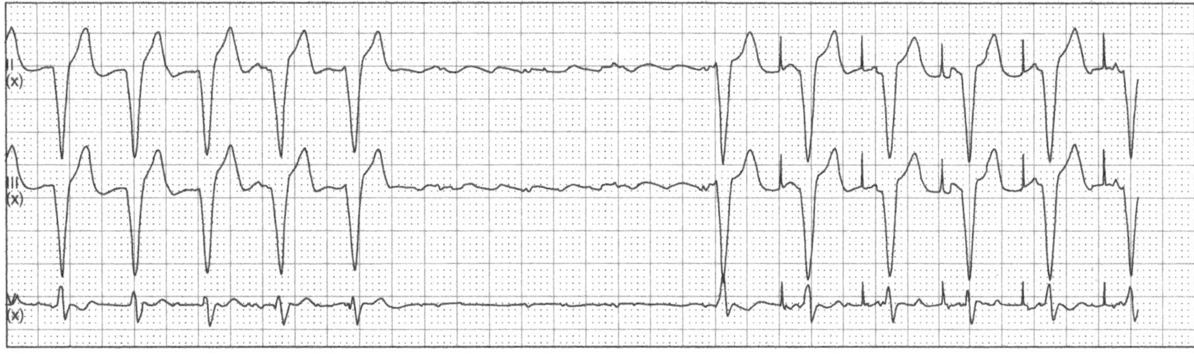

Figure 2.6 Pacemaker responding to bradycardia in a patient with a 3-s pause. Note the atrial pacemaker spikes present before the QRS complexes after the pause.

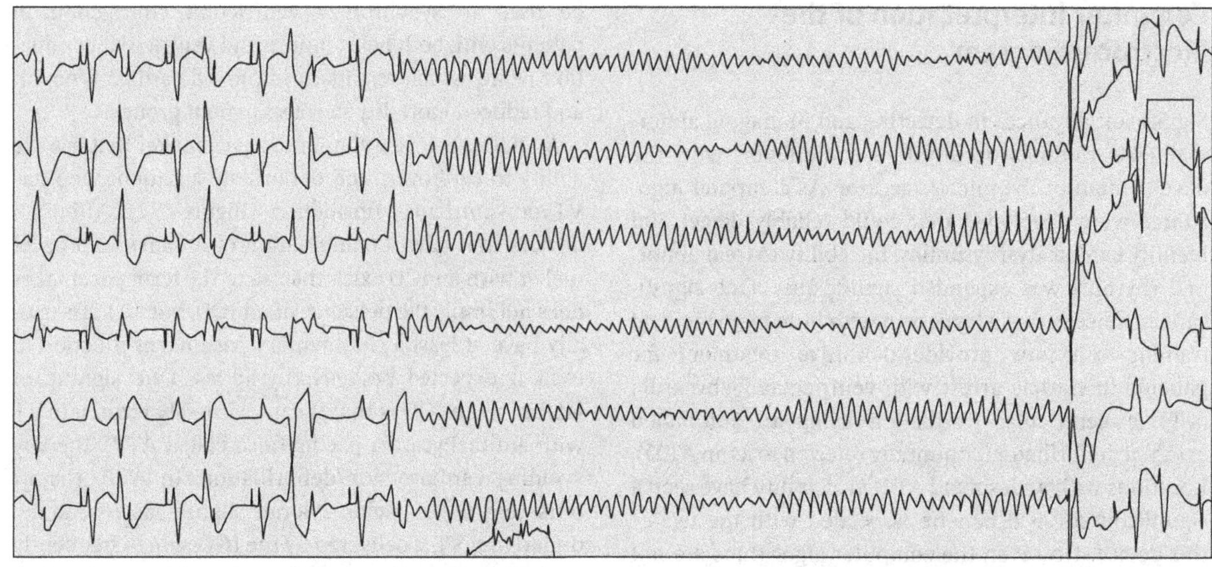

Figure 2.7 Patient with a dual-chamber pacemaker/ICD who develops ventricular bigeminy and ventricular fibrillation with successful defibrillation by their ICD.

programmed, placing a magnet over a pacemaker will most commonly cause it to revert to a simplistic mode where it continuously paces asynchronously and is not inhibited by sensed beats. Placing a magnet over an ICD will typically inhibit defibrillation but will not inhibit the pacemaker feature. Inhibition is especially useful for a patient who is being shocked inappropriately or for a patient with VT storm to delay cardioversion or defibrillation until adequate sedation can be administered.

3
Interpretation of the Electrocardiogram – Single-, Multi-, and 12-Lead Analysis

Robert C. Reiser[1], *Robert C. Schutt*[2], *Korin B. Hudson*[3], *and William J. Brady*[4]

[1] *Department of Emergency Medicine, University of Virginia School of Medicine, Charlottesville, VA, USA*
[2] *Department of Cardiology, Ascension Medical Group, Austin, TX, USA*
[3] *Department of Emergency Medicine, Georgetown University School of Medicine, Medstar Health, Washington, DC, USA*
[4] *Department of Emergency Medicine and Medicine, University of Virginia School of Medicine, Charlottesville, VA, USA*

Introduction

Interpretation of the electrocardiogram (ECG) must be done systematically, and the essential components need to be examined and synthesized into a coherent analysis. No single interpretation strategy is correct; in fact, many approaches can be used, considering patient needs, interpreter ability, the clinical setting, and the purpose of ECG. Regardless of the chosen method, efficiency and accuracy of interpretation are vital issues common to all such strategies of ECG review. The clinician is encouraged to develop his/her own style of approach, considering these issues and stressing these goals.

It cannot be overemphasized that a systematic (or "check-list") approach is absolutely necessary even for experienced clinicians. A systematic approach needs to be strictly followed with every ECG; however, it is especially important with a 12-lead ECG, where the goal is not only to determine the rhythm but also to identify the underlying pathology. One recommended strategy is to consider the ECG in a stepwise manner, determining the rate, rhythm and regularity, axis, intervals, and morphology and then summarizing findings in a final interpretation.

In many cases, particularly with critically ill patients, following a systematic approach is understandably challenging because the clinician is simultaneously managing the airway, securing intravenous access, and ordering medications and other studies, in addition to obtaining and interpreting the ECG. In this instance, an initial rhythm interpretation followed by a careful systematic review of the ECG is a reasonable approach. The most important point in this interpretation is that every ECG obtained is carefully studied because a glaring and obvious finding can divert attention from a different but critical and more subtle finding that is easily missed if a systematic approach is not used. The ECG can provide important clinical information, involving not only the patient's rhythm but also the cardiac and non-cardiac conditions. Each ECG should be reviewed carefully looking for signs of disease such as pathologic rhythms, dysfunction of the conduction system, acute coronary ischemia, or infarction, and the impact of various toxins, electrolytes, and other disease states. Reviewing the individual ECG in an orderly manner by evaluating the rate, rhythm, axis, intervals, and morphology will help ensure that all abnormalities are recognized rapidly and efficiently.

The use of the ECG in a single- or multilead analysis mode is most appropriate for rhythm evaluation. In the hospital setting this is often readily available with bedside monitoring devices. When thinking about the difference between single-lead monitoring and the multilead ECG (including the 12-lead ECG), it is important to remember that the real value of the multilead ECG is that each lead provides a simultaneous yet different view of the same heart beat (Figure 3.1). Figure 3.1 demonstrates an analogy comparing two views of an automobile involved in a motor vehicle collision (MVC); from one perspective, the automobile does not appear to be significantly damaged, while a different view reveals significant damage to the car. The 12-lead ECG in a suspected acute coronary syndrome (ACS) presentation demonstrates similar varying perspectives: one lead demonstrates a non-worrisome ST segment contour, while another lead reveals ST segment elevation myocardial infarction (STEMI).

In most cases, the 12-lead ECG offers little additional information about rhythm identification and has little

The Electrocardiogram in Emergency and Acute Care, First Edition.
Edited by Korin B. Hudson, Amita Sudhir, George Glass, and William J. Brady.

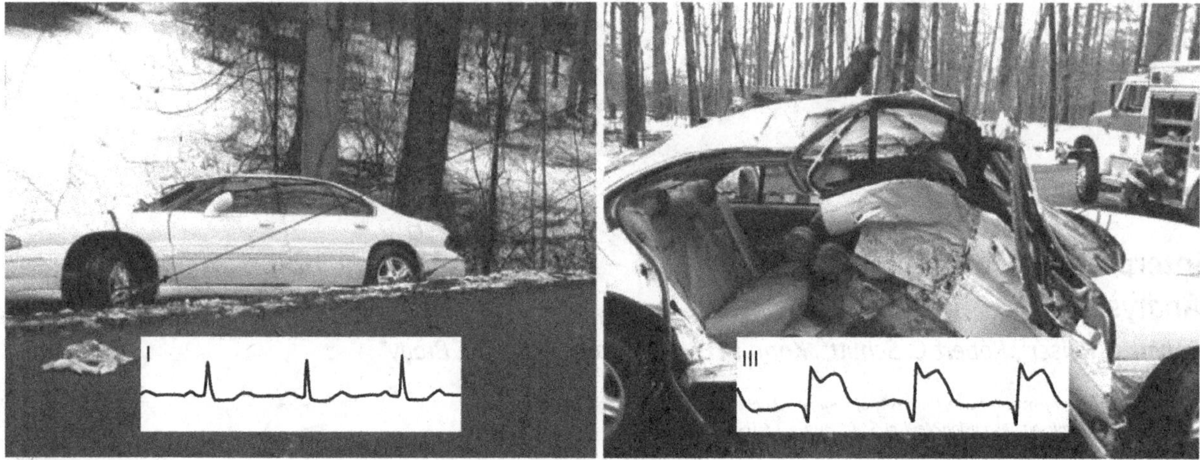

Figure 3.1 A much different perspective about injury is evident depending on what angle either the car or heart is viewed from.

immediate impact on patient management. However, in the setting of potential acute coronary syndrome (ACS), the 12-lead ECG can provide important information critical for the diagnosis of ACS and also guide therapy, predict risk, and suggest alternative diagnoses. For ACS, the use of the 12-lead ECG in "diagnostic mode" is the most appropriate electrocardiographic tool. Single-lead monitoring remains important, however, for the detection of cardiac arrhythmias that frequently complicate ACS. Though the use of single-lead rhythm monitoring is less valuable for diagnosing ACS because evaluation of the ST segment can be affected by device algorithms designed to reduce artifact.

Most single-lead monitors are programmed by default to display lead II, as typically all elements essential to rhythm interpretation (P, QRS, and T) are well seen in this lead. Although the majority of rhythms can be determined by looking at only one lead, the experienced provider knows that at times it can be helpful to look at other leads if a particular element of the ECG is not well seen or the ECG does not match the patient condition (Figure 3.2). All monitors with basic limb leads can at least view leads I, II, and III, and it is always reasonable to look at another lead when presented when faced with a challenging rhythm. In the case shown in Figure 3.2, lead I appears to demonstrate asystole or fine ventricular fibrillation, while simultaneous leads II and III reveal a widened QRS complex, consistent with ventricular tachycardia.

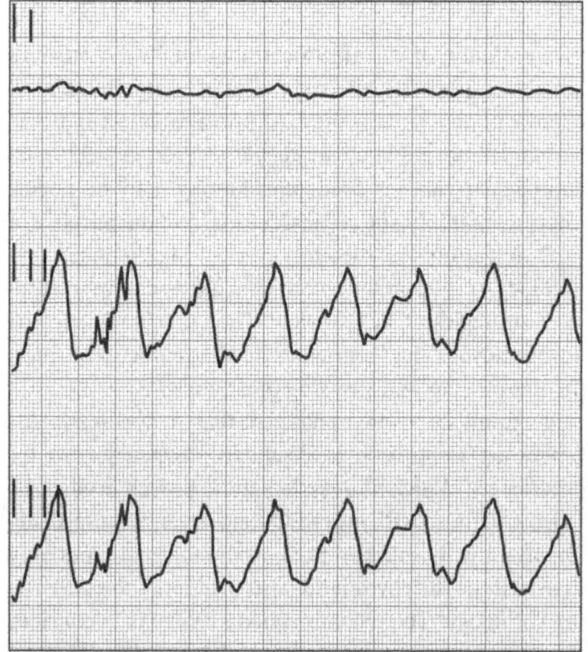

Figure 3.2 If only lead I was monitored, it would be quite possible to falsely conclude that the patient was in asystole, whereas clearly leads II and III tell a different story with ventricular tachycardia. For this reason, historically it was taught that any time asystole was diagnosed, it should be confirmed in a separate lead.

Rate

The heart rate is expressed in beats per minute (bpm). In a normally conducted beat, every atrial contraction is followed by a ventricular contraction; thus, the atrial and ventricular rates are equal. If a dysrhythmia is present, these rates may not be identical and each must be calculated separately.

The following approach can be used to calculate both the atrial and the ventricular rates. To calculate the rates, the clinician must be familiar with the format of standard electrocardiographic paper and recording

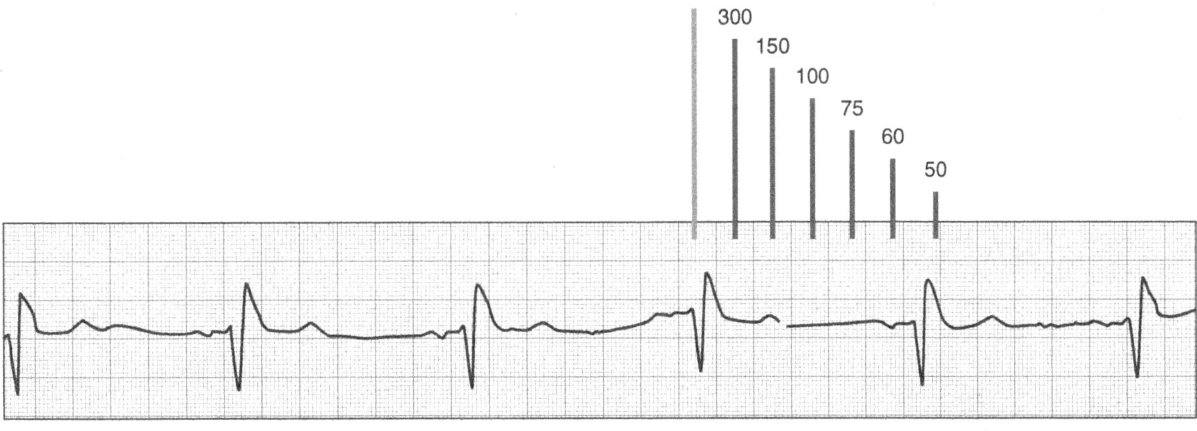

Figure 3.3 Comparison of the "6-s method" and "thick line counting" method for estimating heart rate. The 6-s method estimates the rate at 60 bpm (six QRS complexes × 10 = 60 bpm); the thick line counting method estimates the rate between 50 and 60 bpm; the actual rate measured by counting pulse for one minute was 54 bpm.

techniques. Electrocardiographic paper is divided into a grid by a series of horizontal and vertical lines. The thin lines are separated by 1 mm and thick lines by 5 mm segments. The ECG tracing is recorded at a standard rate of 25 mm/s. Considering both the paper formatting and ECG machine recording speed, one can determine that each thin vertical line represents 0.04 s and each thick vertical line represents 0.2 s. Using these time measurements, the rate can be calculated in two ways (Figure 3.3).

The "Thick Line" Calculation

- Start with a QRS complex that occurs on or near a thick vertical line. Assuming that the rhythm is regular, simply count the number of thick lines to the next complex.
- Because each thick line represents 0.2 s, there are 300 such lines in one minute.
- Divide 300 by the number of thick lines, with the result being the rate expressed as "bpm."

A simplified method using this approach involves the use of the rates associated with corresponding numbers of thick vertical lines. Moving from a QRS complex on a thick vertical line to the next QRS complex and its relation to the next vertical line, the clinician can rapidly estimate the rate. Moving from the QRS complex to the next and using the thick vertical lines, the rate decreases as follows: 300, 150, 100, 75, 60, 50, 42, 38 bpm, and so on.

The "6-s" Average Technique

The second method of calculating the rate is to count the number of complexes in 6 s and multiply by 10. This approach is best used if the rhythm is irregular (Figure 3.4).

Inaccuracy is most problematic in patients with atrial fibrillation, as this rhythm has significant beat-to-beat variability and both the 6-s and thick line counting methods may produce estimates that vary significantly from the actual heart rate. In most circumstances, a normal heart rate is defined as between 60 and 100 bpm in the healthy adult. The normal heart rate in children varies considerably with respect to age with neonates averaging 180 bpm, the infant and toddler ranging from 140 to 100 bpm, and the adolescent assuming "adult values" of 100–70 bpm. One must be mindful, however, to interpret the heart rate in light of the patient's age and overall condition. Because the normal heart rate decreases with age, a normal neonate can have a heart rate of 180 bpm, while a heart rate of 95 may be relatively tachycardic in an 80-year-old patient.

Rhythm

The identification of the P wave and the QRS complex is the first step in rhythm interpretation; the occurrence of each of these structures and their regularity can provide important clues to the rhythm. The relationship of the P wave to the QRS complex is also vital. For instance, is there a single P wave for each QRS complex? Certainly, the absence of either structure will provide important clues to the rhythm diagnosis. While it is not uncommon to encounter rhythms lacking the P wave (i.e. junctional rhythm or atrial fibrillation), the absence of the QRS complex is not compatible with life and will be

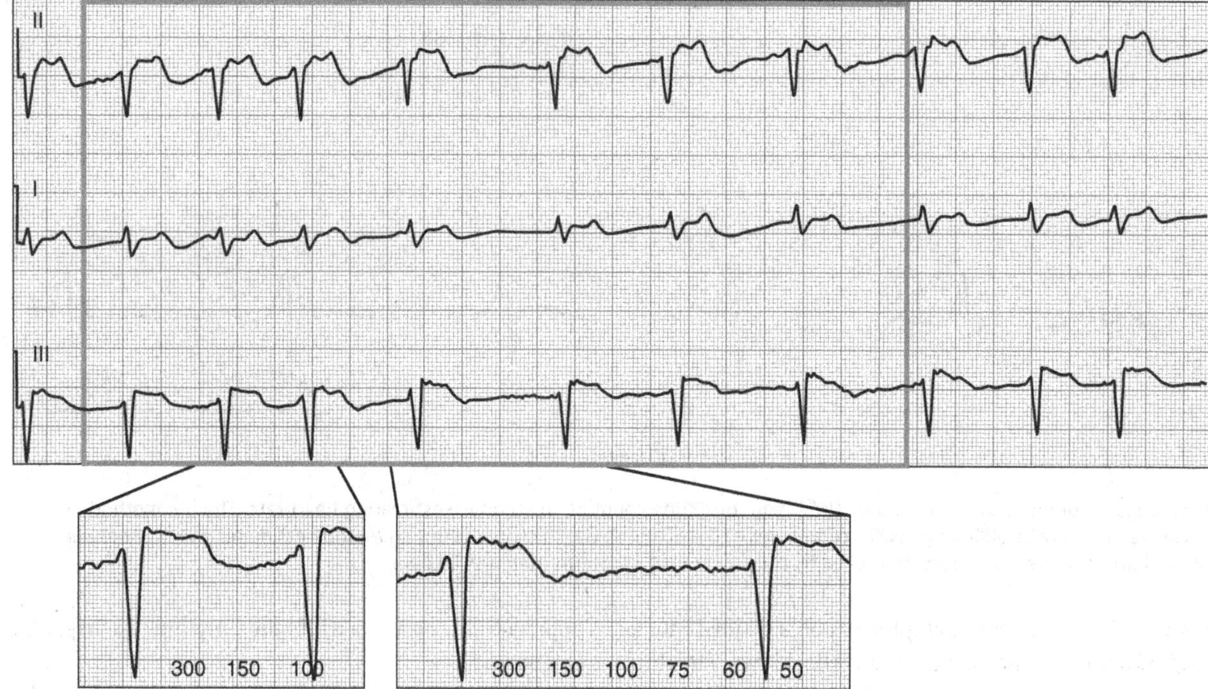

Figure 3.4 This ECG demonstrates that the thick line counting method is especially inaccurate for estimating heart rate in the setting of atrial fibrillation. The estimated rate varies from 55 to 100 bpm depending on which interval is measured. Actual heart rate counted over one minute was 66 bpm. The box marks 6 s and estimates the rate at 70 bpm.

seen only in the cardiac arrest situation involving asystole and ventricular fibrillation. The regular occurrence of these structures can be determined in many ways but measuring the R–R interval is the most accurate, easiest approach to do so.

The R–R interval (time from one R wave to the next) throughout a rhythm strip can be helpful for determining the cardiac rhythm. The rhythm may be regular, regular with occasional extra beats, regularly irregular, or irregularly irregular. Regular rhythms will have a uniform R–R interval throughout the entire strip. Occasionally, there may be one or more extra beats on top of an otherwise regular rhythm. These may be caused by premature atrial contractions or premature ventricular contractions. Regularly irregular rhythms are those with a variable, but predictable R–R interval. An example is the trigeminy pattern in which there is a premature beat for every two regular QRS complexes. The overall R–R interval in such cases is variable, but there is a pattern to the R–R interval that repeats throughout the strip such that the timing of the next QRS is easily predicted. Irregularly irregular rhythms are those with widely variable and unpredictable R–R intervals. Atrial fibrillation is a good example of an R–R interval that is irregular and not predictable.

Axis

The axis is the average direction of electrical charge during cardiac cycle. The axis of any of the various ECG structures (i.e. P wave, QTS complex, and T wave) can be determined; however, from a practical perspective determining the axis of the QRS complex is most important. The action of the heart may be normal (direction of charge down the heart and to the left), leftward deviated, or rightward deviated.

There are many methods to determine the axis. Perhaps the easiest approach is to evaluate the polarity, or main direction, of the QRS complex in leads I, II, and III. If the QRS complex is oriented positively (i.e. mainly upright) in these three leads, the axis is normal (between 0° and 90°). If the QRS complex is positive in lead I and negative (i.e. mainly downward) in leads II and III, the axis is leftward deviated (<0°), and left axis deviation is said to be present. Right axis deviation (>90°), or a rightward axis, is noted when the QRS complex is negative in lead I and positive in lead III; lead II is variable, meaning that it can be either positive or negative. An indeterminate axis, either extreme right or left axis deviation, is seen when the QRS complex is negative in all three leads.

An abnormal axis can be seen in a number of situations including past and current cardiac diseases as well as non-cardiac illness affecting the heart's function.

Intervals

Once rhythm, rate, and axis have been determined, it is important to measure the timing of each portion of the cardiac cycle. This determination can be accomplished by calculating the PR interval length, the QRS complex width, and the QT interval length. These determinations, particularly the PR interval and QRS complex width, will factor significantly into the final interpretation of the ECG.

The PR interval is calculated by measuring the time from the beginning of the P wave to the beginning of the QRS complex. Simply, this interval should not be greater than one large box and no less than three small boxes (between 120 and 200 ms [milliseconds]). The PR interval is an important determinant for many rhythm disorders and other diagnoses; for instance, the PR interval provides pivotal information with regard to atrioventricular block and the Wolff–Parkinson–White syndrome (Figure 3.5).

QRS complex width is calculated by measuring the time from the beginning to the end of the QRS complex; this interval should be less than three small boxes (<80–120 ms). Certain authorities note that a normal QRS complex width is less than 80 ms, while others note that the duration can range up to 120 ms. The normal duration of the QRS complex depends on the age and sex of the patient. This variability is problematic; however, from a practical perspective, nearly all clinicians will agree that a QRS complex duration greater than 120 ms is prolonged, and many will consider a QRS complex duration greater than 100 as prolonged. We recommend the use of 110 ms as the upper range of normal for the QRS complex duration for any patient older than 16 years of age. As is true with all ECG measured and calculated parameters, pediatric normal values are age- and body size-appropriate. Abnormal widening of the QRS complex can indicate a range of pathologic conditions, including intraventricular conduction abnormality (i.e. bundle branch block) and dysrhythmia (supraventricular tachycardia with aberrant ventricular conduction or ventricular tachycardia).

The QT interval is calculated by measuring the time from the beginning of the QRS complex to the end of the T wave. The QT interval normal value varies depending on the heart rate. In general, the QT interval should be no more than half that of the accompanying R–R interval. Such a comparison can be performed rapidly and easily at the bedside to determine if the QT interval is appropriate for that rate. This comparison, however, is only appropriately performed for supraventricular rhythms at rates between 60 and 100 bpm.

In a more precise sense, the QT interval is often corrected for the rate using a number of an equation, termed *Bazett's formula*. Bazett's formula equates the QTc interval (corrected QT interval) to the QT interval divided by the square root of the accompanying R–R interval. A normal QTc interval should be between 300 and 440 ms, although it may go up to 460 ms in women.

Morphology

Once all of the basic determinations have been evaluated as outlined above, the morphology of the P wave, the QRS complex, the ST segment, and the T wave should be considered.

Normal P waves (i.e. those P waves seen in normal sinus rhythm) appear as a single-rounded wave before the QRS complex. The P wave should be upright in all leads except lead aVR. P waves should be rounded and monophasic with a height no greater than 2.5 small boxes (0.25 mV [mV]) and a width no greater than 2¾ small boxes (110 ms). Abnormalities of the P wave are noted if the P wave is pointed, biphasic, tall, wide, or flattened.

Besides determining the width of the QRS complex as noted above, one should consider its morphology. It is important to note that the term *QRS complex* does not

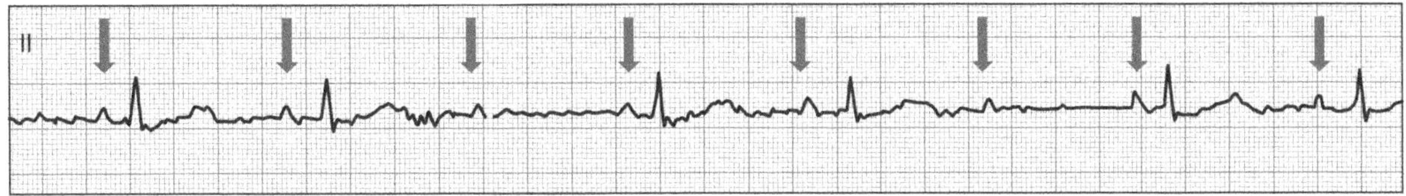

Figure 3.5 Second-degree type I atrioventricular heart block (also called Mobitz I or Wenckebach). The arrows mark the P waves.

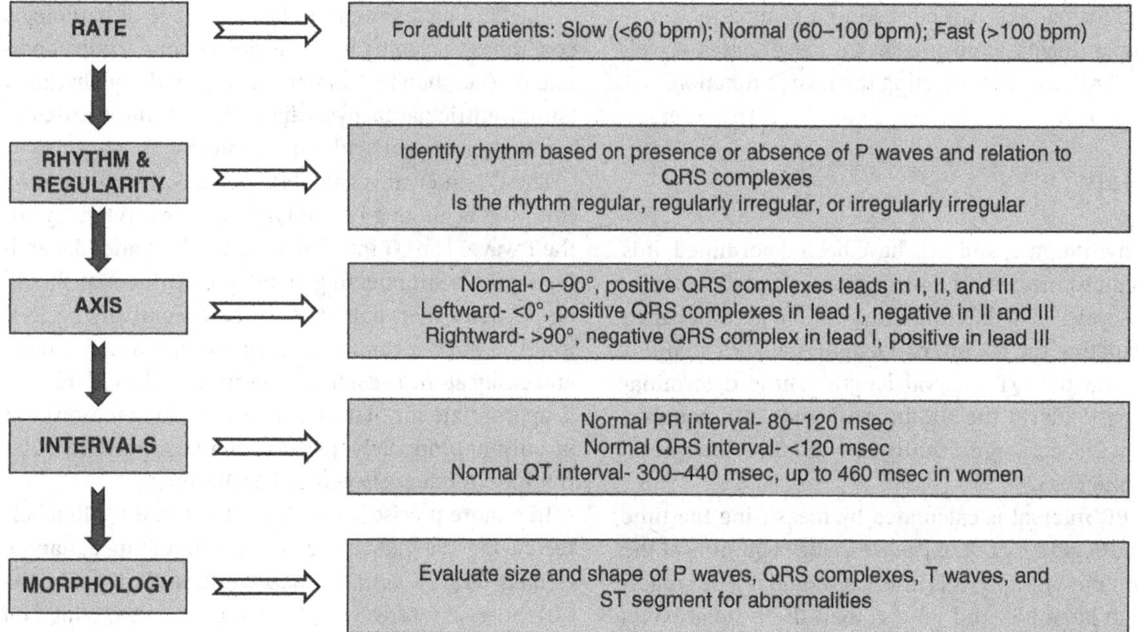

RATE
For adult patients: Slow (<60 bpm); Normal (60–100 bpm); Fast (>100 bpm)
RHYTHM & REGULARITY
Identify rhythm based on presence or absence of P waves and relation to QRS complexes
Is the rhythm regular, regularly irregular, or irregularly irregular
AXIS
Normal- 0–90°, positive QRS complexes leads in I, II, and III
Leftward- <0°, positive QRS complexes in lead I, negative in II and III
Rightward- >90°, negative QRS complex in lead I, positive in lead III
INTERVALS
Normal PR interval- 80–120 msec
Normal QRS interval- <120 msec
Normal QT interval- 300–440 msec, up to 460 msec in women
MORPHOLOGY
Evaluate size and shape of P waves, QRS complexes, T waves, and ST segment for abnormalities

Figure 3.6 Algorithm for interpretation of the ECG.

morphologically describe the QRS complex. The following discussion focuses on the morphology of the QRS complex. A Q wave is defined as an initial negative deflection of the QRS complex. The R wave is the initial positive deflection of the QRS complex; it can be the initial structure of the QRS complex (i.e. there may be no preceding Q wave) or follow the negative deflection of a Q wave. A second negative deflection is termed the *S wave*; it can occur as the sole negative deflection following an R wave or as the second negative deflection following sequential Q and R waves.

The clinician should evaluate for the presence of Q waves, "double" R waves (the R and R′ waves), abnormally tall R or deep S waves, and abnormal progression of R waves from lead V1 to V6. Non-pathologic, that is, "normal," Q waves can be seen in leads I, III, AVF, V5, and V6. These non-pathologic Q waves should be less than ¼ the height of the related R wave and no greater than one small box in width (<40 ms). Q waves differing from this morphology or present in other leads may be an indicator of cardiac disease.

Abnormalities of the R wave focus on the appearance of two positive deflections. Two positive deflections of the QRS complex can also occur with the first positive deflection termed the *R wave* and the second positive deflection the *R' wave*. The presence of a second R wave after the S wave may indicate the presence of an intraventricular conduction delay such as fascicular blocks or bundle branch blocks.

Abnormalities of the ST segment and T wave require careful consideration. ST segments which are elevated as compared to the isoelectric baseline may indicate ischemic disease. ST segments which are depressed compared to the isoelectric baseline may represent reciprocal change, further reflecting ischemia or infarction. Abnormalities of the T wave can indicate electrolyte abnormalities, toxidromes, or changes associated with ischemic disease.

Figure 3.6 reviews the algorithm that provides a systematic approach to the review of the ECG. Abnormalities of any of these ECG features can be indicative of a range of cardiac and systemic events. The various features will be discussed throughout the text of this book.

4
Variants of the Normal, Lead Misplacement, and Electrocardiographic Artifact Encountered in Clinical Practice

Robert C. Reiser[1], Robert C. Schutt[2], Korin B. Hudson[3], and William J. Brady[4]

[1] *Department of Emergency Medicine, University of Virginia School of Medicine, Charlottesville, VA, USA*
[2] *Department of Cardiology, Ascension Medical Group, Austin, TX, USA*
[3] *Department of Emergency Medicine, Georgetown University Hospital, Medstar Health, Washington, DC, USA*
[4] *Departments of Emergency Medicine and Medicine, University of Virginia School of Medicine, Charlottesville, VA, USA*

There are a variety of variants to the normal electrocardiogram (ECG). The term *variant* indicates that the particular ECG finding can be considered a normal finding – despite its abnormal appearance. It is important to be familiar with these since they may be confused with pathologic conditions, resulting in improper treatment. Patients with a significantly abnormal ECG often keep a copy of their ECG with them in their wallet or purse in case they require emergency care to help prevent unnecessary evaluation. ECG lead misplacement and electrocardiographic artifact can also mimic findings encountered in illness. The ECG in such cases should always be correlated with the history and clinical appearance of the patient; in other words, the clinician must interpret the ECG within the clinical context of the particular patient's presentation.

Benign Early Repolarization

Benign early repolarization (BER) is a phenomenon that causes ST segment elevation in about 1% of the population, and does not represent any type of conduction or other cardiac abnormality. While the appearance of ST segment elevation is normally a cause for concern, familiarity with the ECG criteria for BER (Figure 4.1) can help the provider identify low-risk cases. These criteria are as follows:

While the appearance of ST segment elevation is normally a cause for concern, familiarity with the ECG criteria for BER can help the provider identify low-risk cases. These criteria are as follows (Figure 4.1):

1) *Widespread ST segment elevation beginning at the "J point"*
   The J point is the junction of the QRS complex and the ST segment. It is usually minimal with less than 2 mm deflection, yet it may be as high as 5 mm.
2) *Concavity of the ST segment*
   The ST segment appears to have been moved upwards from the baseline to a higher point while keeping its normal concavity intact, unlike the ST segment elevation typical of ST segment elevation myocardial infarction (STEMI), where the segment appears either flat or upsloping (convex).
3) *Notching of the J point*
   The terminal portion of the QRS complex at the J point appears notched or irregular in contour.
4) *Prominent, concordant T waves*
   The T waves, especially in the precordial leads, are large in amplitude, may appear peaked, and are concordant with the QRS complex.
5) *Relatively fixed/constant pattern*
   The ST segment elevation of BER is seen consistently in a patient's ECGs over time.
6) *ECG distribution*
   ST segment elevation is usually seen in the right to midprecordial leads (leads V1–V4); it is also seen concurrently in the inferior leads. It is very rare to encounter such ST segment changes in the inferior leads when it is not present in the anterior leads.

The Electrocardiogram in Emergency and Acute Care, First Edition.
Edited by Korin B. Hudson, Amita Sudhir, George Glass, and William J. Brady.

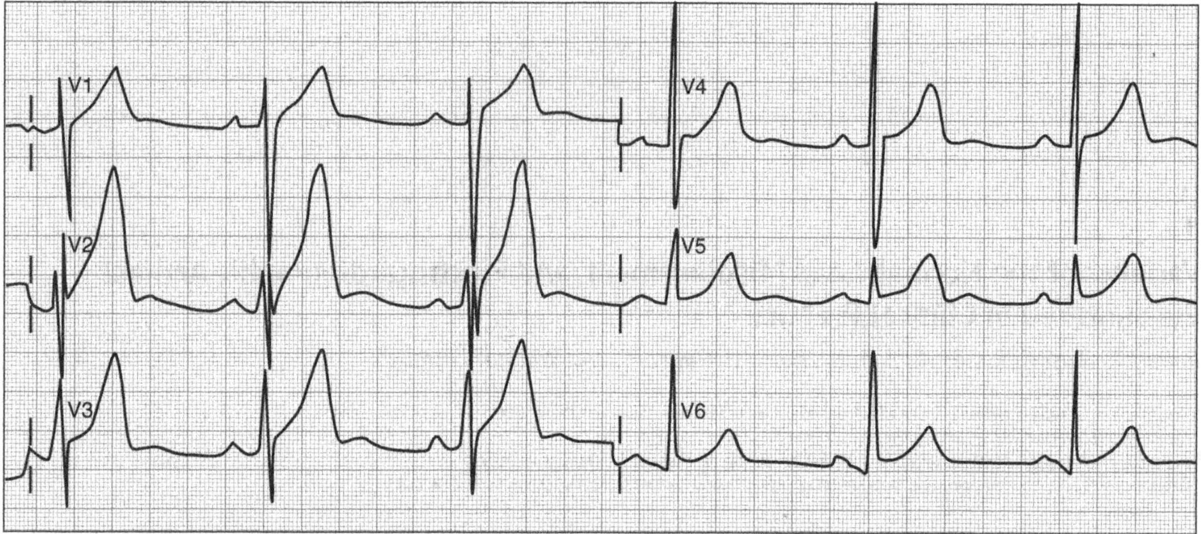

Figure 4.1 BER – This ECG demonstrates benign early repolarization with approximately 1 mm of concave J point elevation with ST segment elevation in most leads and large amplitude, prominent T waves in the precordial leads.

The demographics of the BER pattern are important to consider when the clinician considers this ECG diagnosis. The majority of patients with BER are young with an average age range of 20–30 years. As patients age, the degree of ST segment elevation resulting from BER tends to decrease – in fact, BER is an uncommon finding after age 50. Although it is present in about 1% of the population, it is more common in certain subsets, such as athletes and males.

Although knowing that a patient has BER can be reassuring, the astute clinician provider should always err on the side of caution when determining the cause of ST segment elevation, assuming the worst-case scenario, such as STEMI. Patients with ST segment elevation who have a concerning or unclear clinical picture should be treated with the urgency of a potential life-threatening condition.

Sinus Arrhythmia

In some patients, particularly young healthy individuals, a sinus arrhythmia may be evident on ECG. The ECG shows normal, identical P waves followed by a normal appearing QRS, but the rate varies with respiration, increasing with inspiration and decreasing with expiration, resulting in an irregular appearing rhythm with its origin in the sinoatrial (SA) node. Thus, sinus arrhythmia is normal sinus rhythm with irregular R–R intervals. See Figure 4.2.

Conditions Encountered in Athletes

The ECG of highly conditioned athletes, especially endurance athletes, can demonstrate certain changes that may be confused with pathologic abnormalities. These findings are described in Table 4.1 and include very slow heart rates, prolongation of the PR interval, large QRS complexes, and ST segment elevation. If these ECG findings are present, the history and clinical picture are important in determining if these are pathologic findings or physiologic changes in the heart of an athlete (Figure 4.3). Caution must be exercised in these cases and a broad differential diagnosis should be considered and, if concern for serious etiology exists, the clinician should consider the changes to be potentially pathologic.

T Wave Inversion

While T wave inversion or flattening can be a sign of acute coronary syndrome (ACS) or other systemic events, it can also be normal in certain leads and certain patients. The T wave may be inverted in leads III, aVL, and V1 in normal, healthy patients; lead aVR also frequently demonstrates T wave inversion in the normal patient.

In children, the right precordial leads V1–V4 may exhibit inverted T waves. Some adults do not lose the inverted T waves in these leads after childhood, a

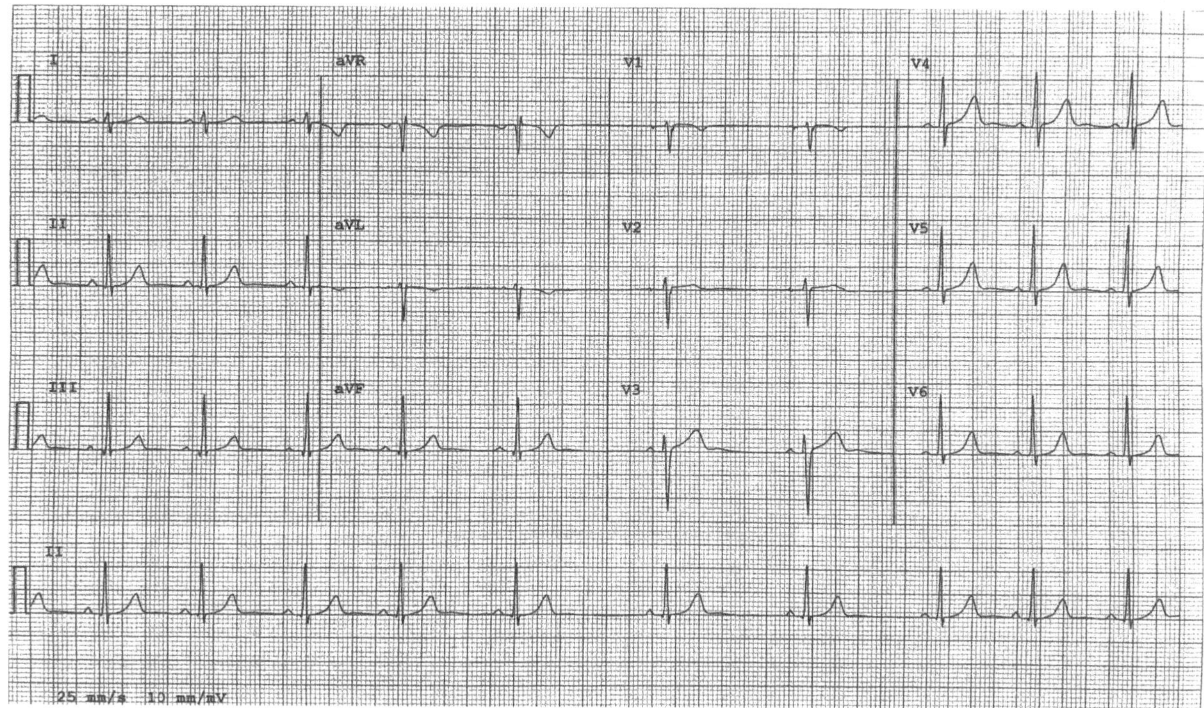

Figure 4.2 Sinus arrhythmia – note the beat to beat variation in the R–R intervals. *Source:* cardiogram from Dr. A. Shah, MedStar Union Memorial Hospital.

Table 4.1 ECG findings associated with athletic heart.

Bradycardia: The resting heart rate of an athlete may be well below 60 bpm and may demonstrate a junctional rhythm. Athletes are also more likely to have sinus arrhythmia.
First- and second-degree type I atrioventricular (AV) block: due to increased parasympathetic tone, may also be a normal variant in the non-athlete.
Increased QRS complex amplitude: may be mistaken for the left ventricular hypertrophy pattern. Changes are due to the increased muscle mass of the heart coupled with a relatively thin chest wall.
J point elevation: largely appearing as ST segment elevation, is similar to that seen in BER; this finding is relatively common in athletes.

phenomenon known as persistent juvenile pattern (PJP). This finding is most commonly seen in leads V2 and V3 (Figure 4.4).

The T wave may also appear inverted if the ECG is performed with the patient in a semi-upright (i.e. non-supine) position. Numerous other "benign" scenarios can produce T wave inversion, including the recent ingestion of a large meal, particularly in leads I, II, and V2–V4; anxiety, fear, and hyperventilation may also cause the T waves to become inverted. Similar to ST segment elevation mentioned in the BER section, if the clinical picture is concerning for ACS or systemic events, T wave inversions should not be dismissed lightly.

Lead Misplacement

It is not uncommon for ECG leads to be placed in incorrect positions, which can lead to an abnormal appearing ECG in an otherwise normal patient. If the ECG appears different than prior tracings from the same patient and the clinical picture has not changed, lead misplacement should be suspected. Similarly, if abnormalities in the ECG cannot be explained by the clinical picture, position of the leads should be checked.

It is important to be able to recognize some common signs of lead reversal. One common problem is the reversal of the right and left arm leads. On the ECG, right arm–left arm reversal is identified when leads I and aVL appear to be the inverse of V5 and V6 and there is an inverted P wave in lead I (or significantly abnormal P wave axis). The other finding easy to identify is the "pseudoasystole" or flat wave in lead III that occurs

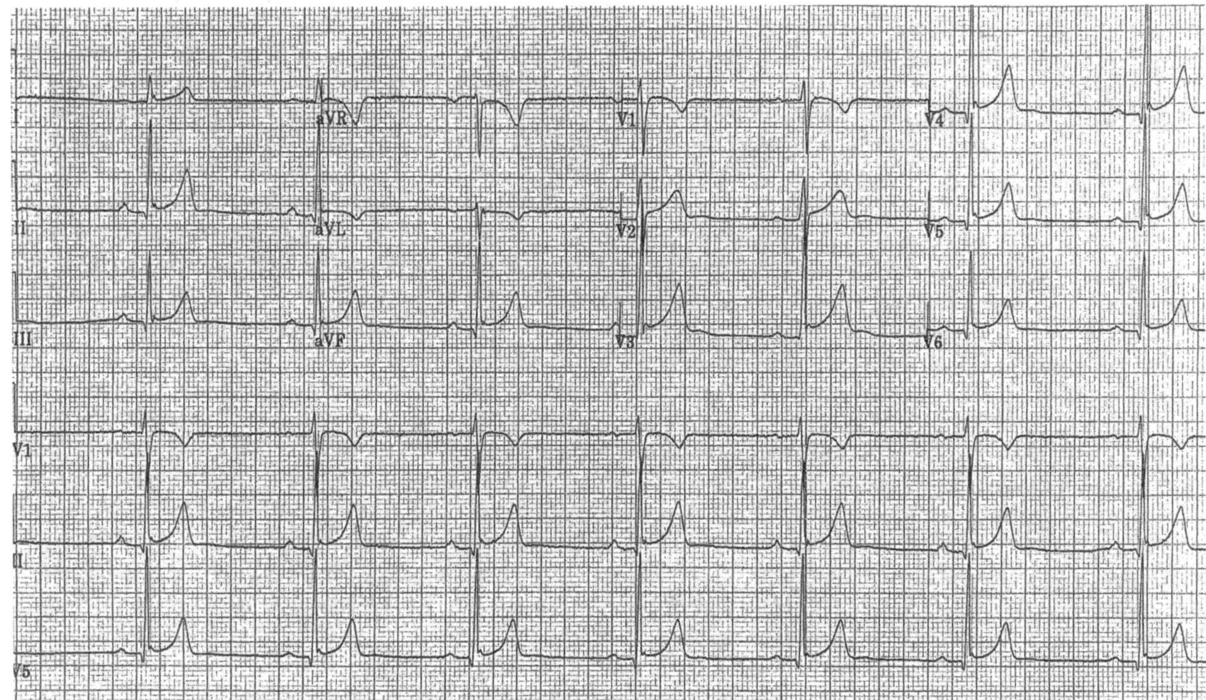

Figure 4.3 ECG findings associated with athletic heart – in this ECG, note bradycardia, large QRS amplitudes, and J-point elevation. *Source:* cardiogram from Dr. A. Shah, MedStar Union Memorial Hospital.

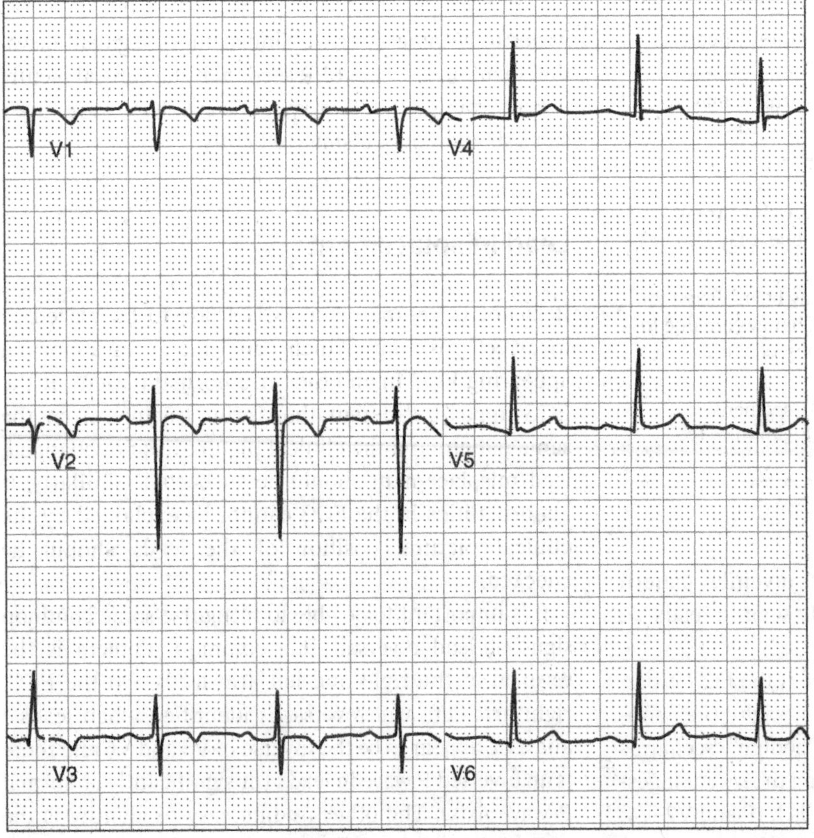

Figure 4.4 Persistent T wave inversions in the precordial leads in an older adolescent or young adult can represent the *persistent juvenile T wave inversion*.

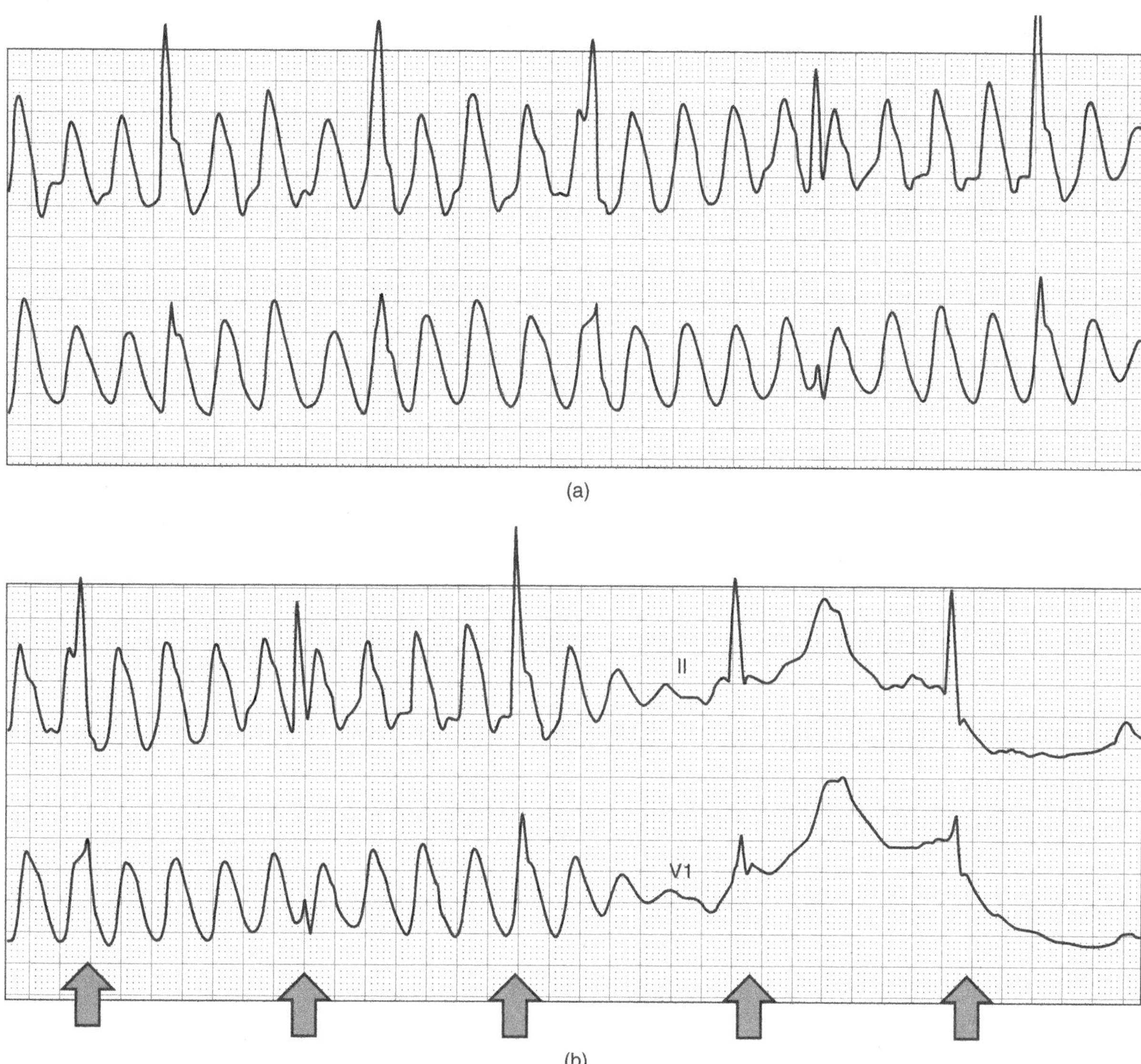

Figure 4.5 "Toothbrush tachycardia" is a common source of telemetry alarms (a). The clue that this is not VT is from the arrows that mark the native QRS complex, clearly evident when the patient stops brushing his or her teeth (b).

with the reversal of the left arm and right leg. Reversal of the right and left leg leads is common; however, fortunately this does not cause significant changes to the ECG.

Artifact

It is possible to see a pathologic ECG that is caused by an artifact. For example, a patient brushing his or her teeth is a classic cause of an artifact resembling ventricular tachycardia (VT) (Figure 4.5). An artifact generally simulates dysrhythmias or produces a disrupted baseline and is unlikely to mimic ischemia.

There are two different types of artifacts: internal artifacts caused by something intrinsic to the patient and external artifacts caused by something external or not related to the patient. An internal artifact can include tremor, shivering, body movements, or coughing; this internal artifact can interfere with skin-to-electrode contact and thus produce electrical transmissions, which can affect the baseline or even create complexes that appear to be abnormal QRS complexes. Furthermore, skeletal muscle contraction produces electrical potentials, which can mimic cardiac activity. An external artifact may be caused by nearby sources of alternating current (the ECG machine should normally filter this out), malfunction of the ECG machine, wires, or electrodes, or static electricity. Electrode malfunction is commonly caused by poor skin-to-electrode contact, such as due to inadequate gel; excessive body hair; or significant perspiration. These electrode-based problems can affect proper electrode adherence to the skin.

If a patient has a significant abnormality on ECG, but appears well and the clinical picture does not fit the ECG findings, the provider should ensure that the ECG findings are not caused by an artifact before embarking on any potentially dangerous interventions.

Section II

Cardiac Rhythms and Cardiac Dysrhythmias

5

Cardiac Rhythms with Normal Rates

Korin B. Hudson[1] *and William J. Brady*[2]

[1] *Department of Emergency Medicine, Medstar Georgetown University Hospital, Washington, DC, USA*
[2] *Departments of Emergency Medicine and Medicine, University of Virginia School of Medicine, Charlottesville, VA, USA*

This section reviews dysrhythmias with normal heart rates – in other words, non-sinus rhythms with rates in the normal range of 60–100 bpm. These dysrhythmias are commonly encountered during the delivery of emergency care and not infrequently cause signs and symptoms that lead patients to seek assistance.

Healthcare providers have many reasons to obtain a surface electrocardiogram (ECG) during the provision of care, which could be a single-lead ECG (rhythm strip), multilead monitoring, or a 12-lead ECG. In some cases, the ECG may be obtained in order to seek a specific etiology of the patient's complaint (i.e. chest pain or shortness of breath); in other cases, it may be performed as part of routine evaluation and monitoring of an ill or injured patient.

Not infrequently, patients present with normal heart rates, defined here as 60–100 bpm for adults and within defined, age-specific ranges for children (Table 5.1). A normal heart rate neither rules in, nor rules out, serious underlying conditions. Certain "normal rate" ECG tracings can immediately indicate a diagnosis – for instance, the 12-lead ECG that reveals normal sinus rhythm with ST segment elevation indicative of a ST segment elevation myocardial infarction (STEMI) or single-lead rhythm strip that shows atrial fibrillation with a controlled ventricular response (i.e. heart rate <100 bpm). However, in many cases, "normal rate" single- and multilead ECGs merely provide additional information to the emergency care provider without indicating a specific diagnosis.

Normal sinus rhythm is a common finding. This rhythm (Figure 5.1) is identified by its rate, P wave morphology, PR interval, QRS complex, relationship of the P wave to the QRS complex, and regularity of the QRS complexes. The normal rate for an adult is between 60 and 100 bpm; of course, children demonstrate age-related differences in rate. Normal P wave morphology refers to a single, consistent P wave, which is upright in the limb leads I, II, and III. The PR interval (0.12–0.20 s) and QRS complex (<0.12 s) are normal in width. Each P wave is associated with a QRS complex, and every QRS complex has a preceding P wave. The rhythm is regular as determined by consistent and identical P–P and R–R intervals. It is important to emphasize that by itself, a finding of normal sinus rhythm neither confirms nor rules out any acute process or injury.

Sinus arrhythmia has all the hallmarks of normal sinus rhythm except that while the P waves and QRS complexes are normal and identical from beat to beat, the P–P and R–R intervals vary (Figure 5.2). This variation is often caused by changes in intrathoracic pressure and may be seen during the normal respiratory cycle. This rhythm is frequently found in healthy young patients and does not necessarily indicate pathology.

Atrial fibrillation is a rhythm that is most commonly described as "irregularly irregular." In atrial fibrillation, multiple electrical foci in the atria discharge simultaneously and in rapid succession, producing "electrical chaos." While the atrial rate may approach 600 bpm, it is not possible to observe this many discharges on the ECG. Rather, there is an absence of a consistent P wave and the chaotic electrical activity in the atria is manifested through the presence of a disorganized baseline that is observed between QRS complexes.

The atrioventricular (AV) node allows only a certain number of atrial impulses per unit time to pass through to the ventricular conduction system, thus protecting the ventricle from excessively rapid rates. At any given time,

The Electrocardiogram in Emergency and Acute Care, First Edition.
Edited by Korin B. Hudson, Amita Sudhir, George Glass, and William J. Brady.

Table 5.1 Age-related normal heart rate ranges for children.

Age	Normal heart rate (bpm)
<12 mo	100–170
1–2 yr	90–150
2–5 yr	80–140
6–12 yr	70–110
>12 yr	60–100

only a single electrical impulse is transmitted through the AV node, leading to depolarization of the ventricles. In atrial fibrillation, this transmission of the atrial impulses is irregular in occurrence, producing no discernible pattern and resulting in irregularly occurring QRS complexes. Therefore, the R–R interval is highly variable from beat to beat. Unless the patient has underlying conduction system abnormalities, the QRS duration in atrial fibrillation will be normal and narrow (<0.12 s). Thus, atrial fibrillation is defined by the absence of discernible P waves and irregularly irregular QRS complexes (Figure 5.3).

In many cases of atrial fibrillation, the ventricular rate is rapid with a rate greater than 100 bpm; this is generally referred to as *atrial fibrillation with rapid ventricular response* (RVR). In other situations, the ventricular rate may be rather slow, less than 60 bpm, and is termed *atrial fibrillation with slow ventricular response.* In situations involving coexistent conduction system disease and/or the use of AV-node-blocking medications (e.g. β-adrenergic and calcium-channel-blocking agents), the ventricular rate may be within the normal range for the adult patient (i.e. ventricular rates of 60–100 bpm). In such situations, the rhythm is termed *atrial fibrillation with controlled (or normal) ventricular response.* Refer to Box 5.1 for further clinical and management issues for atrial fibrillation with a normal heart rate.

Atrial flutter is another common atrial dysrhythmia. Unlike atrial fibrillation, atrial flutter is most frequently regular and paroxysmal; that is to say that it is often intermittent and rarely lasts for more than a few hours at a time. In atrial flutter (unlike the atrial electrical chaos seen in atrial fibrillation), a single ectopic atrial focus produces rapid atrial depolarizations. A single and consistent P wave is noted, which is typically regular in occurrence, occurring at a rate of 250–350 bpm, and is termed a *flutter wave.* Flutter waves have a distinct morphology with a uniform "saw-tooth" pattern that is evident between QRS complexes (Figure 5.4). These "saw-tooth" waves are most evident in the inferior leads (leads II, III, and aVF).

As with atrial fibrillation, the ventricular response in atrial flutter is controlled by the atrioventricular node (AVN). Several flutter waves occur for each conducted impulse, which produces a QRS complex. The ratio of flutter waves to QRS complexes may vary widely but is most commonly seen in ratios of 4 : 1, 3 : 1, or to 2 : 1. Because the flutter waves are so regular, it is assumed that a flutter wave is also occurring simultaneously with the QRS complex. Therefore, by convention, the ratio of flutter waves to QRS complexes is defined by the

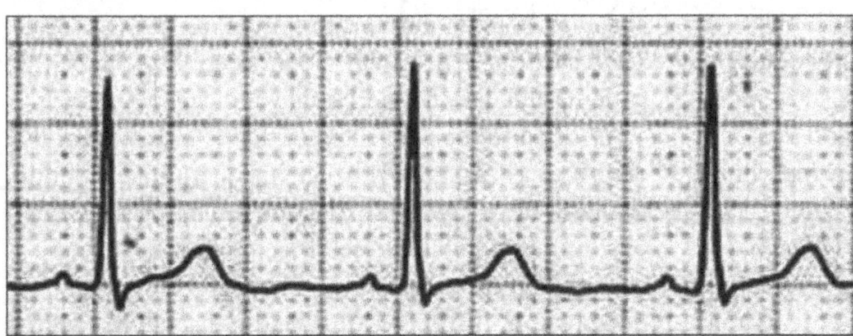

Figure 5.1 Normal sinus rhythm.

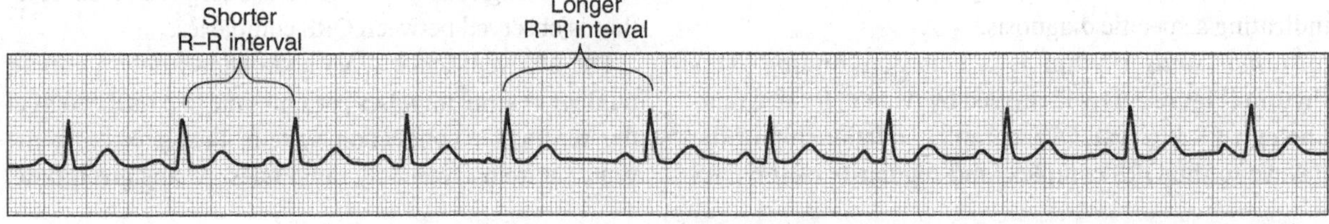

Figure 5.2 Sinus arrhythmia. Note the normal morphology of P wave, QRS complex, and T wave, yet the variable R–R interval.

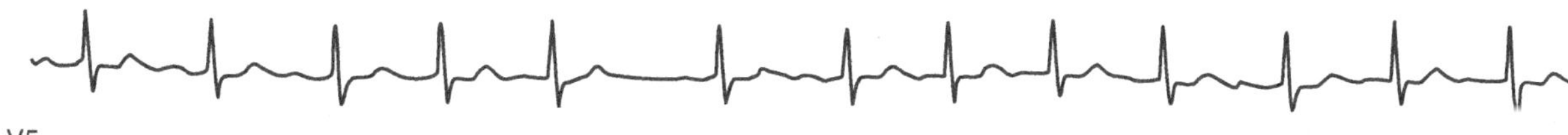

Figure 5.3 Atrial fibrillation. Note the absence of P waves and irregular R–R intervals with an irregularly irregular rhythm with a "random occurrence" of QRS complexes. The average ventricular rate is normal (i.e. between 60 and 100 bpm) and thus is termed *atrial fibrillation* with controlled ventricular response.

Box 5.1 Potential Clinical Features of Atrial Fibrillation with Controlled (or Normal) Ventricular Response

Potential clinical features seen in atrial fibrillation are as follows:

- Chest discomfort
- Shortness of breath
- Weakness/dizziness
- Pulmonary edema
- Hypotension

Patients do not tolerate atrial fibrillation because of two issues:

- Rapid ventricular rate can produce an acute decompensation.
- Loss of concerted atrial contraction/contribution to ventricular filling (loss of the "atrial kick") can produce a chronic decompensation.

"Normal rate" atrial fibrillation:

- Rarely causes acute decompensation (hypotension/pulmonary edema)
- Rarely requires emergency treatment

Atrial fibrillation can cause subacute/chronic decompensation (weakness/dyspnea).

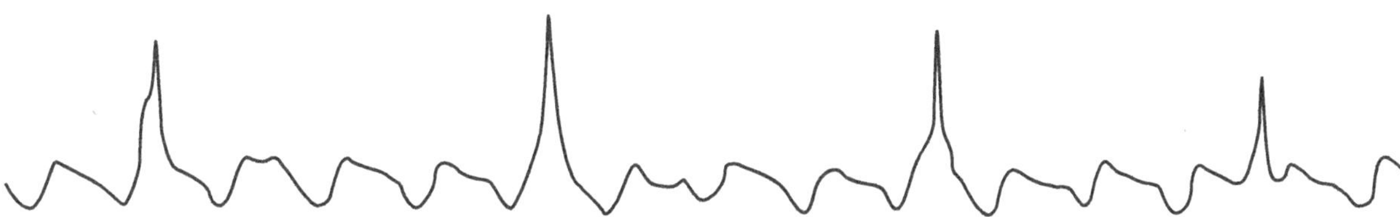

Figure 5.4 Atrial flutter with 4 : 1 conduction. Note the regularly occurring P waves in a "saw-tooth" pattern.

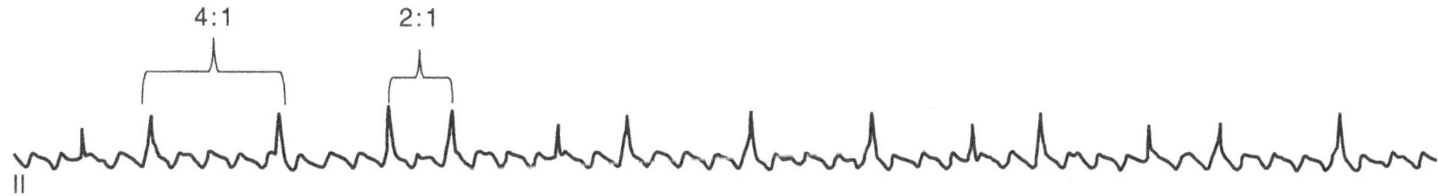

Figure 5.5 Atrial flutter with variable conduction. Note the varying ratio of flutter waves to each QRS complex from beat to beat, ranging from 4 : 1 to 2 : 1.

number of flutter waves seen *between* the QRS complexes plus one. This ratio may change within even a short rhythm strip (Figure 5.5), leading to QRS complexes with varying R–R intervals; this is referred to as *atrial flutter with variable conduction*. It is also possible for atrial fibrillation and atrial flutter to be evident in a single rhythm strip. This entity may be caused by one dominant ectopic atrial focus competing with the impulses from several other ectopic foci, leading to an irregular rhythm that demonstrates characteristics of atrial fibrillation and atrial flutter in different beats (Figure 5.6).

There are several other rhythms that are defined and described in the following chapters that may also be seen with normal ventricular rates. However, the ECG characteristics of these rhythms lead us to group them into broad

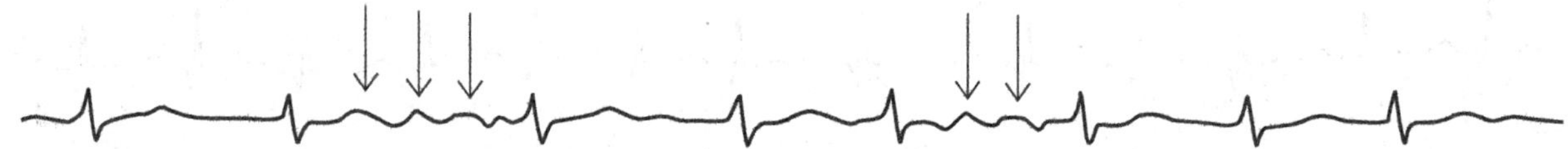

Figure 5.6 Atrial fibrillation/atrial flutter. Note the irregularly irregular R–R intervals and the presence of flutter waves (arrows) between some, but not all, QRS complexes.

categories according to the rate as we have done here. In addition, other ECG phenomena such as intraventricular blocks and atrial and ventricular ectopy may be seen at any rate and are discussed at length in later chapters.

Further Reading

Brady, W. and Truwit, J. (2009). *Critical Decisions in Emergency Medicine and Acute Care Electrocardiography*. Oxford, UK: Blackwell Publishing Ltd.

Chan, T., Brady, W.J., Harrigan, R.A. et al. (2005). *ECG in Emergency Medicine and Acute Care*. Philadelphia: Elsevier Inc.

6

Narrow QRS Complex Tachycardia

Courtney B. Saunders[1] *and Jeffrey D. Ferguson*[2]

[1] *Department of Cardiology, Vidant Health, Greenville, NC, USA*
[2] *Department of Emergency Medicine, Virginia Commonwealth University, Richmond, VA, USA*

Normal activation of the ventricles occurs after an impulse, generated in the sinoatrial (SA) node, is conducted through the atrioventricular (AV) node, and travels through the specialized conduction tissues of the His–Purkinje system. This conducted impulse leads to a rapid depolarization of the ventricles. This normal activation pattern results in the surface electrocardiogram (ECG) showing normal (narrow) QRS complex morphology with duration of less than 0.12 s (three small boxes on standard ECG paper recorded at 25 mm/s). A rhythm is considered narrow complex tachycardia (NCT) if the following two features are encountered: a ventricular rate above 100 bpm and a QRS complex width less than 0.12 s. While these criteria apply to adult patients, children have age-related norms for both rate and QRS duration that are used to make the diagnosis of NCT.

NCTs are further classified as either regular or irregular. Regular NCTs (those having a consistent R–R interval) include sinus tachycardia (ST), atrial tachycardia, AV junctional tachycardia, atrial flutter with fixed AV conduction, and paroxysmal supraventricular tachycardia (PSVT). Rhythms that have consistently irregular R–R intervals throughout are considered irregular NCTs and include atrial fibrillation, atrial flutter with variable AV conduction, and multifocal atrial tachycardia (MAT). Rhythms that have generally consistent, regular R–R intervals but also have occasional irregular beats are likely to be one of the regular rhythms listed above with occasional premature or ectopic beats. Figure 6.1 demonstrates the use of the R–R interval to determine regularity.

Figure 6.2 depicts a decision pathway based on the presence or absence of regular R–R intervals and the presence of ectopic beats. In most cases, a diligent search for the P wave and general knowledge of the cardiac conduction system will lead to appropriate identification of the rhythm. One caveat to the recognition of NCTs is that the presence of a bundle branch block can lead any of the rhythms discussed here to appear as wide complex tachycardia.

Regular Narrow Complex Tachycardia

ST is the most commonly encountered NCT. ST originates from the SA node at a rate greater than 100 bpm (Figure 6.3). Although ST may often be extremely fast in young children, it is rarely seen at rates greater than 200 bpm in older children and adults. Electrical impulses in ST are conducted through the normal cardiac conduction system in the usual manner. The ECG should always include a normal P wave associated with every QRS complex. The QRS complexes are narrow, and the intervals are all normal. Simply put, ST is a normal sinus rhythm at a rapid rate. Importantly, ST should be considered a reactive rhythm, resulting from an abnormal physiologic event; refer Box 6.1 for further information regarding ST.

Atrial tachycardia is a term used to describe an arrhythmia that originates in the atrial myocardium but outside of the SA node with rates greater than 100 bpm. These rhythms may be paroxysmal or sustained, and they may arise from any one of many etiologies including re-entry pathways and adverse effects related to medications. Atrial tachycardias may be further classified as unifocal or multifocal depending on the number of foci within the atrial myocardium that give rise to

The Electrocardiogram in Emergency and Acute Care, First Edition.
Edited by Korin B. Hudson, Amita Sudhir, George Glass, and William J. Brady.

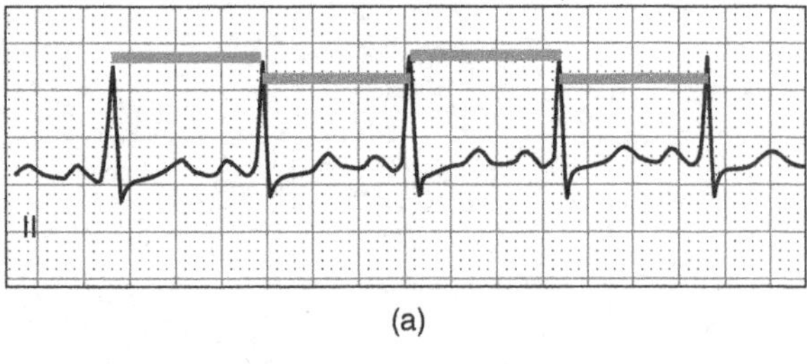

(a)

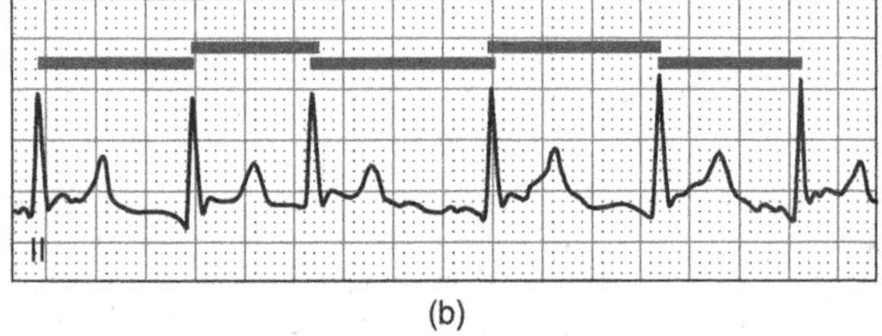

(b)

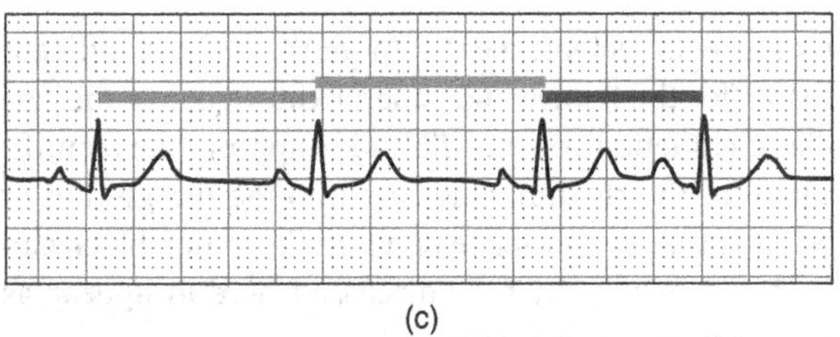

(c)

Figure 6.1 Using R–R interval to determine rhythm regularity. Sinus tachycardia with (a) consistent and regular R–R intervals. (b) Atrial fibrillation with irregular R–R intervals. (c) Normal sinus rhythm with premature atrial contraction (PAC) showing an irregular/ectopic beat in a rhythm with otherwise consistent and regular R–R intervals. In certain regions of this rhythm strip, the addition of the PACs will appear to increase the rate of the NSR, producing an apparent tachycardia.

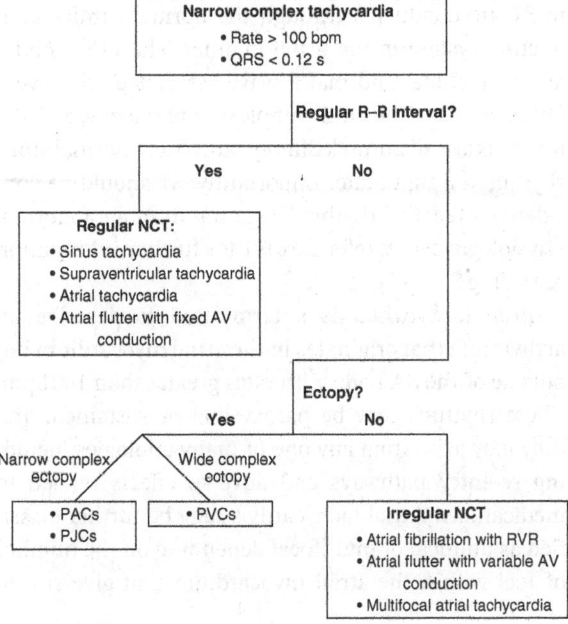

Figure 6.2 Decision pathway for narrow complex tachycardia. RVR, rapid ventricular response.

conducted beats. MAT can produce an irregular rhythm and is discussed with the irregular NCTs later in this chapter.

Unifocal atrial tachycardia is characterized by atrial depolarizations that are generated by the same atrial ectopic focus for at least three consecutive beats and occur at an atrial rate of 100–240 bpm. Atrial tachycardia may occur intermittently with sudden initiation and termination, and it may be difficult to identify the arrhythmia without a long rhythm strip. Depending on the location of the ectopic atrial focus, the surface ECG or rhythm strip may show P waves that are upright or inverted. These P waves may precede the QRS complex, be buried in the QRS complex (either not visualized, or causing a change in the QRS morphology), or appear immediately after the QRS complex. Symptoms associated with the arrhythmia are also often sudden and intermittent.

In atrial tachycardia, the AV conduction ratio is often 1 : 1. At rates less than 160 bpm, it may be difficult to distinguish atrial tachycardia from ST. However, if a conduction delay exists between the atria and ventricles, the atrial rate will be faster than the ventricular rate. The ratio of atrial contractions to ventricular contractions may be consistent (Figure 6.4) or it may vary (Figure 6.5). Unifocal atrial tachycardia in the presence of AV conduction delay can be difficult to differentiate from atrial flutter. However, unifocal atrial tachycardia should have clear P waves with a distinct isoelectric baseline between P waves rather than the characteristic saw-tooth waves of atrial flutter.

Supraventricular tachycardia (SVT) is a term that refers to a variety of NCTs with electrical origins proximal to the ventricle including impulses that originate in the SA node, atrial tissue, the AV node, or the His bundle. While the term PSVT includes any of the regular NCTs that occur intermittently as described above, it is commonly and most correctly used to describe atrioventricular nodal re-entrant tachycardia (AVNRT) and atrioventricular re-entrant tachycardia (AVRT). AVNRT and AVRT are the most frequently encountered types of PSVT.

Both AVNRT and AVRT are rhythms that rely on conduction pathways in and around the AV node that may transmit electrical impulses, not only anterograde (from the atria to the ventricles) but also retrograde (from the ventricles back up toward the atria). These multiple pathways may form a "loop" or re-entry circuit in which electrical activity proceeds in a circular manner, leading to rapid depolarization of the atria and the ventricles. These impulses bypass the usual conduction pathway and do not have typical refractory periods. In order for these rhythms to be maintained, a functioning AV node

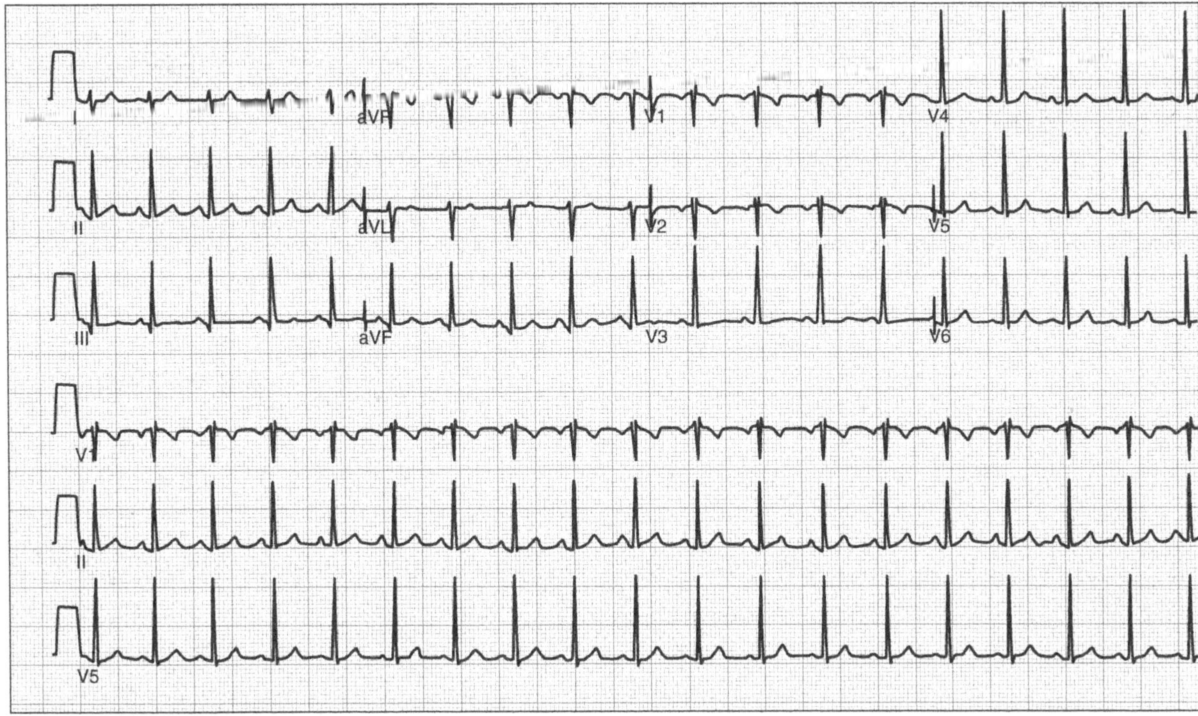

Figure 6.3 Sinus tachycardia.

Box 6.1 Sinus Tachycardia: Clinical Presentation and Management

Sinus tachycardia (ST) is rarely a primary rhythm disturbance; rather, it is most often a sign of another underlying condition; considerations include the following:

- Hypovolemia
- Hypoxia
- Fever
- Pain
- Anxiety
- Medication/chemical agent pharmacologic effect

Presenting symptoms can include the following:

- Palpitations
- Shortness of breath
- Chest discomfort

Symptoms are likely a result of the underlying condition/are not generally *caused by* the dysrhythmia.
Supportive care with attention to the underlying cause of ST is most appropriate (e.g. oxygen therapy, intravenous fluid, antipyretic agents, pain management, etc.).

must be present as part of the re-entry circuit. Therefore, these rhythms are referred to as *AV nodal dependent*. AVNRT occurs with a "microscopic" loop, with both the anterograde and retrograde pathways lying within the AV node, while AVRT demonstrates a "macroscopic" loop with one electrical pathway lying within the AV node and the other in the adjacent tissues; AVRT is most often seen in patients with ventricular preexcitation syndromes such as the Wolff–Parkinson–White (WPW) syndrome; WPW is discussed in Chapter 21.

In AVNRT (Box 6.2), the tachydysrhythmia is triggered when an atrial impulse conducts through the anterograde pathway and proceeds to the ventricles, while simultaneously the impulse is conducted back up to the atria via the retrograde pathway – all within the AV node. This re-entry circuit propagates the impulse leading to rapid, nearly simultaneous depolarization of the atria and the ventricles. When seen on the ECG, AVNRT typically has a rate between 130 and 250 bpm and, in the absence of aberrant conduction or a bundle branch block, manifests as a narrow QRS complex. Most often P waves cannot be identified because depolarization of the atria and ventricles occurs simultaneously. This results in P waves that are masked by the QRS complexes. Two examples of AVNRT are shown in Figure 6.6.

While AVRT is less common than AVNRT, this rhythm also requires the presence of an anatomic

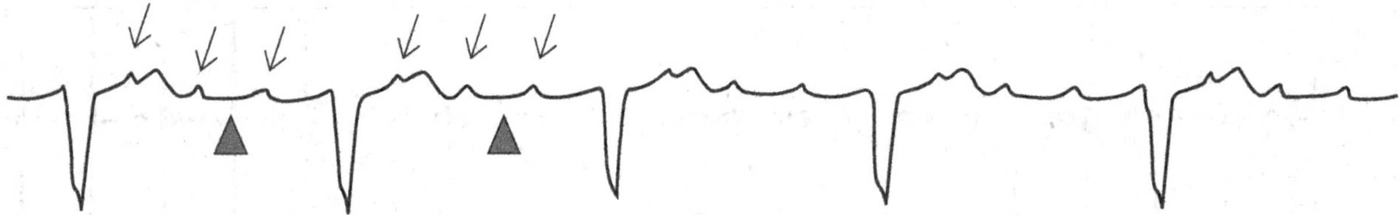

Figure 6.4 Atrial tachycardia. Note the P waves (arrows) denoting a fast underlying atrial rhythm, although each P wave is not conducted through the AV node. There is a clear isoelectric baseline (arrow heads) between P waves unlike atrial flutter.

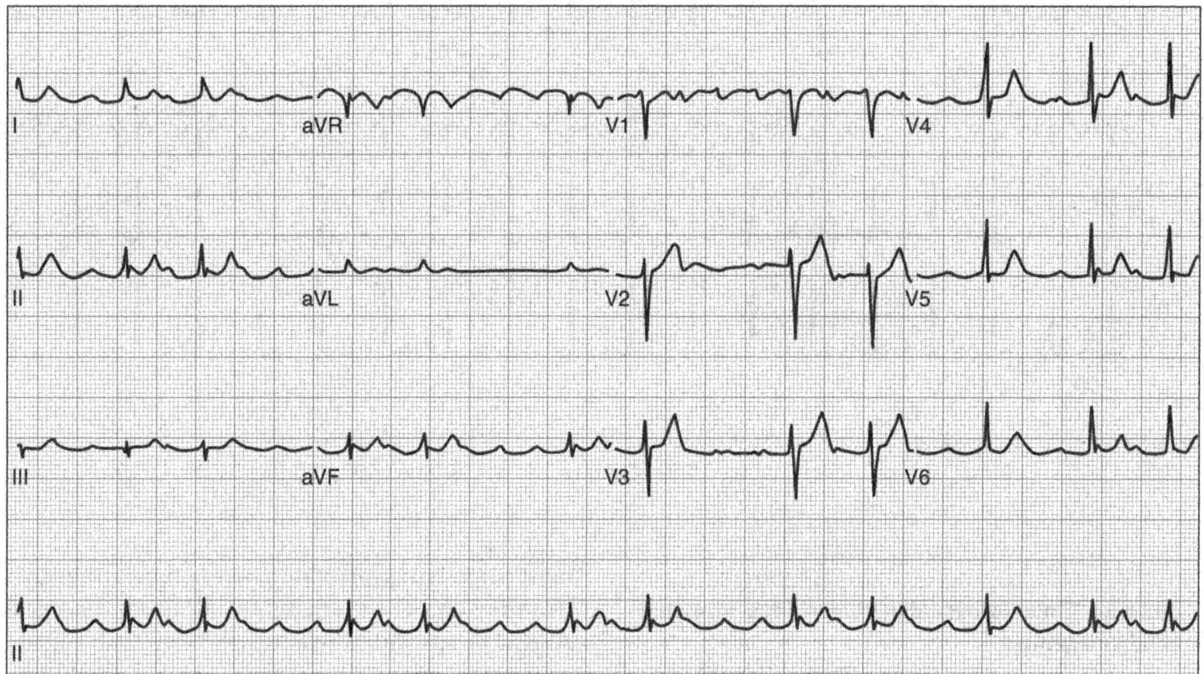

Figure 6.5 Atrial tachycardia with variable AV conduction. Identical, regular P waves indicate a single electrical focus in the atria. The atrial rate is 200 bpm. Varying nodal transmission accounts for the lower ventricular rate of 70. *Source:* Mattu and Brady, 2003, Reprinted with permission from John Wiley & Sons.

accessory conduction pathway between the atria and the ventricles that allows electrical impulses to bypass the AV node. The accessory pathway does not have the intrinsic delay that is present within the AV node and even during sinus rhythm, depolarization of the ventricles may begin via this accessory pathway before normal transmission through the AV node has occurred. This phenomenon is referred to as *ventricular preexcitation* and, when the patient is in normal sinus rhythm, may be seen on the ECG as a slurred upstroke of the initial portion of the QRS complex (referred to as a *delta wave*).

The WPW syndrome is the most common of the accessory pathway syndromes and represents a classic example of AVRT. A tachyarrhythmia that results from WPW can proceed as a circuit, using the accessory pathway and AV node, in either an orthodromic or antidromic manner. In orthodromic rhythms, anterograde conduction occurs from atria to ventricles through the AV node, then the impulse is transmitted in a retrograde manner from ventricles to atria via the accessory pathway. In antidromic rhythms, the impulse from atria to ventricles is conducted anterograde via the accessory pathway, and the impulse is then transmitted in a retrograde manner from the ventricles to atria through the AV node. Figure 6.7 shows both orthodromic and antidromic conduction pathways.

Most often in WPW, impulses originating in the SA node or atrial myocardium proceed in an orthodromic manner as the initial impulse travels through the AV node into the Bundle of His, producing a narrow QRS complex. However, the electrical impulse also travels in a retrograde manner up the accessory pathway, as described above, and reactivates the atria and then the AV node again. This circuit (Figure 6.7a) continues to conduct in a rapid manner leading to regular NCT (Figure 6.8a).

Box 6.2 Atrioventricular Nodal Reentrant Tachycardia (Also Known as PSVT): Clinical Presentation and Management

AVNRT most often occurs in young, otherwise healthy individuals with structurally normal hearts.

Presenting symptoms

- Palpitations
- Shortness of breath
- Diaphoresis
- Dizziness/light-headedness
- Chest pain/discomfort

AVNRT is paroxysmal (brief and intermittent) in nature/frequently self-terminating.

Treatment options include the following:

- Vagal maneuvers
- Adenosine
- β-Adrenergic blocker
- Calcium antagonist
- Synchronized direct current (electrical) cardioversion

WPW-related tachycardia with antidromic conduction takes the opposite pathway. The impulse initiated in the atrium conducts first through the accessory pathway stimulating the ventricular myocardium directly, causing ventricular depolarization in a delayed manner, bypassing the Bundle of His, and resulting in a wide QRS complex (Figures 6.7b and 6.8b). The re-entry circuit is completed when the impulse propagates in a retrograde manner through the AV node to the atria and then back through the accessory pathway once more. Antidromic conduction occurs when the refractory period of the accessory pathway is shorter than the refractory period in the AV node.

Atrial flutter (Figure 6.9) is characterized by rapid, regular atrial depolarizations that occur at rate of 240–340 atrial bpm. The atrial rate may be faster in children or slower in patients taking rate-controlling medications or in patients with dilated atria. The atrial flutter waves, or "flutter waves," are commonly seen as a sawtooth pattern, which is best seen in lead V1.

Owing to the refractory period, the electrical impulses from the atria are only intermittently conducted through the AV node. From the AV node, conduction proceeds through the usual conduction pathways, resulting in a narrow QRS complex on the ECG (assuming a patient has no underlying interventricular conduction abnormalities). The T wave may or may not be evident, given the presence of flutter waves. When seen, the T wave may alter the morphology of the flutter wave that appears directly after the QRS complex.

Atrial flutter is generally described by the ratio of the number of atrial depolarizations to ventricular depolarizations. This ratio is usually fixed, leading to a regular rhythm with a fixed R–R interval. However, varying ratios lead to a rapid, irregular, narrow complex rhythm referred to as *atrial flutter with variable conduction*. By convention, the ratio is described by the number of flutter waves seen between QRS complexes plus one, assumed to be "buried" in the QRS. Ratios of 2:1 and 3:1 conduction are most common; a ratio of 4 : 1 or greater suggests

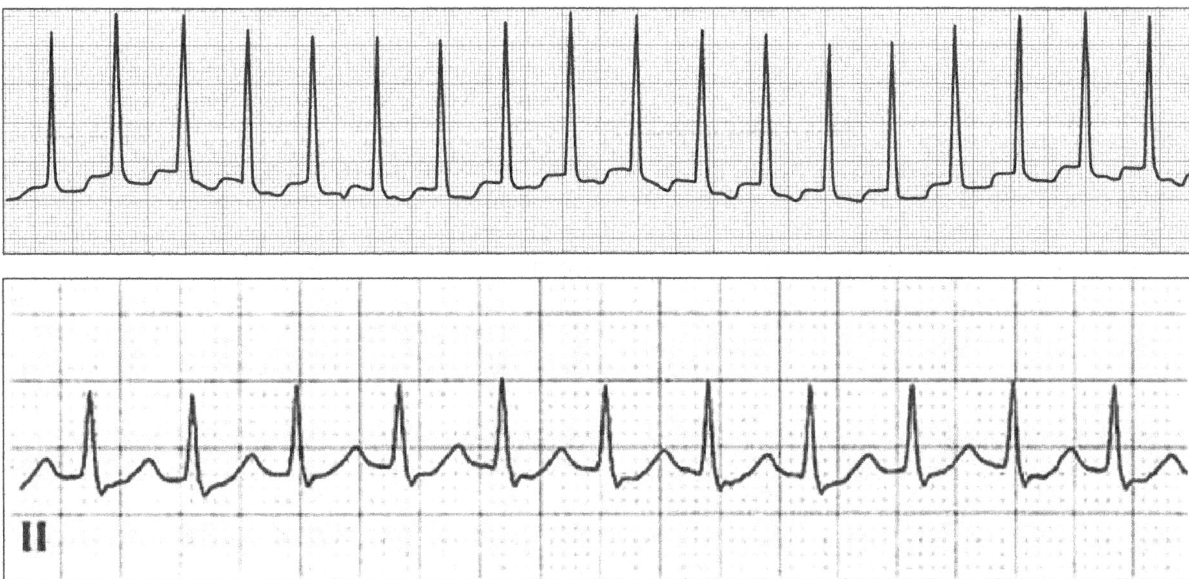

Figure 6.6 Two examples of AVNRT-type supraventricular tachycardia (also known as PSVT).

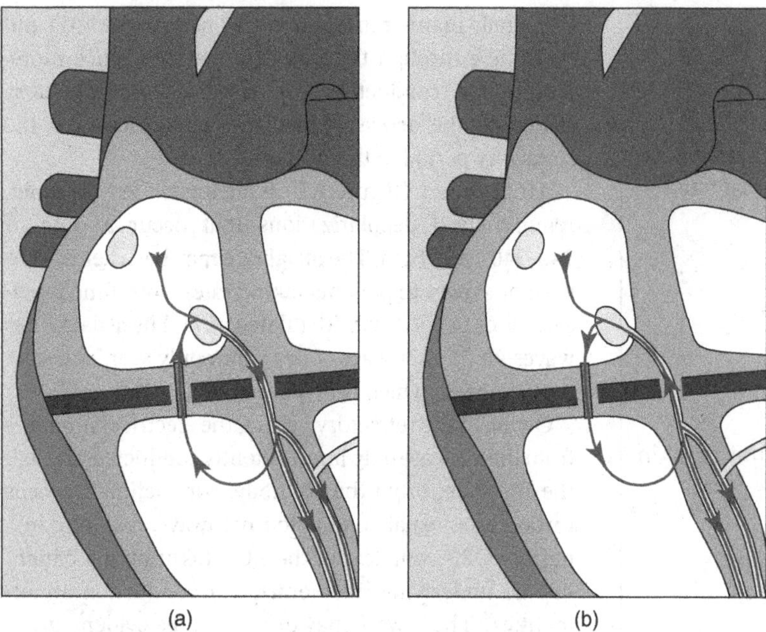

Figure 6.7 Mechanisms for (a) orthodromic and (b) antidromic atrioventricular re-entrant tachycardia (AVRT). *Source:* Reprinted from Morris et al., ABC of Clinical Electrocardiography, Second Edition, 2008 with permission from John Wiley & Sons Ltd.

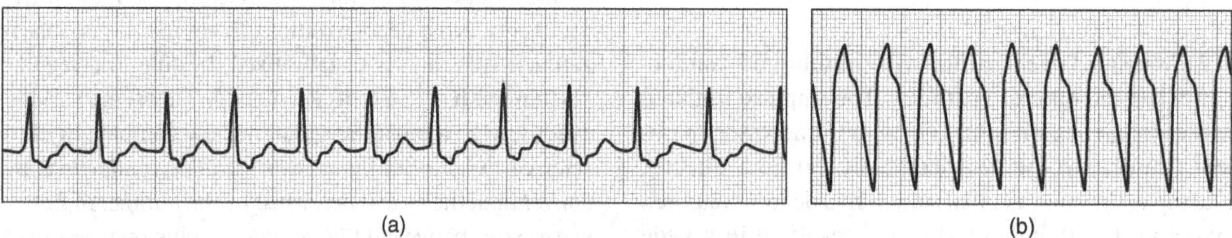

Figure 6.8 WPW re-entrant tachycardia. (a) Orthodromic AVRT with clearly visible P waves, the so-called retrograde P waves, that follow the QRS complex. (b) Antidromic AVRT with wide QRS complexes. *Source:* Reprinted from Morris et al., ABC of Clinical Electrocardiography, Second Edition, 2008 with permission from John Wiley & Sons Ltd.

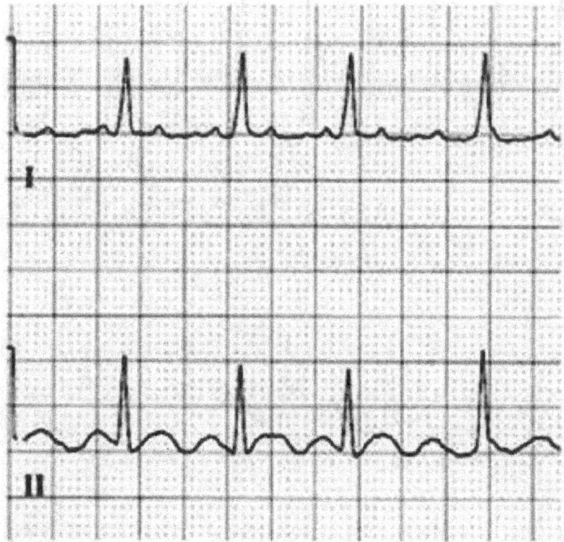

Figure 6.9 Atrial flutter. While distinct P waves can be seen in lead I, lead II shows the characteristic "saw-tooth" pattern.

that the patient is taking AV nodal blocking medications or has underlying intrinsic conduction disease.

Infrequently, 1 : 1 atrioventricular conduction may occur, leading to ventricular rates of approximately 300 bpm and, in the presence of intraventricular conduction abnormalities, a wide QRS complex that may be difficult to differentiate from ventricular tachycardia. Valsalva maneuvers or the administration of AV nodal blocking medication may reveal flutter waves, easing rhythm determination in cases with a high rate of ventricular conduction. However, caution is advised in the administration of AV nodal blocking agents in the setting of a wide complex tachycardia.

Irregular Narrow Complex Tachycardias

Atrial fibrillation (Figure 6.10) is the most common sustained dysrhythmia seen by emergency medical services (EMS) and hospital-based providers. The source of

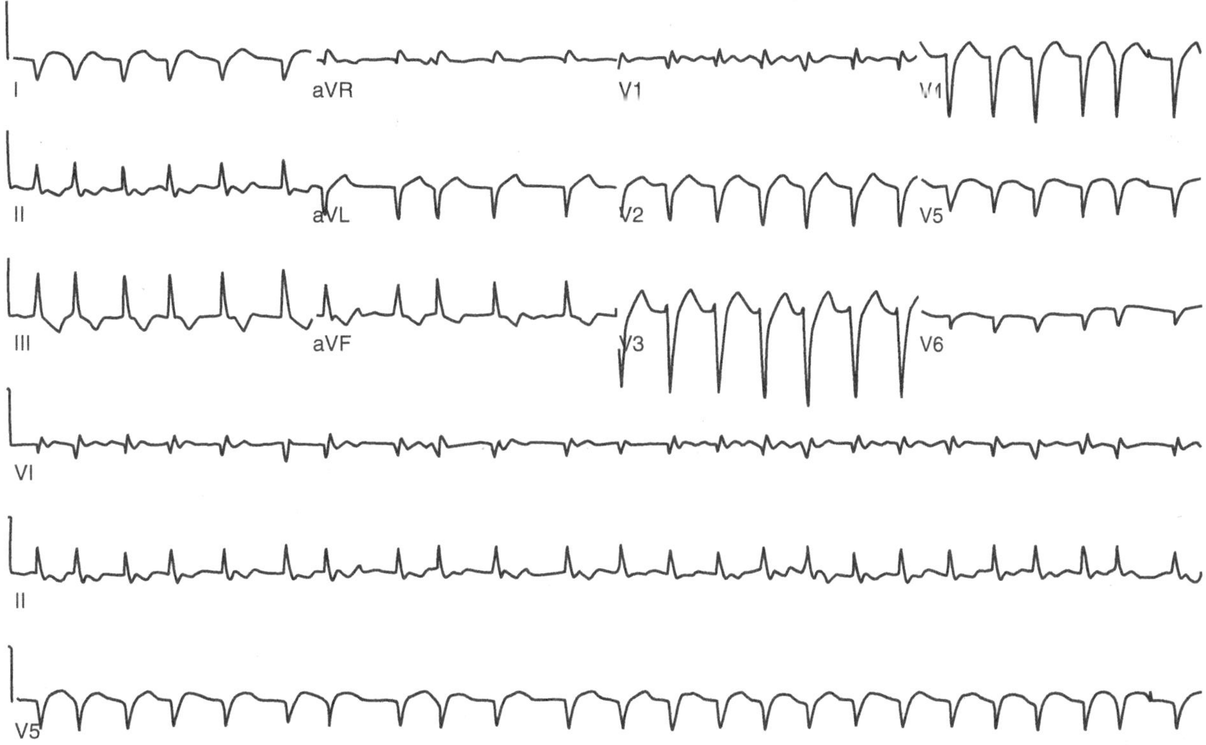

Figure 6.10 Atrial fibrillation with rapid ventricular response.

electrical impulse in atrial fibrillation comes from multiple atrial foci separate from the SA node. These foci may fire independently at rates that can approach 600 depolarizations per minute, not infrequently leading to an irregular, jumpy baseline on the ECG – which is indicative of the irregular, chaotic atrial electrical activity. The chaotic baseline does not reveal distinct P waves and is often best seen in leads V1, V2, II, III, and aVF. Typically, the rhythm conducts through the AV node and His–Purkinje system in a normal manner, resulting in narrow QRS complexes, occurring with irregular R–R intervals.

Atrial fibrillation typically produces an irregularly irregular ventricular rhythm as conduction to the ventricles is dependent on the refractory nature of the AV node. The ventricular rate is variable, but frequently ranges between 100 and 180 bpm. As ventricular rates exceed 150 bpm, atrial fibrillation may be difficult to distinguish from other NCTs. Measuring, or "marching out," the R–R interval with marked paper or calipers will reveal the irregular ventricular rhythm with constant beat-to-beat variability. Some of the most common causes of atrial fibrillation and atrial flutter are listed in Figure 6.11.

MAT is a rhythm that is characterized by P waves with three or more distinct morphologies (Figure 6.12). These P waves arise from competing foci of electrical

- Hypertension
- Post-op CABG (30%)
- Mitral valve disease
- Organic heart disease
- Myocardial infarction
- Thyrotoxicosis
- Pulmonary embolism
- Atrial septal defect
- WPW syndrome
- Sick sinus syndrome
- Alchohol
- Chronic lung disease
- Hypoxia

Figure 6.11 Common causes of atrial fibrillation and atrial flutter. CABG, coronary artery bypass graft.

activity within the atria in the absence of a consistent impulse arising from the SA node. In addition to differing P wave morphologies, the different atrial foci give rise to varied PR intervals and, therefore varied P–P intervals. However, the various atrial impulses are all conducted via the AV node to the ventricles via the normal conduction pathways, resulting in a narrow QRS

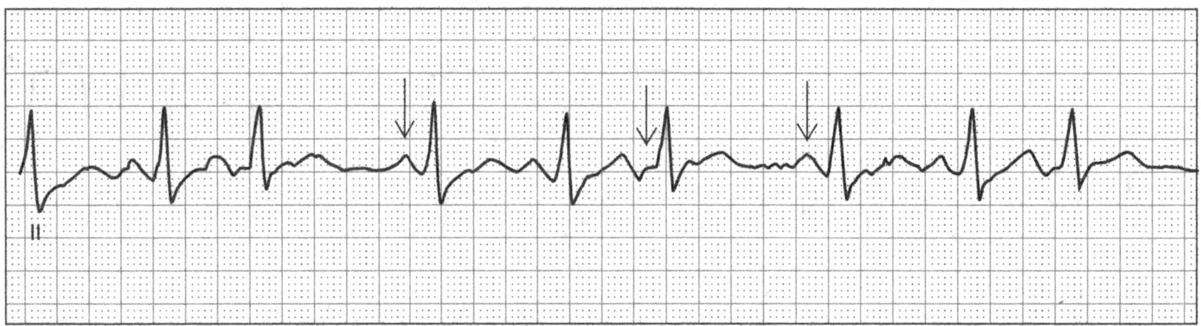

Figure 6.12 Multifocal atrial tachycardia. Note the multiple P wave morphologies (arrows) and distinct isoelectric baseline.

Box 6.3 Multifocal Atrial Tachycardia: Clinical Presentation and Management

Common causes of MAT include the following:

- Chronic obstructive pulmonary disease (acute exacerbation)
- Pneumonia
- Hypoxia
- Fever
- Aminophylline and β-agonist medications
- Acute heart failure (acute exacerbation of congestive heart failure [CHF]/pulmonary edema)
- Cor pulmonale (right-sided heart failure)
- Other forms of organic heart disease with acute event
- Postoperative period
- Sepsis

Presenting symptoms may/may not have direct relationship to underlying cause.
Treatment involves identification of underlying cause with appropriate management.
Many causes of MAT are pulmonary in origin, thus the common mantra "treat the lungs."

complex with a ventricular rate that is often greater than 100 bpm. Refer to Box 6.3 for additional information regarding MAT.

It may be difficult to differentiate between MAT, ST with multifocal premature atrial contractions (PACs), and atrial fibrillation or atrial flutter. In many cases, rhythm recognition may be aided by examining a long single- or multilead rhythm strip. Recall that ST with multifocal PACs will demonstrate a dominant atrial pacemaker (specifically the SA node) with consistent P wave morphology, whereas MAT will have no dominant pacemaker and thus multiple P wave morphologies. Furthermore, MAT should demonstrate an isoelectric baseline with evident P waves, while atrial fibrillation and atrial flutter have neither an isoelectric baseline nor clear P waves.

Further Reading

Fox, D.J., Wolfram, S., Desourza, I.S. et al. (2008). Supraventricular tachycardia: diagnosis and management. *Mayo Clinic Proc.* 83 (12): 1400–1411.

Mattu, A. and Brady, W.J. (2003). *ECGs for the Emergency Physician 1*. London, UK: Blackwell Publishing.

Morris, F., Brady, W.J., and Camm, J. (2008). *ABC of Clinical Electrocardiography*, Second edition. London, UK: BMJ Books.

7

Wide QRS Complex Tachycardia

Michael Levy and Francis X. Nolan Jr†

Anchorage Areawide EMS, Anchorage, Alaska, USA

The normal activation of the ventricles occurs after impulse generation in the sinoatrial (SA) node and conduction through atria and the atrioventricular (AV) node, and then through the specialized conduction tissues of the His–Purkinje system. This conduction system leads to rapid depolarization of the ventricles via their respective bundles. This normal activation pattern results in the surface electrocardiogram (ECG) showing normal (narrow) QRS complex morphology with duration of less than 0.12 s. When a rhythm is found to have a QRS complex width greater than 0.12 s in duration and is at a rate greater than 100 bpm (beats per minute), it is referred to as a wide complex tachycardia (WCT). In children, heart rates and QRS complex widths vary with age – consequently, children may present with WCT, including ventricular tachycardia (VT), with QRS duration of less than 0.12 s; age-related values of the QRS complex duration and ventricular rate define WCT in younger children.

WCTs (Box 7.1) may originate from any atrial, nodal, or ventricular site. "Supraventricular" WCTs can originate from cardiac tissues "above the ventricle," including foci in the SA node, atrial tissues, or the AV node. In these cases, the widened QRS complex results from abnormal conduction through the ventricles. "Ventricular" WCTs originate from the ventricular conduction system or ventricular myocardium (i.e. VT), or they may be the result of a ventricular paced rhythm (i.e. an extrinsic pacemaker). In each of these cases, the site of rhythm generation is located lower in the conduction system, leading to a wide QRS complex due to slower, less efficient conduction through the ventricular myocardium.

Ventricular Tachycardia – Monomorphic and Polymorphic

Although not the most common of all WCTs (supraventricular rhythms with aberrant conduction are more common), VT is the most concerning of the wide complex tachydysrthymias (Box 7.2). VT is defined as three or more beats of ventricular origin at a rate of 100 bpm or greater, although generally the rate is less than 200 bpm. While some minimal irregularity may be seen – particularly at the onset – the ECG in VT typically reveals a rhythm with very regular R–R intervals and a widened QRS complex (>0.12 s). "Normal" beats (those correlating to the patient's baseline or underlying rhythm with a narrow QRS complex) may be visible on rhythm strips before the initiation or after the termination of VT.

The morphology of the QRS complexes of VT may be one of two basic types, monomorphic or polymorphic. Monomorphic VT arises from impulses generated by a single ventricular focus, whereas polymorphic VT arises from multiple foci of impulse generation. The monomorphic type is much more common and is characterized by a regular WCT in which each of the QRS complexes in a given lead has the same appearance (Figure 7.1). In contrast, polymorphic VT has a wavy, undulating appearance (Figure 7.2) that indicates several electrical foci, leading to morphology that varies from beat to beat. Torsade de pointes VT (Figure 7.3) is a very specific subtype of polymorphic VT that is encountered in patients with an underlying prolonged QT interval.

Certain electrocardiographic findings can aid in the diagnosis of VT and can differentiate SVT with conduction aberrancy. These include AV dissociation as well as

† Deceased.

The Electrocardiogram in Emergency and Acute Care, First Edition.
Edited by Korin B. Hudson, Amita Sudhir, George Glass, and William J. Brady.

Box 7.1 Wide Complex Tachycardia

- Differential diagnosis of WCT includes supraventricular rhythms with aberrant ventricular conduction and VT.
- Clinical features associated with VT:
  - Age greater than 50 years
  - History of significant congestive heart failure (CHF)
  - History of past myocardial infarction (MI)
- No reliable clinical features are associated with supraventricular tachycardia (SVT) with aberrant conduction.
- ECG diagnosis/distinction is frequently unclear/at times is impossible.
- Stability or instability is not associated with specific rhythm diagnosis in the WCT patient.
- Management issues should focus on patient and ECG findings.

Box 7.2 Ventricular Tachycardia

Clinical manifestations of VT

- Cardiac arrest (i.e. pulseless, apneic, and unresponsiveness)
- Chest pain
- Shortness of breath
- Weakness/dizziness
- Altered mental status
- Hypotension/shock
- Pulmonary edema

Causes of VT

- Acute coronary syndrome/acute MI
- Chronic/past ischemic heart disease
- Moderate-to-severe chronic CHF (left ventricular dysfunction)
- Cardiomyopathy
- Medication toxicity
- Electrolyte abnormality

Management is based on patient presentation.

- Cardiac arrest – electrical defibrillation with resuscitation
- Shock/end-organ hypoperfusion – electrical synchronized cardioversion
- Symptomatic without shock – medical management with electrical cardioversion and resuscitative measures on standby

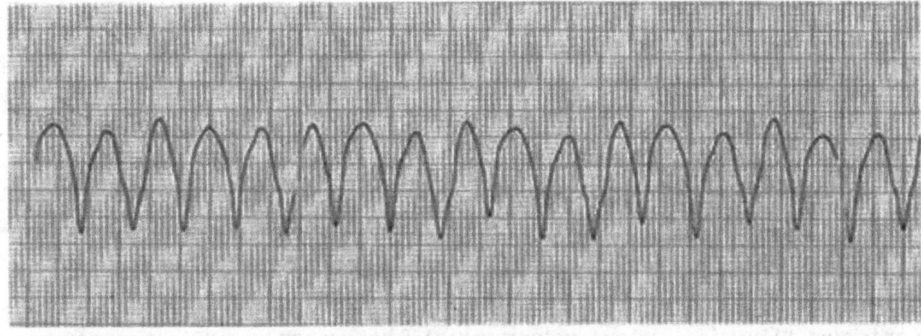

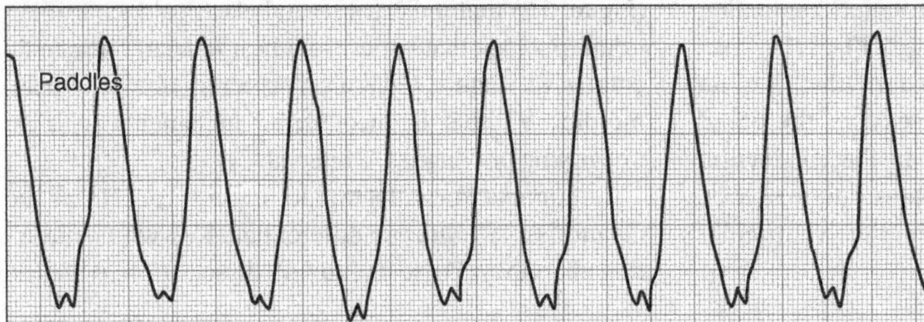

Figure 7.1 Monomorphic ventricular tachycardia. Note the consistent morphology of the QRS complex from beat to beat with a regular rhythm.

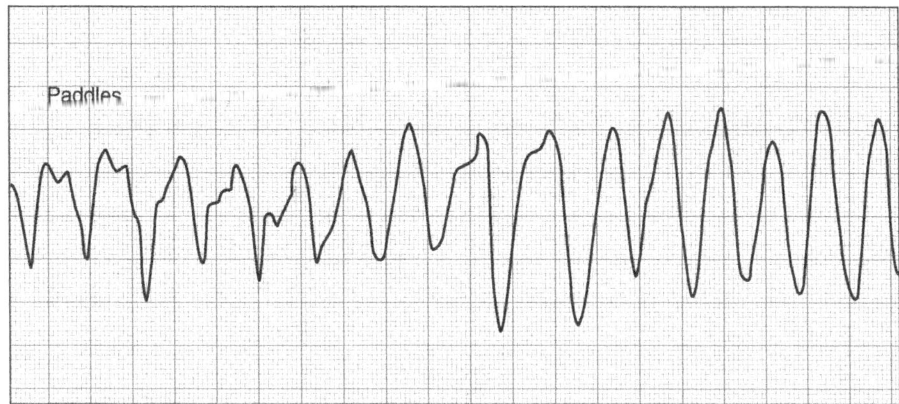

Figure 7.2 Polymorphic ventricular tachycardia. Note the varying QRS complex morphology with variation from one complex to the next and an irregular rhythm.

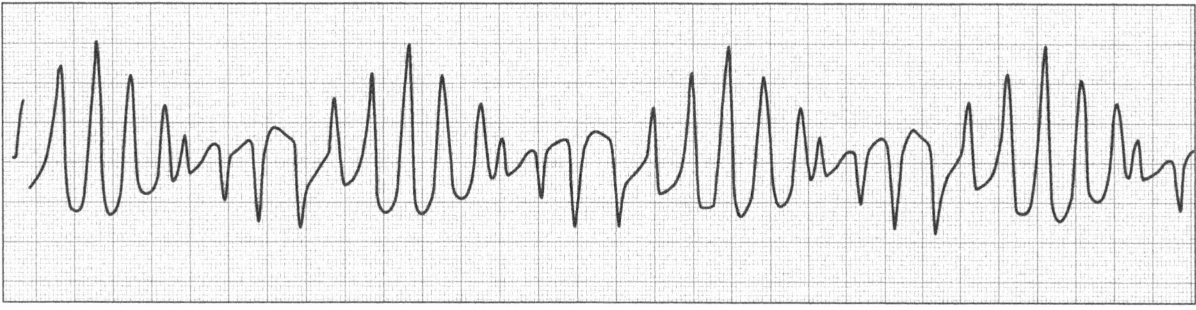

Figure 7.3 Polymorphic ventricular tachycardia, torsade de pointes. Note the gradual change in the amplitude of the QRS complex from maximal to minimal to maximal with repetition of this pattern.

capture beats and/or fusion beats. The presence of these findings provides strong evidence suggesting that the rhythm is VT rather than a supraventricular rhythm with aberrant conduction. Unfortunately, these findings are not always obvious on rhythm strips and 12-lead ECGs; the clinician should review both the standard 12-lead ECG and a longer single-lead rhythm strip for their presence in a patient who presents with WCT.

Atrioventricular dissociation: In VT, the ventricular depolarization typically renders the AV node refractory to normal conduction. However, the atria may continue to depolarize normally, leading to complete dissociation of the P wave and QRS complex. In many cases, the P waves are not visible as they become obscured by the rapid, wide QRS complexes. On some tracings, however, this dissociation can be seen with P waves appearing between QRS complexes but having no obvious fixed relation to the QRS complexes (Figure 7.4).

Capture and fusion beats: Occasionally, an atrial impulse may find the AV node and His–Purkinje system nonrefractory, and the impulse will be conducted through the normal conduction system, arriving at the ventricle and producing a depolarization – a supraventricular depolarization in the overall setting of ventricular depolarizations. In these cases, a normal appearing QRS complex will appear among the otherwise widened QRS complexes. Such a depolarization is known as a *capture beat* in that the supraventricular impulse "electrically captures" the ventricle (Figure 7.5).

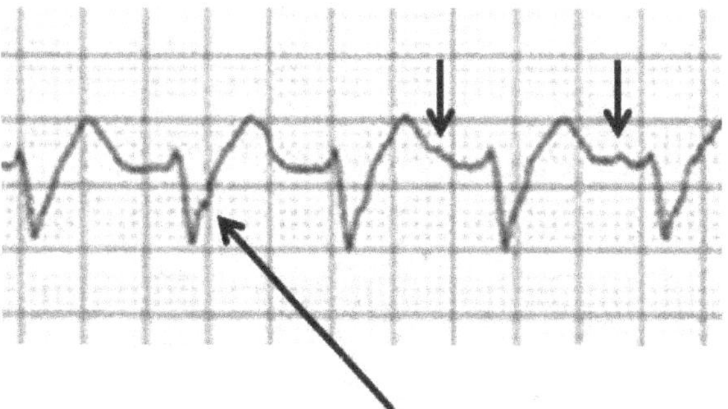

Figure 7.4 Monomorphic ventricular tachycardia with AV dissociation. Note direct evidence of P waves indicated by small arrows and deflections in the QRS complex likely resulting from the presence of a P wave (long arrows). *Source:* Reproduced from Brady WJ & Truwit J, Critical Decisions in Emergency & Acute Care Electrocardiography, 2009, with permission from John Wiley and Sons Ltd.

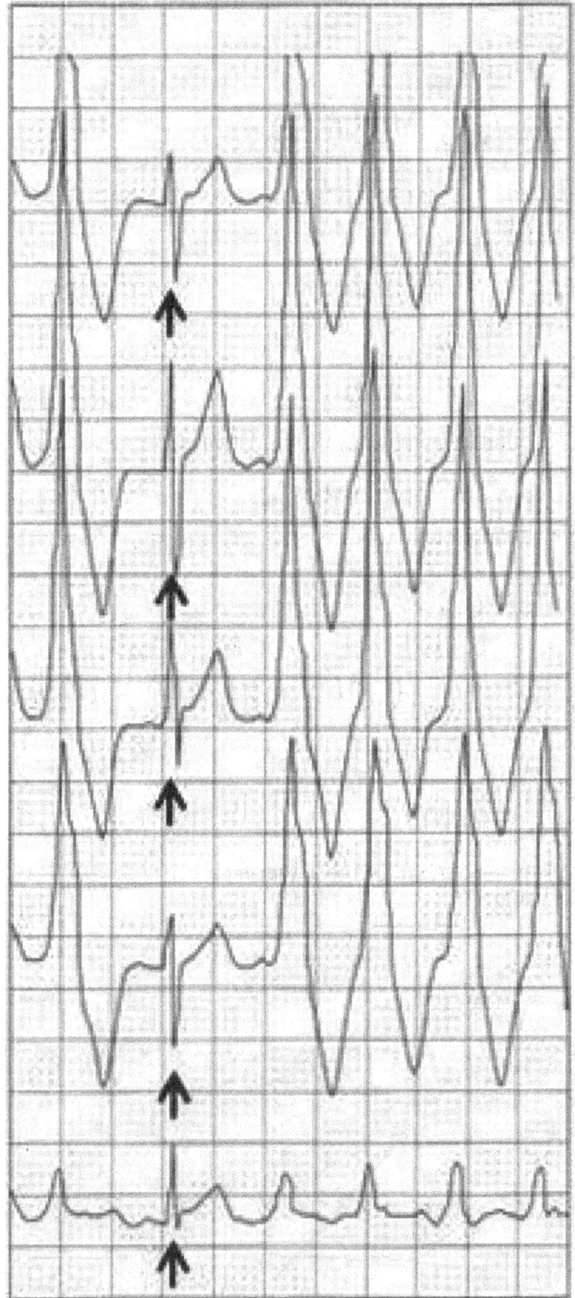

Figure 7.5 Ventricular tachycardia with capture beat. Note that the second beat (arrow) has a very different appearance from the surrounding beats. This narrow QRS complex, a capture beat, suggests that the surrounding wide complex beats represent ventricular tachycardia. *Source:* Reproduced from Brady WJ & Truwit J, Critical Decisions in Emergency & Acute Care Electrocardiography, 2009, with permission from John Wiley and Sons Ltd.

A variation of this electrical capture may occur when there is simultaneous AV transmission of a supraventricular impulse and generation of a ventricular impulse – both impulses electrically fuse, producing an intermediate width QRS complex. This phenomenon is called a *fusion beat*, as it is the combination of two separate ventricular depolarizations merged into a single complex seen on the surface ECG tracing (Figure 7.6).

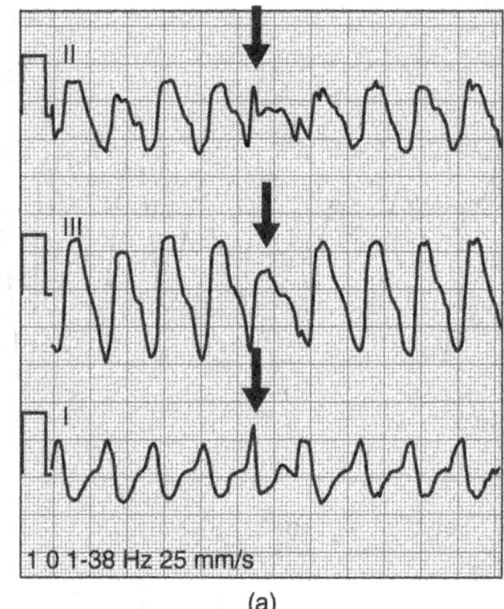

(a)

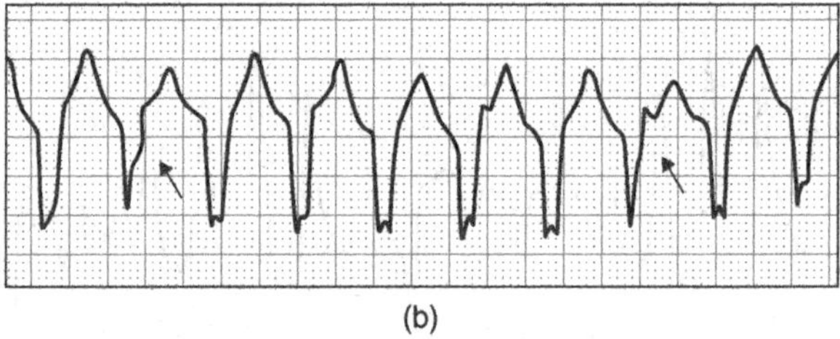

(b)

Figure 7.6 Ventricular tachycardia with fusion beats. Note the intermediate width QRS complex indicated by the arrows in (a) and (b). *Source:* Figure (b) reproduced from Brady WJ & Truwit J, Critical Decisions in Emergency & Acute Care Electrocardiography, 2009, with permission from John Wiley and Sons Ltd.

Marked irregularity of the WCT strongly suggests that the rhythm is supraventricular in origin, specifically atrial fibrillation with aberrant conduction. The opposite statement, however, is not true – marked regularity does not confirm the diagnosis of VT. Other electrocardiographic findings have been suggested to be of value to distinguish SVT with aberrant conduction from VT. These include ventricular rate and features of the QRS complex (width, axis, and morphology). Unfortunately, these findings used either alone or in conjunction are not entirely reliable for ruling in or ruling out VT; furthermore, their use is cumbersome.

Ventricular Fibrillation

Ventricular fibrillation (VF) represents electrical chaos within the ventricles. In VF, conduction through the ventricular system becomes completely disorganized with multiple ectopic ventricular foci competing to direct cardiac conduction. None of these foci are successful because of colliding electrical signals and re-entry loops that are sometimes referred to as *circus re-entry*. The ECG representation of VF is equally chaotic; it has rapid, high-amplitude, inconsistent waveforms that lack any discernible focus. This pattern is called *coarse VF* (Figure 7.7a). Over a short period of time, the coarse pattern decreases to a low-amplitude waveform called *fine VF* (Figure 7.7b) that culminates. Statistically, most resuscitations ultimately result in *asystole*.

Supraventricular Tachycardia with Aberrant Conduction

As described in Chapter 6, SVT most commonly occurs with a narrow QRS complex (normal duration <0.12 s). However, if there is aberrant ventricular conduction, this supraventricular rhythm will present as a WCT. Aberrant conduction most often occurs due to one of the three classic mechanisms of a widened QRS complex: a pre-existing bundle branch block (BBB), a rate-related BBB (a BBB that develops owing to a rapid heart rate affecting the ability of the conduction tissues to repolarize), or dysfunction of the bundle branches due to metabolic (i.e. elevated serum potassium) or medication toxicity (i.e. sodium channel blockade). The ensuing beat will manifest as a widened QRS complex and, in

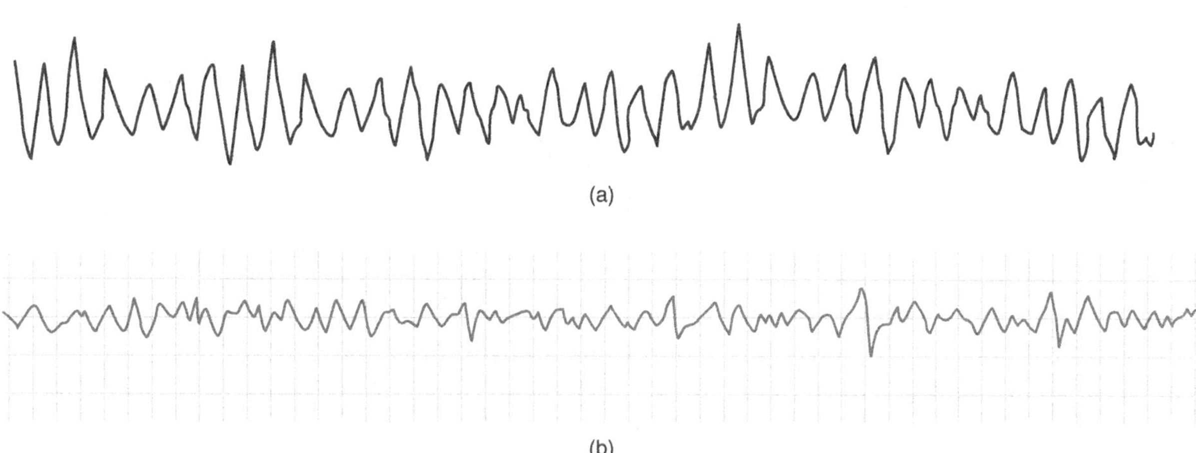

Figure 7.7 Ventricular fibrillation. (a) Coarse ventricular fibrillation. The amplitude of the waveforms is large and varying, producing the coarse pattern. This form of VF can be confused with polymorphic VT. In either case, the patient is pulseless, requiring electrical defibrillation. This form of VF tends to occur early in cardiac arrest. (b) Fine ventricular fibrillation. The amplitude of the waveforms is markedly less, producing a much less coarse waveform.

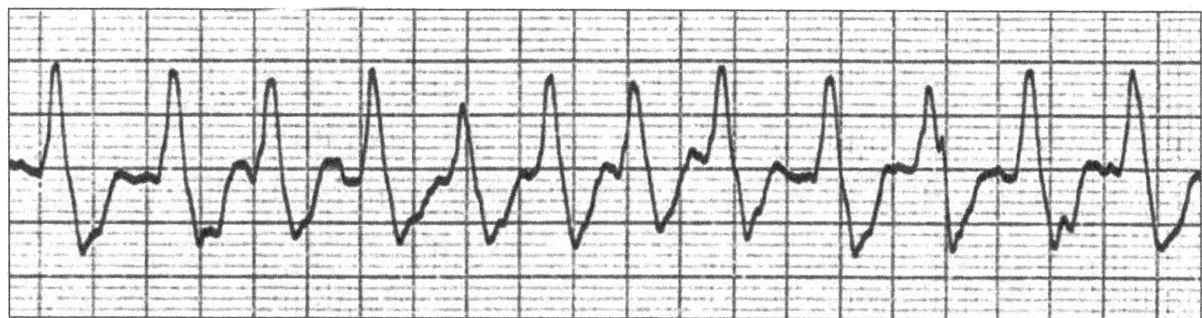

Figure 7.8 Supraventricular tachycardia with aberrant ventricular conduction due to fixed bundle branch block. Atrial fibrillation with bundle branch block.

sustained rhythms, a WCT is generated. WCTs of supraventricular origin may occur as a result of any of the SVTs including sinus tachycardia, atrial tachycardia, atrial flutter, atrial fibrillation, and paroxysmal SVT, if they are associated with aberrant ventricular conduction.

The most frequently encountered mechanism producing the widened QRS complex is the pre-existing BBB. Although an SVT that occurs in a patient with a pre-existing BBB will present as a WCT, the rhythm will retain the certain features of the underlying rhythm (Figures 7.8 and 7.9). The second most frequently encountered mechanism accounting for a widened QRS complex involves the rate-related BBB. This type of intraventricular block is not evident at normal or even mildly accelerated heart rates; rather, it only occurs in the setting of more rapid rates when one of the bundles is slower to repolarize. This delayed repolarization will leave the slower bundle refractory to conduction on subsequent beats, thus slowing the propagation of the electrical impulse and leading to a widened QRS complex (Figure 7.9). These rate-related intraventricular blocks may present as WCT in patients with no previous history of BBB.

The least commonly encountered reason for a widened QRS complex is related to either a metabolic or medication adverse impact on intraventricular conduction (Figure 7.10). In these situations, either an electrolyte disturbance (i.e. hyperkalemia) or medication (i.e. tricyclic antidepressant) alters the conduction system's ability to function, slowing the conduction of electrical impulse and thus producing a widened QRS complex.

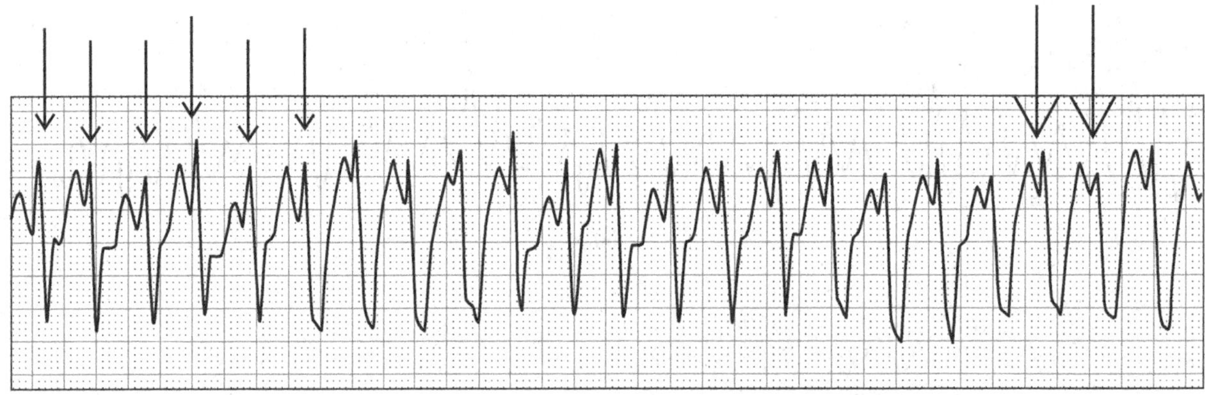

Figure 7.9 Supraventricular tachycardia with aberrant ventricular conduction due to a rate-related bundle branch block. Note small arrows with narrow QRS complex with progressively widening QRS complex (long arrows).

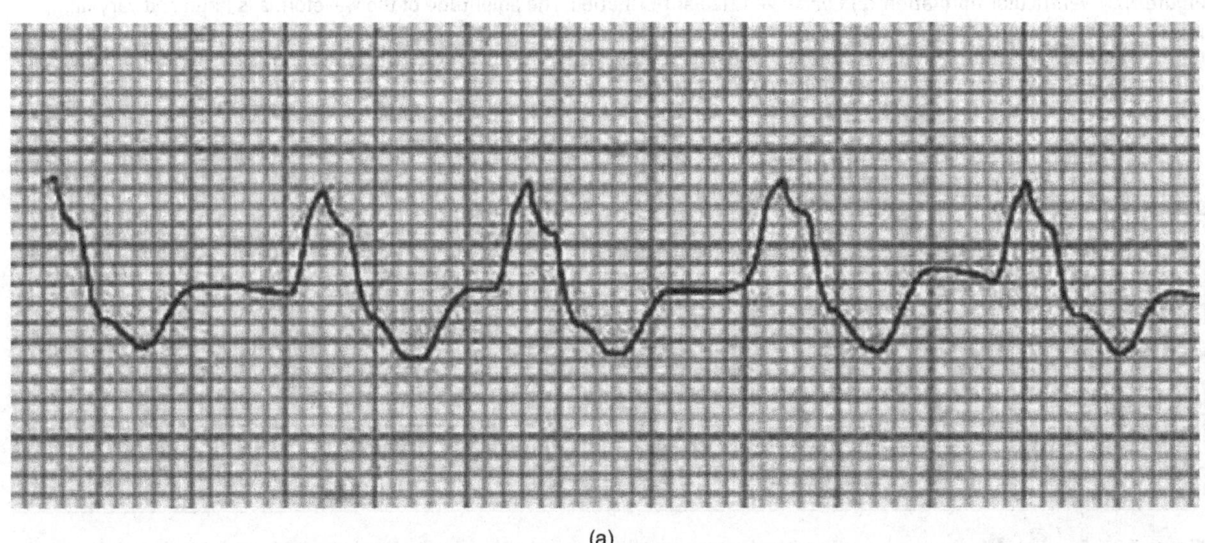

(a)

Figure 7.10 Supraventricular tachycardia with aberrant ventricular conduction due to abnormal intraventricular conduction due to (a) hyperkalemia and (b) medication (sodium channel blockade) toxicity.

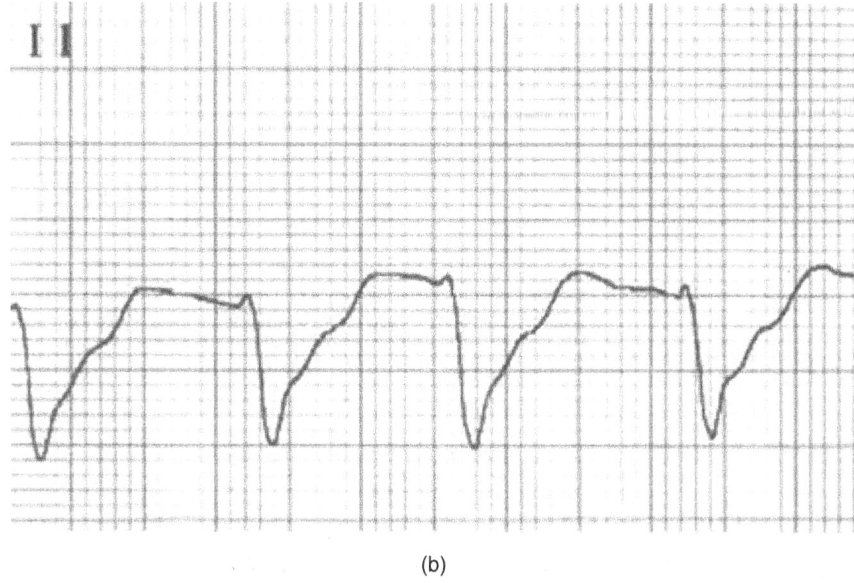

(b)

Figure 7.10 (Continued)

Further Reading

Brady, W. and Truwit, J. (2009). *Critical Decisions in Emergency & Acute Care Electrocardiography*. Oxford, UK: Wiley.

8

Bradycardia

Korin B. Hudson[1], J. Aidan Boswick[2], and William J. Brady[3]

[1] Department of Emergency Medicine, Georgetown University School of Medicine, Med star Health, Washington, DC, USA
[2] Crossix Analytics Services, Veeva Systems Inc., New York, NY, USA
[3] Departments of Emergency Medicine and Medicine, University of Virginia School of Medicine, Charlottesville, VA, USA

Bradycardia is a frequent finding in clinical practice. Simply put, bradycardia refers to any heart rate that is slower than the normal or predicted heart rate for a given patient. For adult patients, the term *bradycardia* typically refers to heart rates slower than 60 bpm (beats per minute). In children, the normal heart rate varies depending on the age of the child.

The correct diagnosis of a bradycardic rhythm is crucial to understanding the clinical significance of that rhythm and choosing the appropriate management strategy (Boxes 8.1 and 8.2). The causes of bradycardia are classified into intrinsic and extrinsic entities (Table 8.1). Intrinsic causes focus on disorders based within the conduction system itself; extrinsic causes result from issues external to the conduction system, most commonly coronary ischemic, respiratory, metabolic, and toxic syndromes. In this chapter, we will discuss the ECG characteristics of the following bradycardic rhythms: sinus bradycardia, sinus arrhythmia, sinoatrial (SA) block, sinus pause/arrest, junctional rhythms, idioventricular rhythms, sinoventricular rhythm, and slow atrial fibrillation. Atrioventricular (AV) blocks, which also often occur at rates less than 60 bpm, are discussed in Chapter 9.

Sinus Bradycardia

The term *sinus bradycardia* simply refers to a regular rhythm of sinus origin that presents with a rate less than 60 bpm in the adult or less than the expected lower limit of normal for the pediatric patient. Sinus bradycardia may be further classified into regular and irregular variations.

Regular sinus bradycardia is defined as *sinus rhythm* with a rate less than 60 bpm (Figure 8.1). This rhythm is generated by the SA node and proceeds through the normal conduction pathways. In essence, sinus rhythm with a rate less than 60 bpm in the adult and less than the lower limit of normal for the pediatric patient is sinus bradycardia. By definition, sinus bradycardia has a P wave of normal morphology and a normal axis (or unchanged from the patient's previous baseline axis). The PR interval (PRI) is consistent and is less than 0.2 s, and the QRS complex is narrow (<0.12 s). There is a P wave before every QRS complex and a QRS complex following every P wave. Note that the QRS duration may be widened when intraventricular conduction is impaired and that AV conduction blocks may also coexist with sinus bradycardia. The rhythm is regular with consistent P–P and R–R intervals and these are equal.

Irregular sinus bradycardias include sinus arrhythmia, SA block, and sinus arrest. Sinus arrhythmia (Figure 8.2) may occur at rates less than 60 bpm and thus may be classified as a form of sinus bradycardia. Sinus arrhythmia is generated by the SA node and conducts through the normal cardiac conduction pathway. It has the same features of sinus bradycardia with the exception of irregularity; in fact, the rhythm has all of the hallmarks of a regular sinus bradycardia except that it is somewhat (and in some cases markedly) irregular owing to varying P–P and R–R intervals. This irregularity is often due to differences in intrathoracic pressure during the respiratory cycle or from intermittent stimulation of the vagus nerve, both of which lead to beat-to-beat variability in the heart rate. Bradycardic sinus arrythmia is frequently found in healthy young patients and does not necessarily

The Electrocardiogram in Emergency and Acute Care, First Edition.
Edited by Korin B. Hudson, Amita Sudhir, George Glass, and William J. Brady.

Box 8.1 Bradycardia: Clinical Presentation

Bradycardia can be:

- An incidental finding or directly related to the patient's complaint.
- Relative bradycardia – hypotension with normal heart rate rather than compensatory tachycardia.
- A normal variant finding, especially in younger endurance athletes.

Symptoms associated with bradycardia can include the following:

- Weakness/decreased exercise tolerance
- Dizziness/light-headedness
- Syncope/near-syncope
- Chest pain
- Shortness of breath
- Feeling "ill"

Signs associated with bradycardia can include the following:

- Hypotension/shock
- Pulmonary edema
- Altered mental status

Underlying causes of bradycardia are classified into either intrinsic (sometimes called *primary* causes) or extrinsic (also referred to as *secondary* causes) entities (Table 8.1).

- Intrinsic factors – damage to the conduction system, often chronic and related to aging.
- Extrinsic factors – etiologies external to the conduction system; the most common extrinsic cause is acute ST segment elevation MI.

Box 8.2 Management of Bradycardia

Management considerations must focus on the rhythm itself and the underlying cause.

Rhythm-based therapy

- Chronotropic agents: atropine, glucagon, epinephrine.
- External pacemaker: transcutaneous and transvenous.

Underlying cause therapy (broad range of causes with broad range of therapies), including oxygen, intravenous (IV) fluids, and management focused on the cause (acute coronary syndrome [ACS], metabolic, toxic, etc.). In general, sinus bradycardia responds more favorably than junctional bradycardia, which responds more favorably than idioventricular bradycardia.

indicate pathology – unless the clinical presentation suggests that decompensation is present.

SA blocks (SA exit blocks) are rhythms generated by the SA node in which there is transient failure of impulse conduction into and through the atria. This failure may cause substantial pauses between beats. The morphology and intervals of the conducted beats are normal. They have normal, upright P waves; short PRI (<0.2 s); normal and narrow QRS complexes (<0.12 s), and normal T waves. However, the P–P and R–R intervals may be intermittently and profoundly lengthened.

The causes of SA block are varied, including normal variant situations (i.e. in young patients and well-conditioned athletes) and presentations with increased vagal tone.

Sinus pause and sinus arrest (Figure 8.3) may be impossible to differentiate from SA block based on ECG alone. In sinus pause or sinus arrest, the SA node intermittently fails to generate an impulse. The impulses that are generated produce a beat through the normal conduction pathway. The conducted beats each have normal P waves, narrow QRS complexes, and normal T waves. The conducted beats are associated with normal intervals. However, as in SA block, there may be substantial pauses between beats when the SA node fails to generate an impulse. Sinus pause refers to short episodes without SA impulse generation, whereas sinus arrest refers to longer failures of the SA node. Without the benefit of the electrophysiology laboratory and advanced studies, it may be impossible to know the difference between SA block and sinus arrest as they appear identical on the surface ECG or single-lead rhythm strip.

Junctional Rhythm

Junctional rhythm (Figure 8.4) is considered an "escape" rhythm because the SA node fails to produce an impulse, and a site in the AV node assumes the role of pacemaker. The pacemaker site is typically supraventricular, often within the AV node itself and the rhythm is regular and frequently slow, between 40 and 60 bpm.

Table 8.1 Causes of bradycardia.

- Idiopathic/degenerative (age related)
- Cardiomyopathy
- Coronary artery disease
  - Infarction/ischemia
- Infectious conditions
  - Pericarditis/myocarditis/endocarditis
  - Lyme disease
  - Chagas disease
- Infiltrative conditions
  - Amyloidosis
  - Sarcoidosis
  - Hemochromatosis
- Autoimmune conditions
  - Lupus
  - Scleroderma
  - Rheumatoid arthritis
- Iatrogenic
  - Radiation related
  - Postoperative
    - Cardiac transplant
    - Valve replacement
    - Correction of congenital heart disease
- Myotonic muscular dystrophy
- Trauma
- Familial
- Autonomic causes
  - Increased vagal tone
  - Carotid sinus hypersensitivity
  - Neurocardiogenic syncope
- Acute MI
- Medications/drugs
  - Antiarrhythmics, class I and class III
  - β-Adrenergic blockers
  - Calcium channel blockers
  - Digoxin
  - Clonidine
  - Lithium
- Metabolic
  - Electrolyte imbalance (especially hyperkalemia)
  - Acidosis
- Hypoxia
- Hypothermia
- Hypothyroidism
- Neurologic conditions that affect the autonomic nervous system
- Increased intracranial pressure
- Sleep apnea

MI, myocardial infarction.

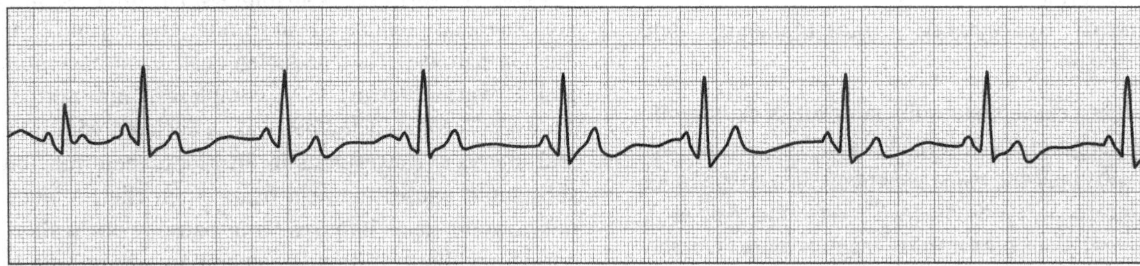

Figure 8.1 Sinus bradycardia. In essence, sinus rhythm with a rate less than 60 bpm in the adult and less than the lower limit of normal for the pediatric patient.

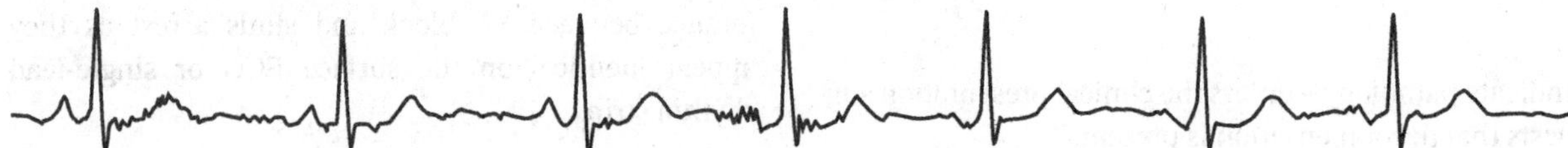

Figure 8.2 Sinus bradycardia with sinus arrhythmia. Note the varying R–R interval.

Junctional rhythms in this rate range should be considered junctional rhythms at a "normal rate," that is, normal for the junctional rhythm. Rates slower than 40 bpm are referred to as *junctional bradycardias*, while rates faster than 60 bpm are described as *accelerated junctional rhythms*.

Recall that the P wave on the surface ECG represents the depolarization of the atria in response to an impulse from the SA node. Therefore, the junctional rhythm often does not demonstrate P waves (as there is no impulse from the SA node; Figure 8.4a). Depending on where the impulse is generated, however, retrograde

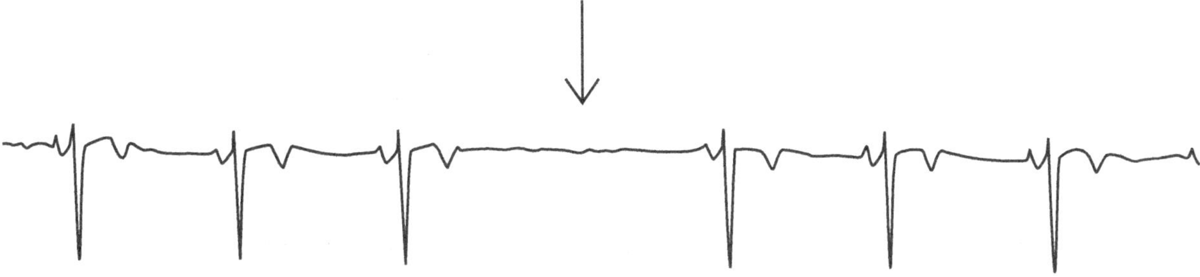

Figure 8.3 Sinus pause/sinus arrest. Note the long pause between conducted beats (arrow).

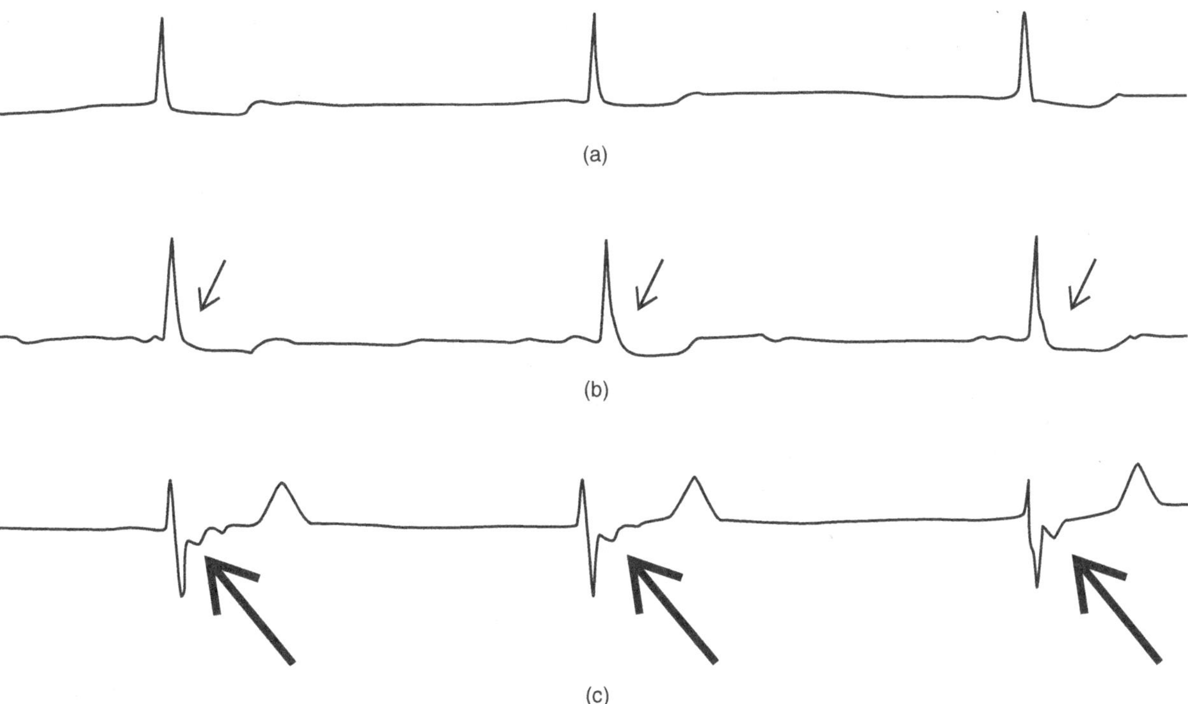

Figure 8.4 Junctional rhythm. (a) Junctional rhythm with no evident P wave; the rhythm is regular with a narrow QRS complex. (b) Junctional rhythm with a P wave "buried" in the terminal portion of the QRS complex (small arrow). (c) Junctional rhythm with an inverted P wave, which is evident after the QRS complex (long arrow).

conduction (i.e. from the AV node retrograde into the atrial tissues) may produce a P wave, which may be either upright or inverted and may be either immediately before the QRS complex (with a shorter than expected PRI) or just after the QRS complex (Figure 8.4b, c). In some cases, a retrograde P wave may become "buried" in the QRS complex (Figure 8.4b), changing the appearance of the QRS complex. The PRI may be non-existent if no P wave is noted; conversely, if a retrograde P wave is seen, the PRI often is quite short or even negative (in the case where the P wave follows the QRS complex [Figure 8.4c]). The QRS complex in junctional rhythms is typically narrow; however, in the presence of a pre-existing bundle branch block (which is discussed in a later chapter), the QRS complex may widen.

Idioventricular Rhythm

An idioventricular rhythm (Figure 8.5) is also considered an "escape rhythm," in that both the SA and AV nodes fail to produce an impulse. In idioventricular rhythms, a pacemaker site in the His–Purkinje system or ventricular myocardium assumes the role of "pacemaker" and generates the rhythm. These rhythms are typically very slow and regular, with rates between 20 and 40 bpm, although faster rhythms may be seen and are considered "accelerated idioventricular rhythms." Idioventricular rhythms typically do not demonstrate P waves, and thus there is no PRI. The QRS complexes are typically wide because of the pacemaker site distal to the AV node. The QT interval is typically normal.

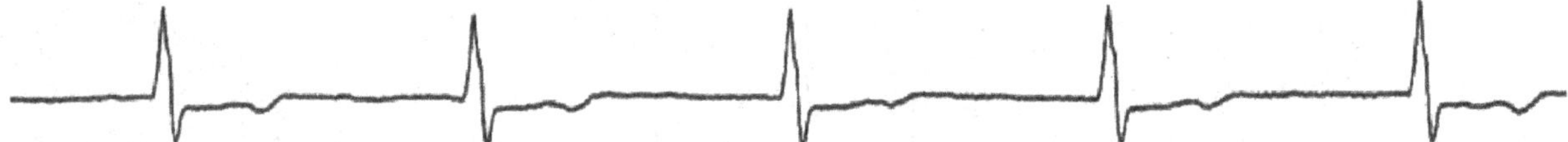

Figure 8.5 Idioventricular rhythm. The rhythm is regular without evidence of P waves; the QRS complex is widened.

The axis may be normal (or unchanged from the patient's baseline) but is often shifted (in either direction) because of the low site of impulse generation. Frequently, a single pacemaker site assumes control, giving the idioventricular rhythm a very regular appearance; if there are multiple competing pacemaker sites, however, the rhythm will have a more irregular and inconsistent appearance.

Sinoventricular Rhythm of Severe Hyperkalemia

Sinoventricular rhythm (Figure 8.6) is a very specific rhythm that is related to severe hyperkalemia (Box 8.3), the clinical syndrome involving significantly elevated serum potassium levels. The rhythm originates from the SA node; yet, owing to the presence of extremely high

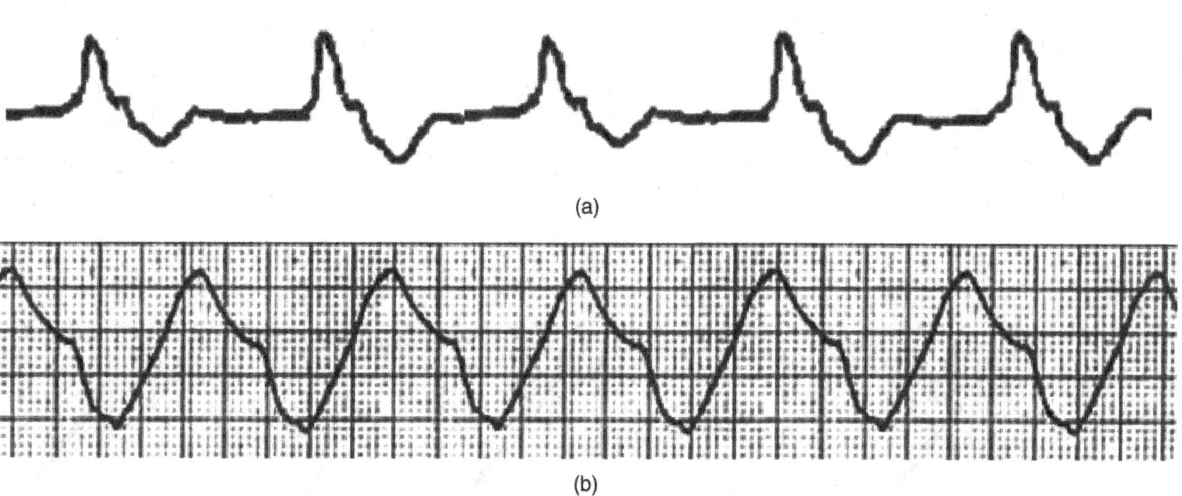

Figure 8.6 Wide QRS complex rhythm in the setting of hyperkalemia. The QRS complex is very broad without evidence of P waves; the rhythm is usually slow and regular. (a) Widened QRS complex; (b) Sinoventricular rhythm of severe hyperkalemia with widened QRS complex with sine wave configuration of the QRS complex.

Box 8.3 Sinoventricular Rhythm and Severe Hyperkalemia

Sinoventricular rhythms are generated in the setting of severe hyperkalemia.

Appearance of the rhythm

- Absolute serum level of potassium is not directly related to rhythm's development.
- Rapidity and chronicity of the serum potassium elevation are related to rhythm's development; rapid increase and/or new onset of hyperkalemia are more likely seen with this rhythm.

Causes of hyperkalemia

- Renal dysfunction (acute kidney injury and chronic renal failure)
- Severe, end-stage liver disease
- Severe, end-stage heart failure
- Potassium-sparing diuretic and other medications
- Excessive potassium replacement
- Salt substitute (potassium chloride) use

Management goals

- Stabilization of cardiac cell membrane: calcium.
- Internal shifting of potassium intracellularly: insulin, glucose, sodium bicarbonate, magnesium sulfate, and albuterol; impact is transient in nature, lasting 20–40 minutes.
- Removal of potassium from the body: gut-binding resins, hemodialysis.

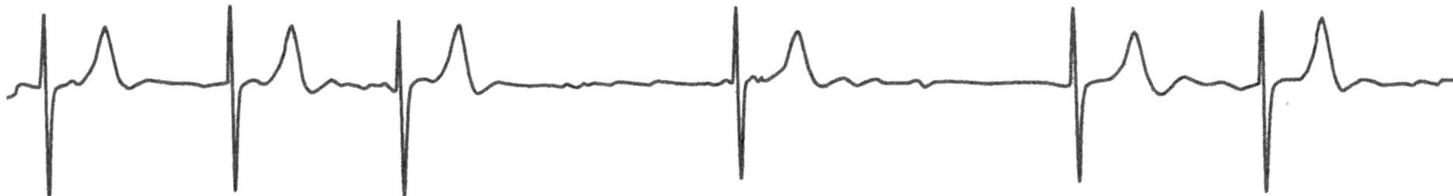

Figure 8.7 Atrial fibrillation with slow ventricular response.

levels of extracellular potassium, the atrial myocardium does not generate a detectable depolarization; thus, this rhythm does not generate a P wave on the surface ECG. Further, conduction through the AV node is also impaired; thus, a ventricular pacemaker assumes control with regard to impulse generation and conduction. Further conduction delay in the ventricles leads to additional widening of the QRS complex. The resulting rhythm has a rate of usually 50–60 bpm – although it can present with markedly faster or slower rates. The QRS complex is quite wide and, if untreated, will further widen, ultimately assuming the appearance of a sine wave. Asystole or ventricular fibrillation will soon follow.

Other Bradycardias

Atrial fibrillation often presents at rates less than 60 bpm (Figure 8.7) and is referred to as *atrial fibrillation with a slow ventricular response*. This rhythm may be very brief, occurring as a single episode; it may be intermittent with frequent recurrences, or may present as a sustained dysrhythmia. Particularly, in cases of chronic atrial fibrillation, which is often treated with medications to maintain the ventricular response, it is not uncommon to encounter patients with an irregularly irregular heart rate that is quite slow (~40–60 bpm).

Further Reading

Brady, W. and Truwit, J. (2009). *Critical Decisions in Emergency Medicine and Acute Care Electrocardiography*. Oxford, UK: Blackwell Publishing Ltd.

Chan, T., Brady, W.J., Harrigan, R.A. et al. (2005). *ECG in Emergency Medicine and Acute Care*. Philadelphia, US: Elsevier Inc.

Harrigan, R.A. and Brady, W.J. (2000). The clinical challenge of bradycardia: diagnosis, evaluation, and intervention in the emergency department. *Emerg. Med. Rep.* 21 (19): 205–215.

Mangrum, J.M. and DiMarco, J.P. (2000). The evaluation and management of bradycardia. *N. Engl. J. Med.* 342 (10): 703–709.

9

Atrioventricular Conduction Block

Steven H. Mitchell[1], *Korin B. Hudson*[2], *and William J. Brady*[3]

[1] *Department of Emergency Medicine, University of Washington School of Medicine, Seattle, WA, USA*
[2] *Department of Emergency Medicine, Medstar Georgetown University Hospital, Washington, DC, USA*
[3] *Departments of Emergency Medicine and Medicine, University of Virginia School of Medicine, Charlottesville, VA, USA*

Atrioventricular (AV) blocks are rhythms in which conduction through the AV node is altered (Box 9.1). In some cases, conduction is only minimally impacted, and thus clinical manifestations of the block may be mild or even absent. However, in other instances, AV conduction is markedly and adversely affected; significant clinical signs and symptoms will be evident. The AV blocks are described on the basis of the PR interval and the relationship between the P waves and the QRS complexes.

First-Degree Atrioventricular Block

First-degree AV block (Figure 9.1 and Box 9.2) is most often generated by an impulse from the sinoatrial (SA) node and produces a normal P wave. Conduction is simply delayed through the AV node. The rhythm is characterized by a prolonged PR interval greater than the normal 0.2 s. Although delayed, each impulse is conducted through the AV node to the ventricle, maintaining a 1 : 1 atrial–ventricular relationship. In other words, each P wave is followed by a QRS complex, and every QRS complex has a corresponding P wave. The PR interval is consistent from one beat to the next and yields consistent and equal P–P and R–R intervals. The axis is usually normal, and, except in cases of pre-existing bundle branch blocks, the QRS complex is normal and narrow (<0.12 s).

While first-degree AV blocks do not directly *cause* bradycardia, patients exhibiting this rhythm often have heart rates less than 60 bpm. This observation is particularly true in patients with other defects of impulse formation and conduction, as well as in patients who are taking medications that decrease heart rate. Furthermore, first-degree AV block may be seen in conjunction with the higher degree blocks, described below, that often occur at slower rates. The altered AV conduction of first-degree heart block rarely, if ever, leads directly to clinical compromise.

Second-Degree Atrioventricular Block

Second-degree AV block is further subcategorized into Mobitz type I (Wenckebach) and Mobitz type II (non-Wenckebach) AV block. These subtypes are defined by the length of the PR interval and the progressive relationship of the P wave to the QRS complex.

Second-degree AV block Mobitz type I (Figure 9.2 and Box 9.2), also known as the *Wenckebach rhythm*, shares some features of the first-degree AV block and may demonstrate either a normal or a slow ventricular rate. Although this rhythm most often occurs in the setting of a prolonged PR interval, the initial PR interval may be normal. The hallmark of the Mobitz type I AV block is the progressive lengthening of the PR interval from one beat to the next. This progressive lengthening continues until there is a beat in which the impulse from the SA node generates a normal P wave, but is then completely blocked at the AV node. Therefore, there is no resulting QRS complex associated with this particular beat (often referred to as a *dropped* beat). This P wave is sometimes referred to as an *orphan P wave*, that is, one with no QRS complex following.

The Electrocardiogram in Emergency and Acute Care, First Edition.
Edited by Korin B. Hudson, Amita Sudhir, George Glass, and William J. Brady.

Box 9.1 Atrioventricular Conduction Blocks

AV blocks may be caused by many entities.

- Primary causes include any intrinsic defect in the generation or conduction of the impulse or structural abnormalities within the conduction system itself.
- Secondary causes, which are extrinsic to the cardiac conduction system but which affect AV nodal conduction.

Potential secondary causes of AV block include the following:

- Ischemic and non-ischemic cardiovascular disease
- Pharmacologic/toxicologic
- Neurologic and reflex-mediated (i.e. vagal stimulation)
- Infectious
- Rheumatologic
- Endocrine
- Metabolic

Acute coronary ischemic events, particularly ST segment elevation myocardial infarction (STEMI), are the most frequent cause of high-grade AV blocks.

Box 9.2 First-Degree and Second-Degree Type I Atrioventricular Blocks

May be a normal variant if no other conduction abnormalities/no other etiology for bradycardia is found.

- To be considered a normal variant, all acute pathologies must be excluded.
- Caution must be exercised in such instances.

Clinical presentation:

- Most patients are asymptomatic.
- Rarely does this rhythm require acute intervention or treatment due to the these forms of AV block.
- If symptomatic, then significant coexisting bradycardia is present.
  - Weakness/fatigue
  - Lightheadedness
  - Syncope/near syncope
  - Chest discomfort
  - Hypoperfusion/shock

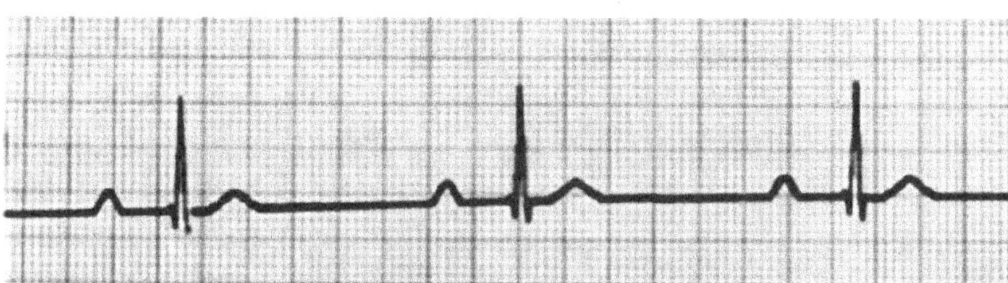

Figure 9.1 First-degree AV block with coexisting sinus bradycardia. Note the prolonged PR interval, which is unchanging from beat to beat.

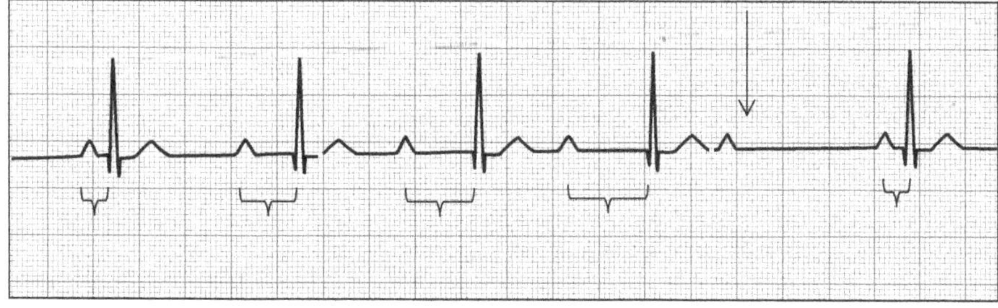

Figure 9.2 Second-degree type I AV block (Mobitz I or Wenckebach). Note progressive lengthening of the PR interval (braces) followed by dropped beat, i.e. no QRS complex (arrow).

In the beat following the dropped QRS complex, the PR interval "resets" and returns to the length of the PR interval in the first conducted beat in the pattern. The following beats demonstrate, once again, progressive lengthening of the PR interval, and ultimately a dropped beat. This pattern may recur in either an intermittent or a continuous manner. The number of conducted beats (i.e. a P wave for each QRS complex) between non-conducted P waves may vary; thus, a long rhythm strip may be necessary to correctly identify the rhythm. The lengthening of the PR interval and subsequent dropped beat lead to a "grouped" configuration of QRS complexes that may become more evident when evaluating a longer rhythm strip; this phenomenon is termed *grouped beating of Wenckebach*.

In the absence of a pre-existing intraventricular conduction delay, the impulses that are conducted through the AV node and His–Purkinje system generate narrow QRS complexes with normal morphology. In the setting of coexistent bundle branch block, however, there is further conduction delay below the AV node and the electrical impulse is aberrantly conducted through the ventricles, yielding a widened QRS complex. Patients with both an AV block and a bundle branch block have a higher risk of progression to third-degree AV block.

Second-degree AV block Mobitz type II (Figures 9.3 and 9.4 and Box 9.3) is characterized by a static, or unchanging, PR interval. In this rhythm, conduction is intermittently blocked at the level of the AV node or the His bundle, resulting in an "orphan" P wave and "dropped" QRS complex. The PR interval "resets" on the following beat, and conduction returns to the previously observed P wave to QRS complex pattern. Unlike Mobitz I blocks, where the conduction is delayed leading to a progressive lengthening of the PR interval, Mobitz II blocks exhibit an "all-or-none" conduction phenomenon. Thus, on the beats in which the conduction proceeds through the AV node, the PR interval remains consistent from beat to beat.

The heart rate in Mobitz II is typically slow, running between 40 and 60 bpm and the number of conducted beats between each dropped beat may vary. It may become necessary to evaluate a long rhythm strip in order to correctly identify the rhythm. Furthermore, roughly 70% of Mobitz II blocks are associated with a concurrent bundle branch block, which produces widened QRS complexes. Thus, second-degree AV block Mobitz type II tends to represent more advanced disease than first-degree or second-degree Mobitz I blocks and is more likely to progress to a more serious form of heart

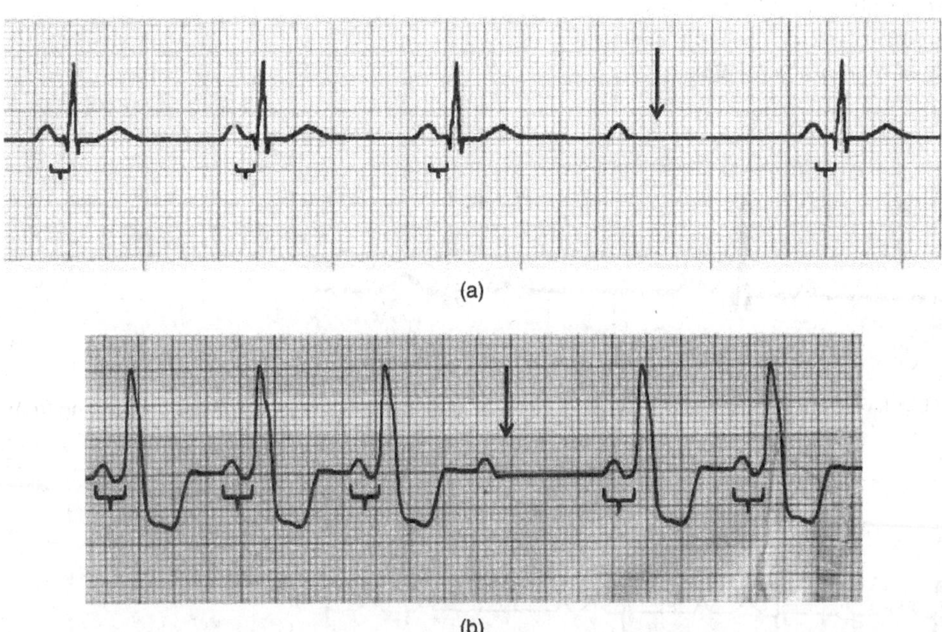

Figure 9.3 Second-degree type II AV block type (Mobitz II). Note the consistent PR interval (braces) followed by an orphan P wave and resultant dropped QRS complex (arrow). (a) Narrow QRS complex; (b) wide QRS complex.

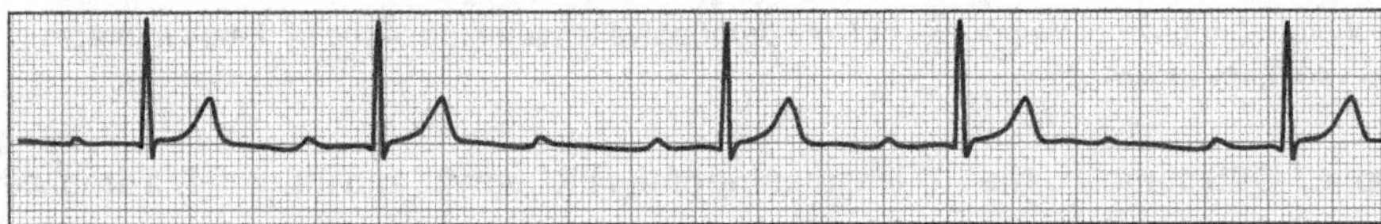

Figure 9.4 Second-degree heart block type II (Mobitz II). Note the prolonged PR interval, indicating a first-degree AV block, and sinus bradycardia as well.

Box 9.3 Second-Degree Type II and Third-Degree (Complete) Atrioventricular Blocks

Usually results from significant primary conduction system disease or secondary event.

- These patterns are never considered normal variants.
- STEMI and cardioactive medication overdose are frequent causes of significant conduction system blockade.

Symptoms associated with significant conduction system blockade:

- Chest discomfort
- Shortness of breath
- Dizzy/light-headedness
- Syncope/near syncope
- Altered mental status
- Hypoperfusion/shock

Management priorities include treatment of primary rhythm disorder and identification/treatment of underlying cause.

- Chronotropic agents – less likely to be beneficial.
- Transcutaneous pacing – likely most effective therapy; considered a bridge to more definitive care.

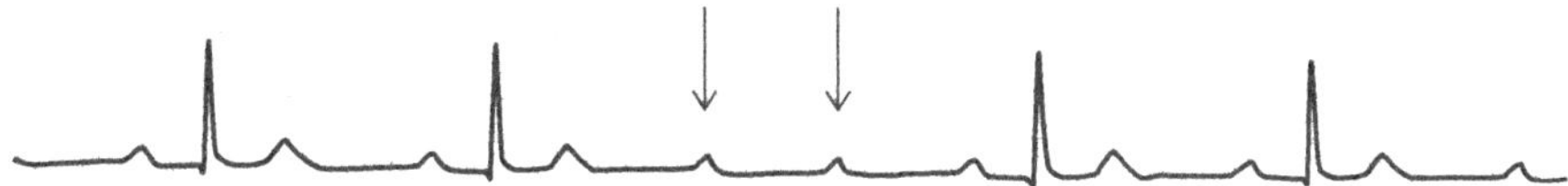

Figure 9.5 Second-degree AV block (Mobitz II) with high-grade block. Note the consecutive blocked P waves (arrows), meaning that more than one non-conducted P wave is noted on the rhythm strip.

block, such as third-degree AV block. This rhythm is always abnormal and should be considered an ominous finding.

Second degree high-grade AV block is a particularly dangerous type of second-degree AV block that occurs when two or more consecutive P waves are not conducted (Figure 9.5). This results in multiple dropped beats. In this setting, the rate of the ventricular beats is typically 20–40 bpm and the QRS complex is often widened. This pattern is a manifestation of advanced conduction system disease and has an extremely high risk of progressing to a third-degree (complete) heart block.

Third-Degree Atrioventricular Block

Third-degree AV block (Figure 9.6 and Box 9.3), also known as *heart block* or *complete heart block*, represents the most worrisome form of AV conduction blockade. Atrial impulses may be generated by the SA node or may be from an ectopic atrial focus. Regardless of their source, atrial impulses are completely blocked at the level of the AV node, and no conduction passes through to generate a ventricular contraction (i.e. QRS complex). If the patient continues to have a perfusing rhythm, ventricular contraction must be initiated by a ventricular escape rhythm. Because the ventricular impulse is generated below the AV node, the QRS complex is most often wide (>0.12 s).

In third-degree AV block, the atria and ventricles depolarize in an independent manner. These two regions of the heart generate their own electrical discharges; thus, the atrial tissues produce a P wave and the ventricular myocardium renders a QRS complex – yet, both events are not related to one another. The atrial rate is typically faster than the ventricular rate, and importantly, the P waves are not associated in any manner with the QRS complexes. While these separate and distinct depolarization patterns from the atria and ventricles generate regular P–P intervals and regular R–R

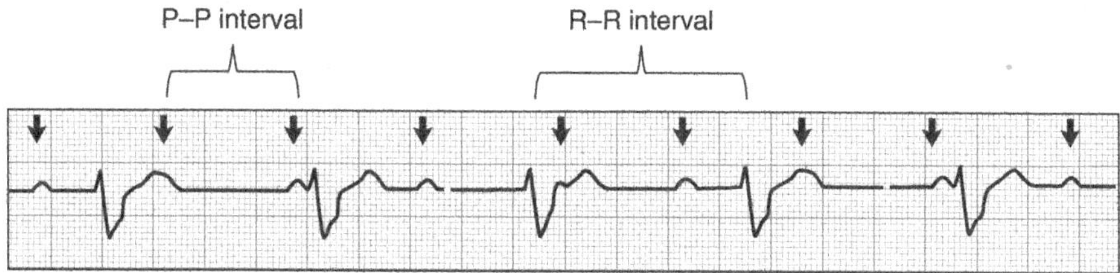

Figure 9.6 Third-degree AV block, or complete heart block. Note the regular P–P and R–R intervals that have no relationship to one another. P waves (arrows) may also be "buried" or superimposed with the QRS–T complex.

intervals, these intervals are not equivalent and they have no relationship with each other.

The QRS complex duration and the ventricular rate in third-degree AV block are dependent on the focus of the ventricular escape beat. If the focus is more distal in the His–Purkinje system or the ventricle, the QRS complexes will be wider and produce rates that are often less than 40 bpm; a more proximal focus will produce a more rapid rate (>40 bpm) and a less widened QRS complex.

Atrioventricular Dissociation

AV dissociation is a term used to describe any rhythm disturbance where the atrial and ventricular pacemakers function independently of each other. The atrial focus can arise from either the SA node or from the atrial myocardium, while the ventricular focus may originate at the AV junction, at any point in the His–Purkinje system, or from the ventricular myocardial tissue. AV dissociation can take three distinct forms based on the atrial and ventricular rates: in complete (third degree) heart block, the atrial rate is greater than the ventricular rate; in ventricular tachycardia (VT), the ventricular rate is greater than the atrial rate; and in isorhythmic AV dissociation, the atrial and ventricular rates are equal. This latter case may be very difficult to identify.

The concept of AV dissociation is a challenging one, given that the two seemingly unrelated rhythms, third-degree AV block and VT, are both examples of this phenomenon. However, it is important that the emergency care provider be able to identify AV dissociation as it represents a significant deviation from normal conduction and without immediate intervention may lead to rapid deterioration of the patient's condition.

10

Intraventricular Conduction Block: Bundle Branch Block and Other Conduction Abnormalities

Steven H. Mitchell[1], *Richard B. Utarnachitt*[2], *and William J. Brady*[3]

[1] *Department of Emergency Medicine, University of Washington School of Medicine, Seattle, WA, USA*
[2] *Airlift Northwest, Harborview Medical Center, University of Washington School of Medicine, Seattle, WA, USA*
[3] *Departments of Emergency Medicine and Medicine, University of Virginia School of Medicine, Charlottesville, VA, USA*

In normal cardiac conduction, an electrical impulse is transmitted through atrioventricular (AV) node to the ventricles via the His bundle, which divides into the right and left bundle branches in the intraventricular septum. Depolarization in the ventricle is accomplished by the progression of the electrical impulse via the right and left bundles. The left bundle further divides into the anterior and posterior fascicles. The left anterior fascicle becomes the Purkinje fibers of the anterior and left free ventricular wall. The left posterior fascicle fans out and terminates in the Purkinje fibers of the inferior and posterior walls of the left ventricle (Figure 10.1).

The ventricular phase of cardiac conduction can be divided into two phases: the first phase involves the depolarization of the intraventricular septum via the left bundle branch, which progresses in an anterior and rightward direction. The second phase follows rapidly, involving the near-simultaneous depolarization of the left and right ventricles. Mechanical contraction of the ventricles occurs immediately after electrical depolarization of the ventricular myocardium.

A bundle branch block (BBB), or intraventricular conduction abnormality (Box 10.1), occurs when this organized transmission through the normal ventricular conduction system is hindered. When a block occurs, there are characteristic changes in the morphology and deflection of the QRS complex. The type and degree of morphologic changes depend on where in the conduction system the blockage occurs. Complete conduction block of either the left or the right bundle branches typically causes a widening of the QRS complex (>0.12 s) leading to either a left bundle branch block (LBBB) or right bundle branch block (RBBB), respectively. Hemiblocks – a blockade of either the anterior or the posterior fascicle of the left bundle branch – typically demonstrate a lesser degree of QRS complex prolongation (0.08–0.12 s). Finally, nonspecific intraventricular conduction abnormalities may occur in cases where there is a blockade of the usual ventricular conduction system but do not fulfill the criteria of either RBBB or LBBB pattern.

The Bundle Branch Blocks

RBBB presents when an electrical impulse is transmitted normally through the bundle of His as well as through the left bundle and its anterior and posterior fascicles to the left side of the heart; yet during conduction, the right bundle is non-functional and transmission of the impulse is "blocked." Therefore, the right ventricle must depolarize via cardiac cell-to-cell transmission. This inefficient pathway gives rise to the characteristic ECG changes that are noted in RBBB (Figure 10.2).

In RBBB, the QRS complex has altered morphology with the deflection representing right ventricular (RV) activation being delayed and becoming very prominent, resulting in a broad R wave in lead V1. This broadened R wave may take any of the following morphologies: monophasic R, biphasic RSR′ ("M"-shaped or "rabbit ears"), or QR formation. In leads I and V6, early intrinsicoid deflection (time to peak deflection and the onset of the R′ wave) and either a wide, shallow S wave or RS wave are seen. QS complexes are often encountered in the inferior leads. The QRS complex duration is prolonged, usually greater than 0.12 s. Marked ST segment changes are often seen including

The Electrocardiogram in Emergency and Acute Care, First Edition.
Edited by Korin B. Hudson, Amita Sudhir, George Glass, and William J. Brady.

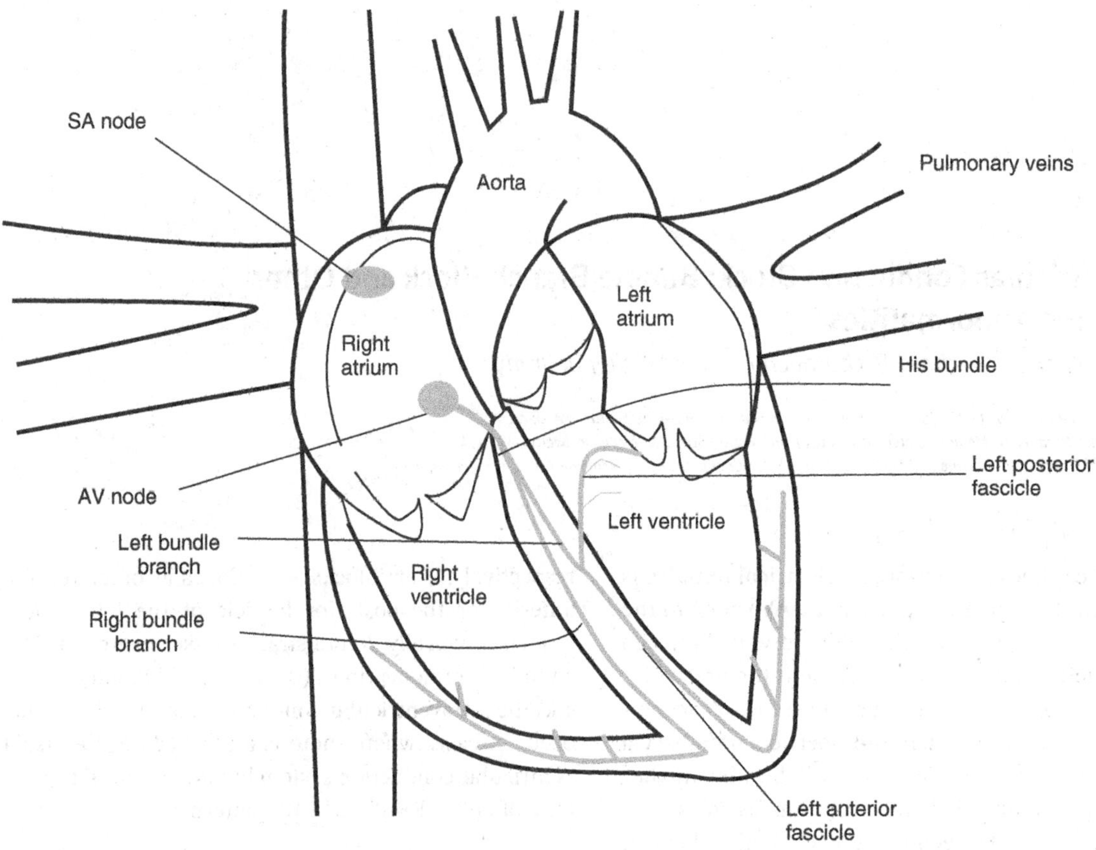

Figure 10.1 The cardiac conduction system. SA, sinoatrial.

Box 10.1 Clinical Issues Associated with Intraventricular Conduction Abnormality

Left bundle branch block

- LBBB pattern is a marker of significant acute and/or chronic left ventricular dysfunction.
- In acute coronary syndrome (ACS) presentations, LBBB is a marker of extreme cardiovascular risk.
- LBBB alters the ECGs ability to detect ST Segment Elevation Myocardial Infarction (STEMI).
- LBBB both confounds STEMI detection via the ECG and mimics findings associated with STEMI.

Right bundle branch block

- RBBB can be considered both a normal variant pattern and a marker of extreme cardiovascular risk.
- RBBB does not confound the ECGs ability to detect STEMI; it does mimic STEMI findings.

ST segment depression and T wave inversion in the right precordial leads (leads V1–V3), associated with the predominantly positive QRS complexes. Further, the ST segment in inferior and left precordial leads is frequently elevated with an upright T wave, with a greater degree of ST segment elevation seen in the inferior leads. These changes represent a "new normal" in the patient with RBBB (Figure 10.3), and do not necessarily indicate an acute ischemic event.

LBBB is either caused by a blocked common left bundle branch or a malfunction of both the anterior and posterior fascicles of the left bundle simultaneously. Rather than conduction through the normal pathway, electrical impulses travel down the right bundle first. This partial depolarization is soon followed by a much slower cell-to-cell depolarization from the right portions to the left segments of the ventricular myocardium. Owing to the inefficient

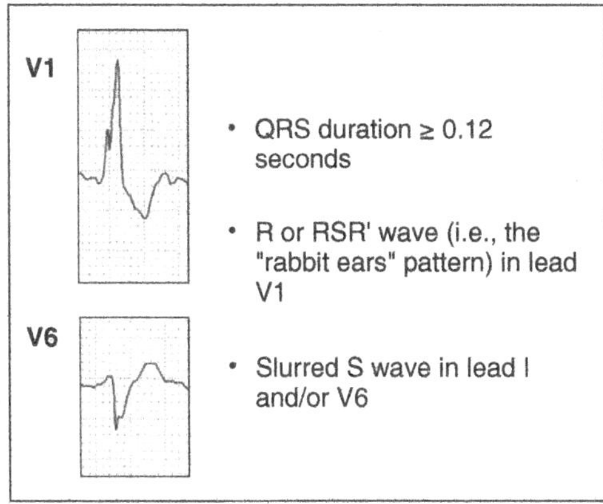

V1
• QRS duration ≥ 0.12 seconds
• R or RSR' wave (i.e., the "rabbit ears" pattern) in lead V1
V6
• Slurred S wave in lead I and/or V6

Figure 10.2 Identifying characteristics of right bundle branch block involving leads V1 and V6.

nature of cell-to-cell transmission, the depolarization becomes markedly longer, leading to a significantly widened QRS complex with characteristic morphology (Figure 10.4).

In the patient with LBBB, the ECG demonstrates broad, mainly negative QS or RS complexes in leads V1–V3. In lead V6, a positive, monophasic R wave is seen in the absence of Q waves; similar structures are also frequently found in leads I and aVL. Poor R wave progression or QS complexes are noted in the right (V1–V2) to mid (V3 – V4) precordial leads, but rarely extend beyond leads V4 or V5. QS complexes may also be encountered in leads III and aVF.

One of the most prominent features of LBBB is a change in the ST segment and T wave. Here, the anticipated or expected ST segment–T wave configurations are discordant, that is, the ST segments are directed opposite from the terminal portion of the QRS complex. As such, leads with either QS or RS, in which the terminal portion of the complex (the S wave) is below the isoelectric baseline, may have markedly elevated ST segments, mimicking acute myocardial infarction. Leads with a large monophasic R wave, in which the terminal portion of the complex is above the

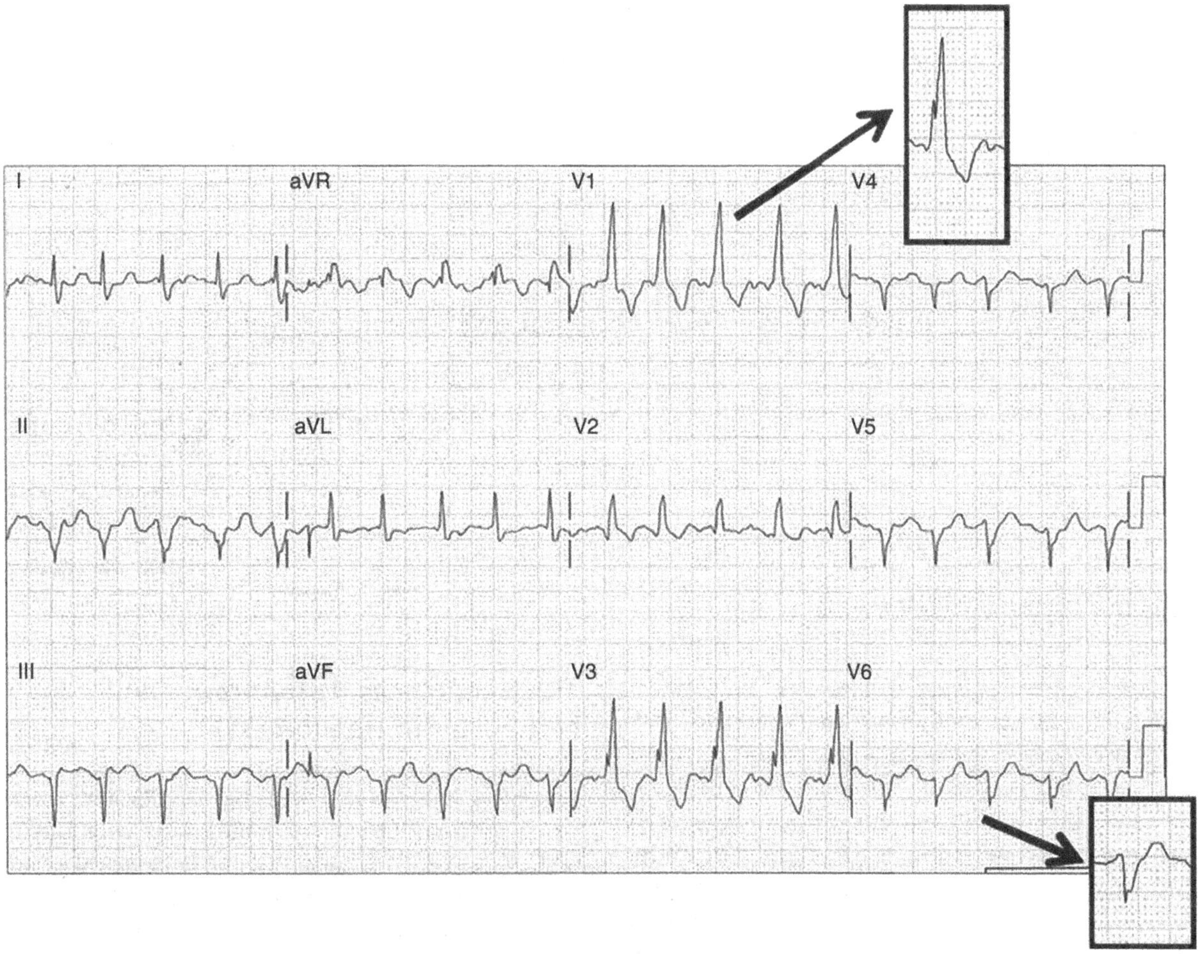

Figure 10.3 Right bundle branch.

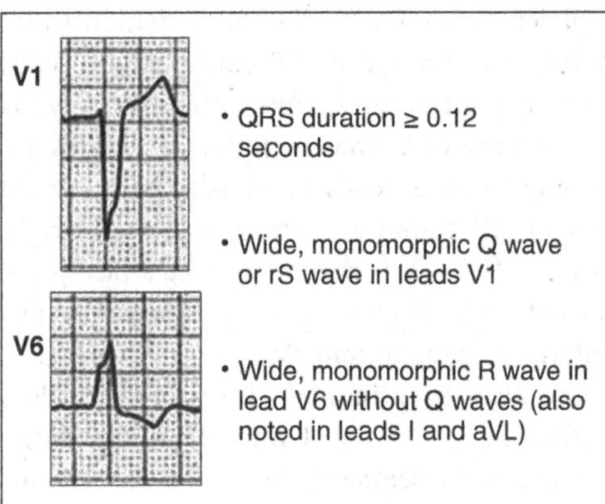

V1
V6
• QRS duration ≥ 0.12 seconds
• Wide, monomorphic Q wave or rS wave in leads V1
• Wide, monomorphic R wave in lead V6 without Q waves (also noted in leads I and aVL)

Figure 10.4 Identifying characteristics of left bundle branch block involving leads V1 and V6.

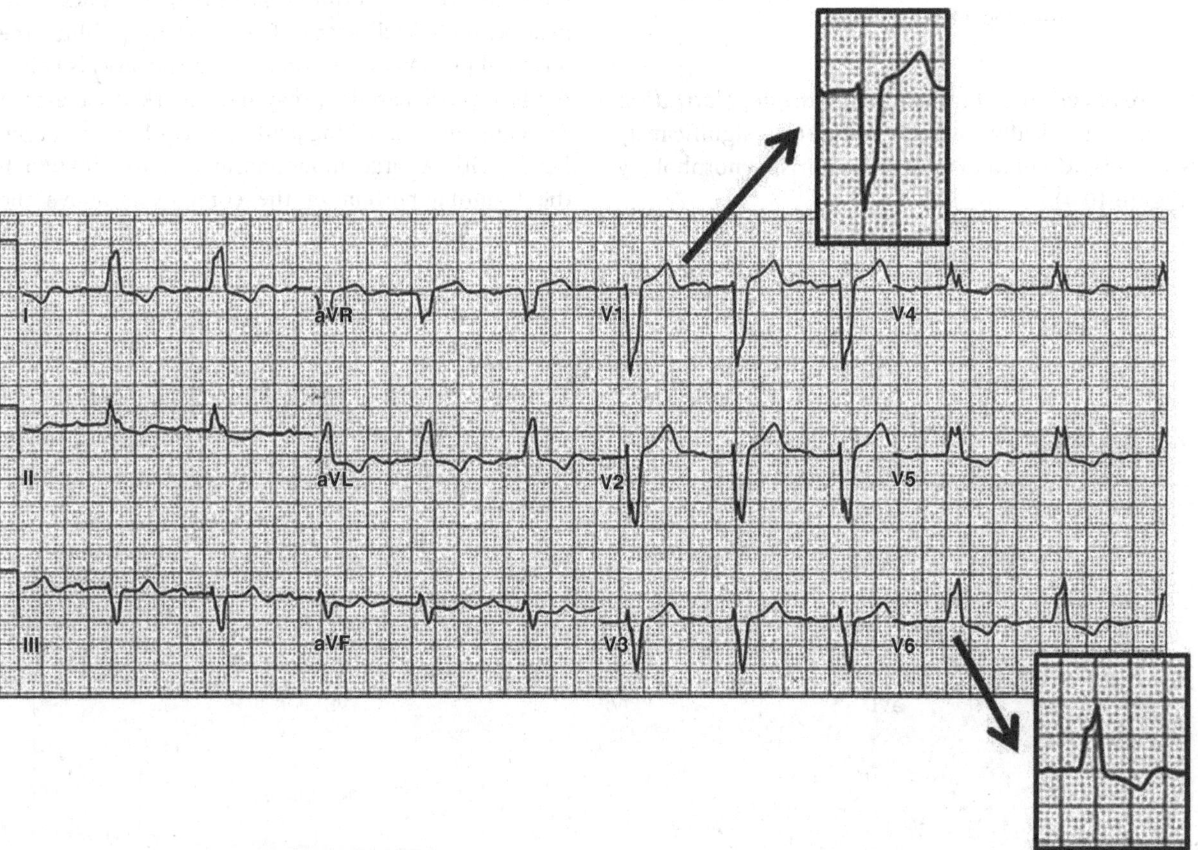

Figure 10.5 Left bundle branch block.

isoelectric baseline, often demonstrate ST segment depression and frequently inverted T waves as well. The T wave, especially in the right to mid-precordial leads, often has a convex upward shape or a tall, vaulting appearance, similar to the hyperacute T wave of early myocardial infarction. However, as with RBBB, these changes may be chronic, representing a "new normal" for the patient, and do not necessarily rule in or rule out acute disease (Figure 10.5), such as acute myocardial infraction.

The Hemiblocks (Left Anterior and Left Posterior Hemiblocks)

Hemiblock is a term that is used to describe any case in which either the left anterior or the left posterior fascicle is blocked. The terms *hemiblock* and *fascicular block* are synonymous. The causes of hemiblocks are the same as those for other BBBs, including both acute and chronic etiologies.

As noted above, the left anterior fascicle branches off the left bundle and eventually forms the Purkinje fibers that depolarize the anterior and lateral walls of the left ventricle. The left posterior fascicle also branches off of the left bundle branch but does not form a discrete fascicle such as the left anterior fascicle. Rather, the fibers of the posterior fascicle "fan out" loosely, depolarizing the inferior and posterior walls of the left ventricle.

Left anterior fascicular block (LAFB) presents with a QRS complex that is relatively narrow because the electrical impulse is proceeding, for the most part, down the normal cardiac conduction pathway. With an isolated LAFB, electrical activity occurs first in the posterior fascicle and is then transmitted in a delayed manner to the anterior portion of the ventricle. Electrical activity is recorded in a "slurred" manner. This posterior-to-anterior sequence of left ventricular activation shifts the QRS complex axis leftward; thus, a left axis deviation is seen. During initial activation of the left bundle branch, the posterior fascicle has unopposed electrical activity, which is manifested at the beginning of the QRS complex in the superior and leftward leads – leads I and aVL – as small, negative Q waves. Subsequent spread of electrical activity toward the anterior fascicle (superior and leftward) is recognized in leads I and aVL as prominent, positive R waves. Conversely, the inferior leads (leads II, III, and aVF) depict small R waves and prominent S waves. Figure 10.6 reviews the characteristic findings of LAFB, and Figure 10.7 depicts LAFB on a 12-lead ECG.

Left posterior fascicular block (LPFB) is much less common than LAFB both because it is less susceptible to ischemic injury (due to its dual blood supply) and because the posterior fascicle fans out extensively making it anatomically less prone to blockage. In LAFB, electrical impulses are transmitted via the AV node to the left and right bundle branches. Depolarization occurs first in the anterior fascicle and is then transmitted in a delayed manner to the posterior portion of ventricle. The anterior-to-posterior sequence of activation of the left ventricle shifts the QRS complex axis rightward. During the initial activation of the left bundle branch, the anterior fascicle has unopposed electrical activity. This unopposed initial activity is recognized at the beginning of the QRS complex as small, negative Q waves in the inferior leads II, III, and aVF. Subsequent spread of electrical activity toward the posterior fascicle is indicated by prominent R waves in lead III (and likely in II and aVF as well). Conversely, leads I and aVL reveal small R waves and prominent S waves. Figure 10.8 reviews the characteristic findings of LPFB, and Figure 10.9 shows LPFB on a 12-lead ECG.

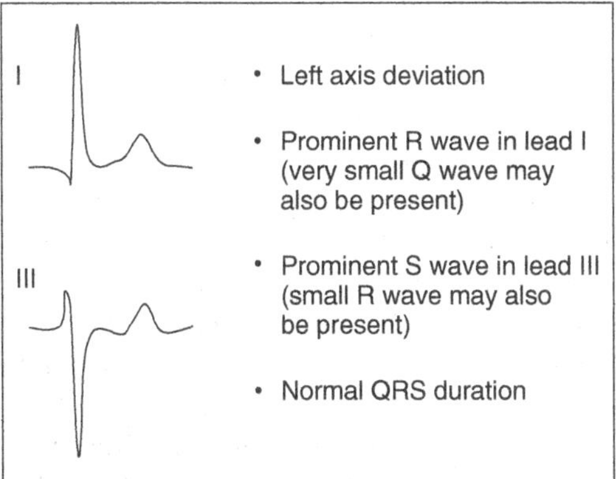

I
III
• Left axis deviation
• Prominent R wave in lead I (very small Q wave may also be present)
• Prominent S wave in lead III (small R wave may also be present)
• Normal QRS duration

Figure 10.6 Identifying characteristics of left anterior fascicular block involving leads I and III as well as a consideration of the QRS complex axis.

Bifascicular and Trifascicular Blocks

The ventricular conduction system disturbances can be classified as unifascicular, bifascicular, or trifascicular blocks based on the site of the lesion or lesions and the number of lesions present. Unifascicular blocks, as described above, consist of a disruption of electrical activity to either the entire right bundle branch or to one fascicle of the left bundle branch or the entire right bundle branch.

Bifascicular blocks consist of disruption of both fascicles of the left bundle branch, LBBB as described above, or disruption of the right bundle branch *plus either* the left anterior *or* the left posterior fascicle. Figure 10.10 reviews the characteristics of bifascicular blocks involving a RBBB and a portion of the left bundle branch system, and Figure 10.11 depicts a 12-lead ECG demonstrating bifascicular block.

The term *trifascicular block* implies RBBB associated with LAFB *and* LPFB (or complete LBBB). However, there is some disagreement as to what constitutes a *trifascicular block.* One interpretation defines a trifascicular block as a bifascicular block in addition to a prolongation of the PR interval, indicating dysfunction at the AV node (first- or second-degree AV block). In this case, "trifascicular block" is a misnomer as the AV node is outside the ventricle and not truly a fascicle. Another definition suggests that a trifascicular block requires a permanent block of one fascicle along with intermittent or alternating blocks in the other two fascicles. In either case, however, trifascicular blocks are an ominous finding as they carry a high risk of progressing to third-degree, or complete, AV block.

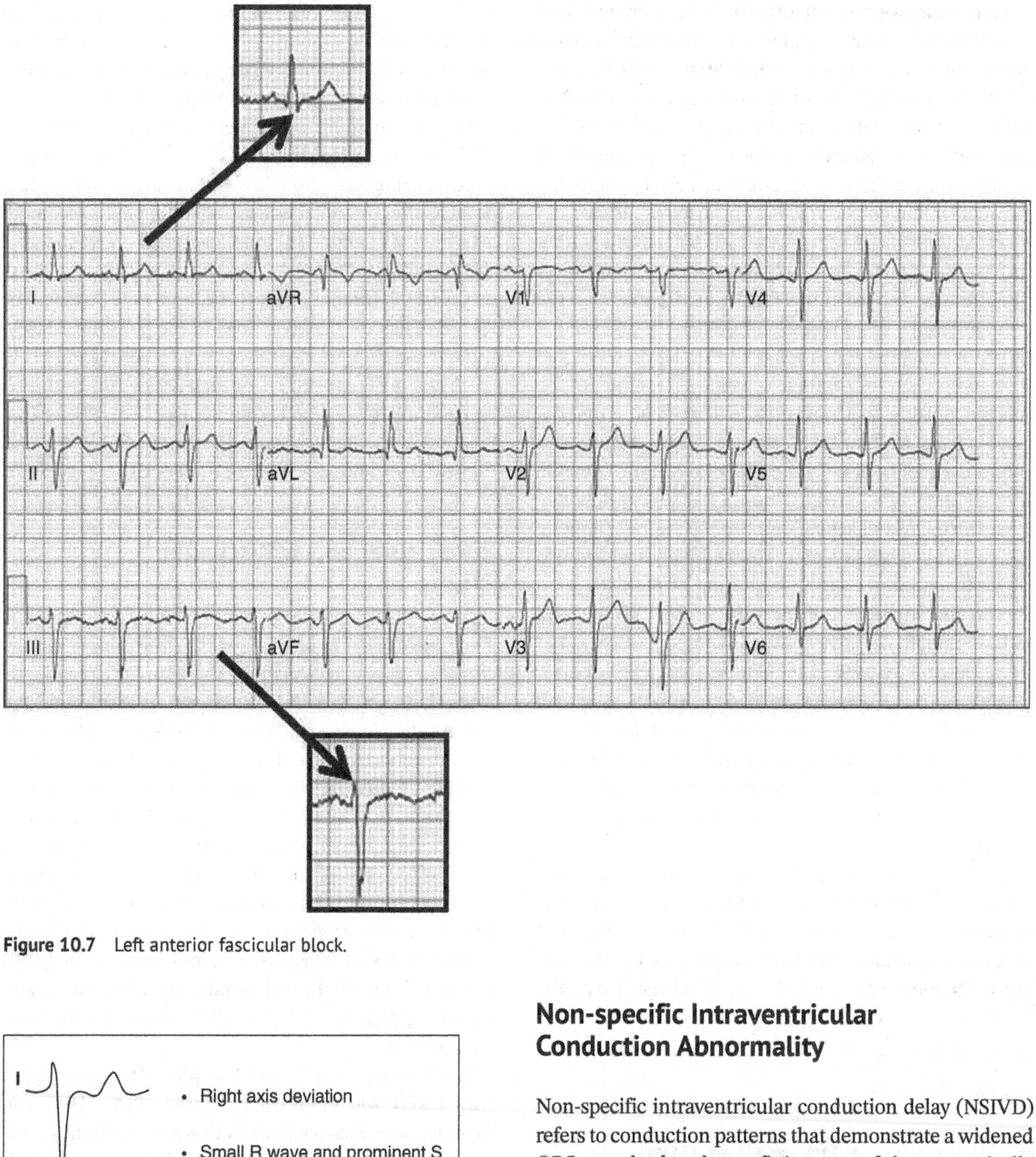

Figure 10.7 Left anterior fascicular block.

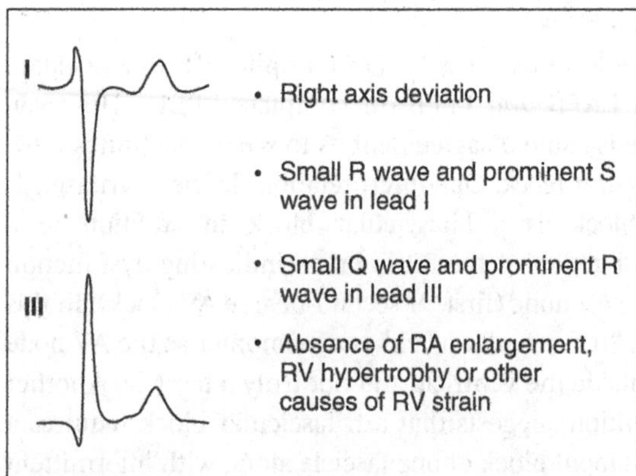

I
III
• Right axis deviation
• Small R wave and prominent S wave in lead I
• Small Q wave and prominent R wave in lead III
• Absence of RA enlargement, RV hypertrophy or other causes of RV strain

Figure 10.8 Identifying characteristics of left posterior fascicular block involving leads I and III as well as a consideration of the QRS complex axis. RA, right atrial; RV, right ventricular.

Non-specific Intraventricular Conduction Abnormality

Non-specific intraventricular conduction delay (NSIVD) refers to conduction patterns that demonstrate a widened QRS complex but do not fit into any of the anatomically defined categories described above. While the QRS complex may be widened to some extent, it is usually not to the extent seen in complete LBBB or RBBB and lacks the characteristic morphology of hemiblocks as described above. The key to understanding and treating NSIVD is to search for the underlying cause of the conduction delay. The most important consideration is an electrolyte imbalance, most notably hyperkalemia (Figure 10.12). Other conditions may cause QRS prolongation including medications (e.g. tricyclic antidepressant medications) as well as some drugs of abuse (e.g. cocaine).

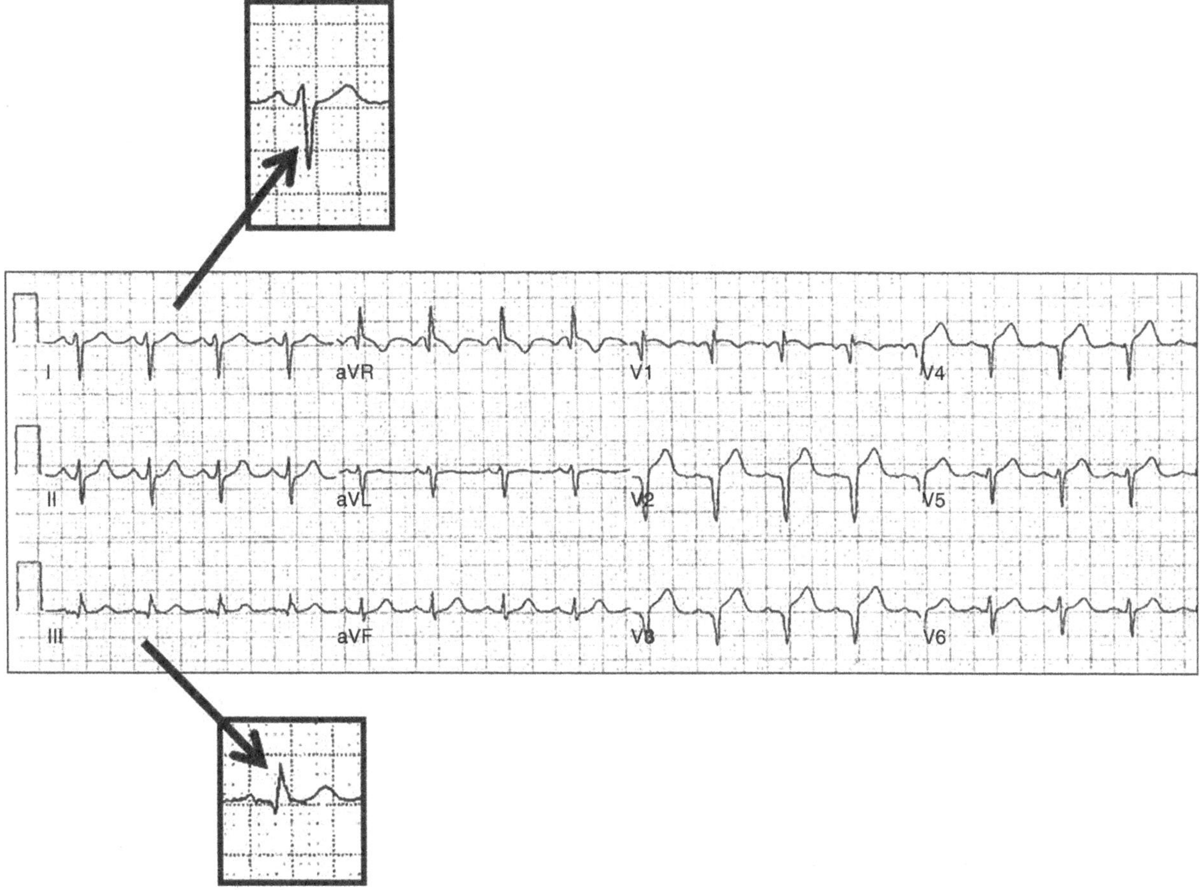

Figure 10.9 Left posterior fascicular block in a patient with anterior wall acute myocardial infraction.

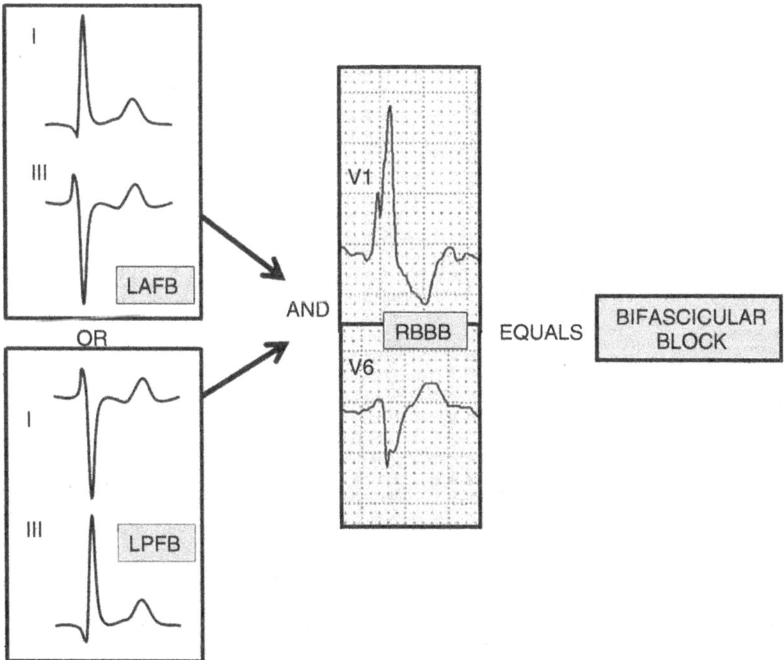

Figure 10.10 Identifying characteristics of bifascicular block involving a RBBB and either left anterior or left posterior fascicular block. Note that another form of bifascicular block is an isolated LBBB (not shown here).

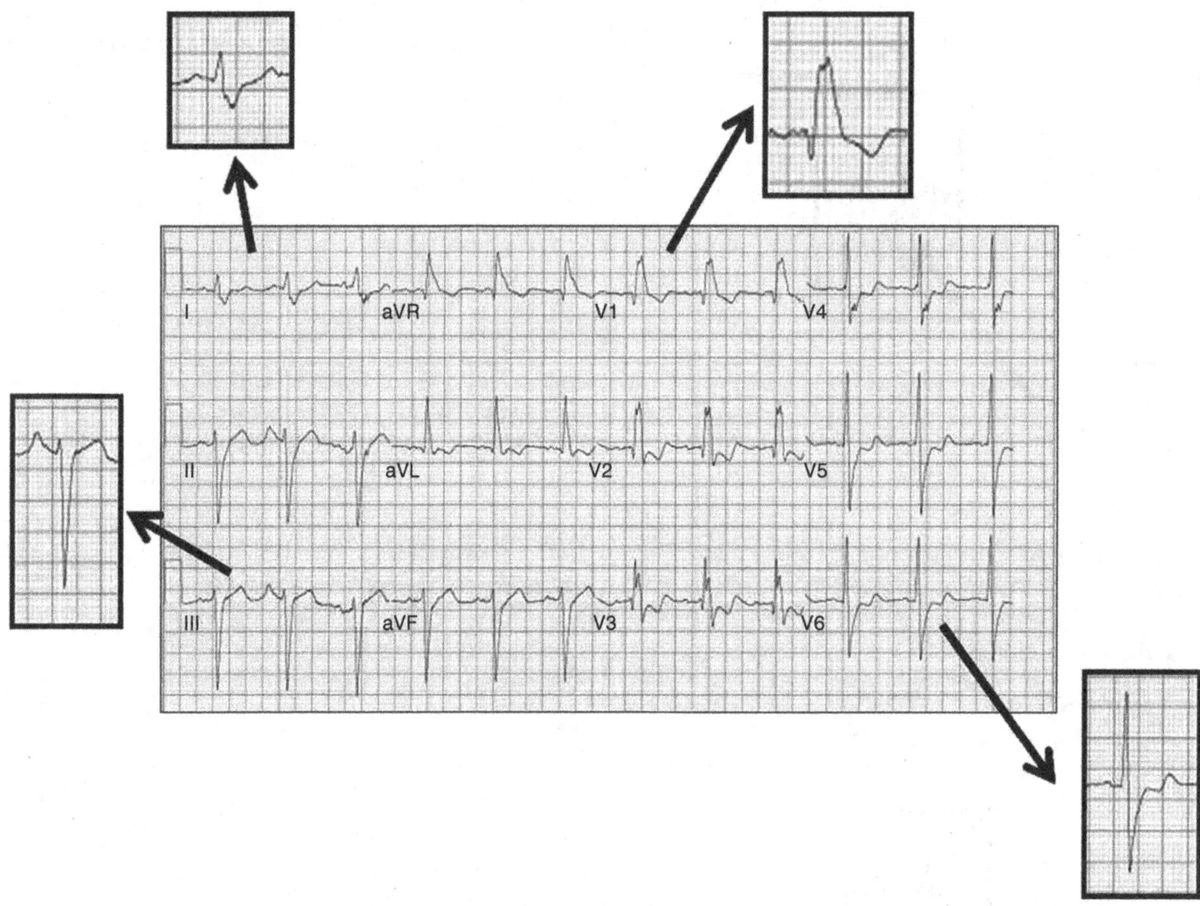

Figure 10.11 Bifascicular block demonstrating characteristics of RBBB (biphasic R wave in lead V1 and R wave with deep S wave in lead V6) and LAFB (R wave in lead I, rS wave in lead III, and left axis deviation).

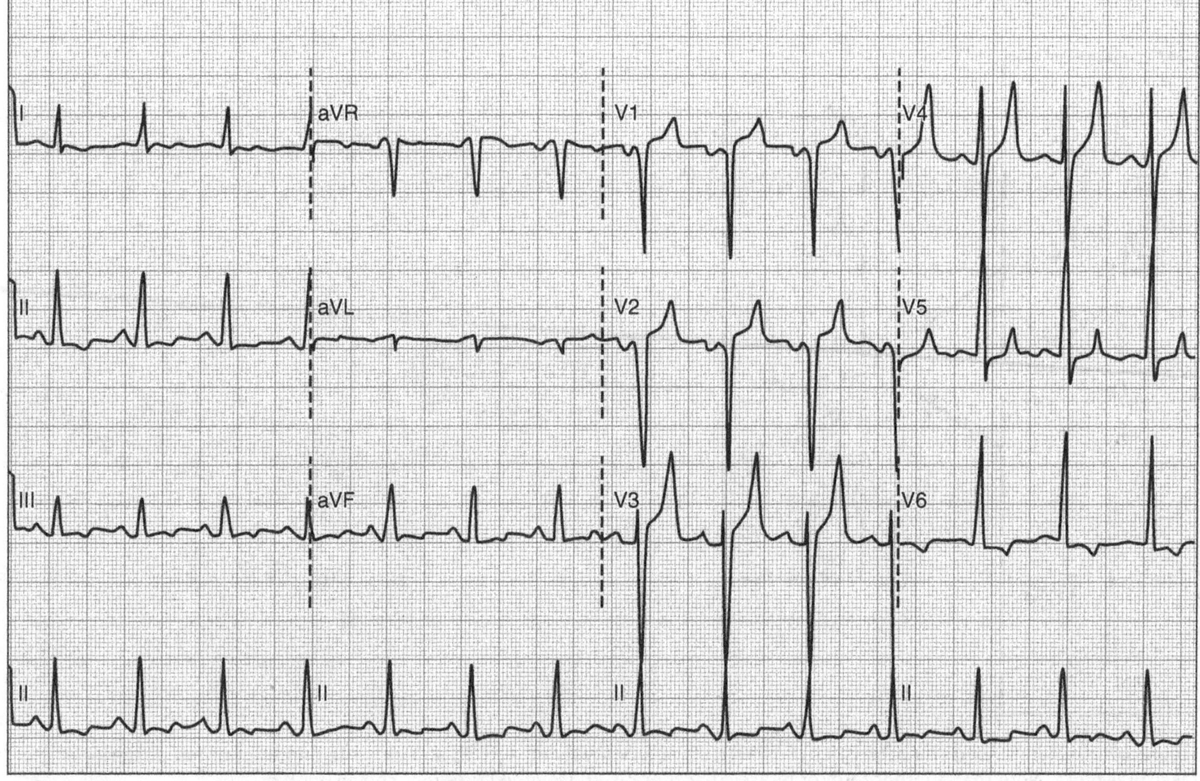

Figure 10.12 Non-specific intraventricular conduction delay. The QRS complex is abnormally widened, yet a consideration of the QRS complex axis and morphologies does not suggest either LAFB, LPFB, LBBB, or RBBB.

11

Atrial and Ventricular Ectopic Beats

Jeffrey D. Ferguson[1], *Michael Levy*[2], *J. Aidan Boswick*[2], *and William J. Brady*[3]

[1] *Department of Emergency Medicine, Virginia Commonwealth University, Richmond, VA, USA*
[2] *Crossix Analytics Services, Veeva Systems Inc, New York, NY, USA*
[3] *Departments of Emergency Medicine and Medicine, University of Virginia School of Medicine, Charlottesville, VA, USA*

In the course of evaluating any electrocardiogram (ECG) or rhythm strip, it may become evident that, while a primary rhythm clearly exists, there are also additional beats that have morphology inconsistent with that underlying rhythm. These abnormal beats are referred to as *ectopy*, or ectopic beats. These ectopic electrical "beats" seen on the ECG or rhythm strip may or may not cause ventricular contraction or a mechanical beat. Because these ectopic beats occur between "normal" beats, however, they disrupt what may otherwise be a regular rhythm and may cause the pulse to feel irregular – at times, this irregularity in rhythm can be detected by the patient and thus become symptomatic.

Ectopy can arise from anywhere in the cardiac conduction system and from many segments of other cardiac tissues; ectopic beats are classified on the basis of where they originate: premature atrial contraction (PACs) with an atrial source, premature junctional contractions (PJCs) with a junctional or atrioventricular (AV) nodal source, and premature ventricular contractions (PVCs) with a ventricular source (Box 11.1). They are termed *premature* contractions because they appear between "normal" beats at a point earlier than one would expect the next beat. This earlier occurrence leads to a short R–R interval on the preceding beat and a long R–R interval on the following beat.

Premature Atrial Contractions

PACs are impulses generated in the atrial myocardial tissue. PACs are characterized by P waves of a different morphology and axis with a shorter than anticipated P–P interval when measured from the preceding beat. The PR interval in a PAC may be the same, shorter, or longer than that of the baseline rhythm, depending on the location of the ectopic atrial focus. Owing to the refractory period in the AV node and the His–Purkinje system, these impulses are not always conducted to the ventricles. When transmitted, however, the impulse follows the normal conduction pathway, resulting in a normal-appearing, narrow QRS complex. PACs typically "reset" the SA node, resulting in a longer R–R interval immediately following the PAC (Figure 11.1).

Premature Junctional Contractions

PJCs arise from the AV node or the most proximal portion of the His–Purkinje system. The beat that follows proceeds through the normal conduction system and produces a narrow QRS complex that often lacks a preceding normal P wave and thus PR interval. Occasionally, however, P waves (often inverted) may be seen within the QRS complex, immediately preceding the QRS complex (with a very short P–R interval), or immediately following the QRS complex because of retrograde depolarization of the atria – producing the so-called retrograde P wave. PJCs may or may not reset the SA node; therefore, the R–R interval immediately following the PJC may either be prolonged or may be consistent with the underlying rhythm (Figure 11.2).

Premature Ventricular Contractions

PVCs occur when an ectopic focus in the ventricular myocardium electrically discharges the ventricles prematurely, usually occurring during the relative refractory

The Electrocardiogram in Emergency and Acute Care, First Edition.
Edited by Korin B. Hudson, Amita Sudhir, George Glass, and William J. Brady.

Box 11.1 Atrial, Junctional, and Ventricular Ectopy

- Both atrial and ventricular ectopic beats often occur without causing symptoms; in fact, ectopic beats do not always indicate underlying cardiac pathology.
- If symptomatic, patients complain of palpitations and irregular heart rates.
- Certain medications or drugs such as alcohol, tobacco, caffeine, or other stimulants may increase the frequency of these ectopic beats.
- Conditions that lead to an irritated myocardium, such as electrolyte abnormalities, ischemia/infarction, cardiomyopathy, or endocrine dysfunction may also lead to increased ectopy.
- Management is rarely indicated in the acute setting for PACs and PJCs; situations in which therapy can be considered for PVCs include the following:
  - Frequent unifocal and/or multifocal PVCs
  - R-on-T PVCs
  - PVCs occurring in the setting of certain acute events, such as acute coronary syndrome (ACS).

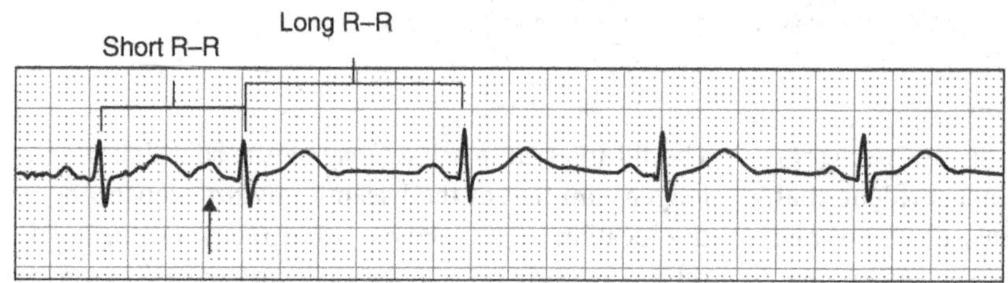

Figure 11.1 Premature atrial contraction. Normal sinus rhythm with premature atrial contraction. Note the different P wave morphology (arrow) compared to the underlying rhythm. Also evident is the shortened R–R interval preceding and the long R–R interval following the ectopic beat.

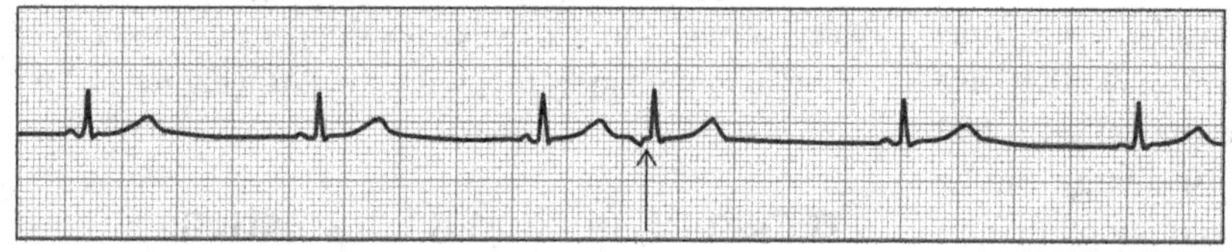

Figure 11.2 Premature junctional contraction. Sinus bradycardia with premature junctional contractions. The arrow indicates an abnormal P wave with an extremely short PR interval.

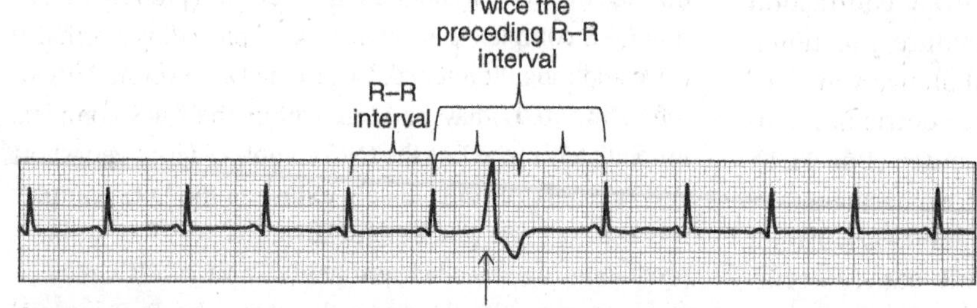

Figure 11.3 Unifocal premature ventricular contraction (indicated by the arrow). The braces show the underlying R–R interval and the complete pause following the PVC. The interval between the R wave preceding the PVC and the R wave following the PVC is exactly twice that of the underlying rhythm.

period of ventricular repolarization. This impulse gives rise to a QRS complex of unusual morphology, which is typically wide (>0.12 s) and lacking a preceding P wave.

One of the distinguishing characteristics of PVCs is that they are followed by a compensatory pause. The PVC does not usually affect or reset the SA node; so, the regular R–R interval is maintained after a pause of a single beat, the PVC. This PVC feature may be recognized by measuring the interval between the R wave on the beat preceding the PVC and the R wave on the beat following the PVC, noting that it is exactly twice as long at the R–R interval of the underlying rhythm (Figure 11.3). If the R–R interval does not “march out,” the suspect complex is not a PVC and may instead be an aberrantly conducted premature beat (i.e. PAC or PJC) from a supraventricular focus (Figure 11.4).

PVCs can present in varying manners. Multiple PVCs in a single ECG strip can be either unifocal or multifocal. Unifocal PVCs share the same morphology and ectopic ventricular focus (Figure 11.5), while multifocal PVCs demonstrate different morphologies and result from two or more different foci (Figure 11.6). Multifocal PVCs are of potentially greater concern because they indicate that the premature beats are coming from more than one ventricular focus and thus represent widespread "irritation" of the ventricular myocardium. This increased irritability may progress to less organized rhythms such as polymorphic ventricular tachycardia (VT) or ventricular fibrillation.

PVCs may also occur as couplets (Figure 11.7), a term that refers to two PVCs back to back. Three or more PVCs in a row are considered to be both a triplet and a "burst" or "run" of VT. Furthermore, PVCs may present in a "regular" manner, occurring every other beat, as bigeminy (Figure 11.8) every third beat as trigeminy (Figure 11.9), and so on. Finally, PVCs may occur

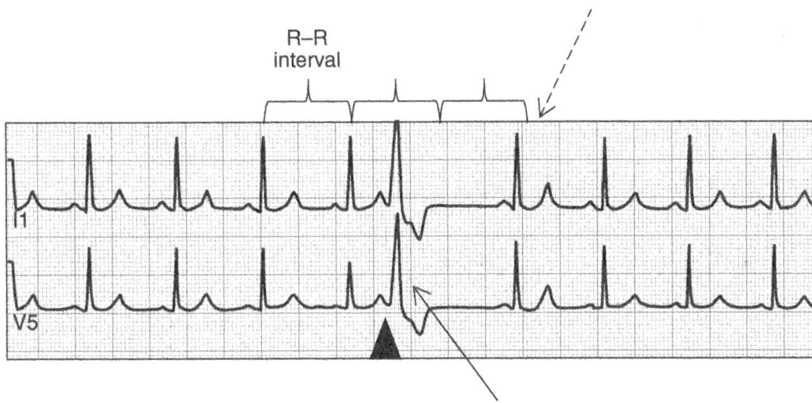

Figure 11.4 The wide complex ectopic beat (arrow) may at first glance appear to be a PVC, but careful examination reveals a P wave (arrow head). Furthermore, the dashed arrow shows that the R wave following the ectopic beat comes earlier than would be expected if it were a PVC. This ectopic beat likely represents a premature supraventricular (atrial or junctional) beat with aberrant intraventricular conduction likely resulting from bundle fatigue.

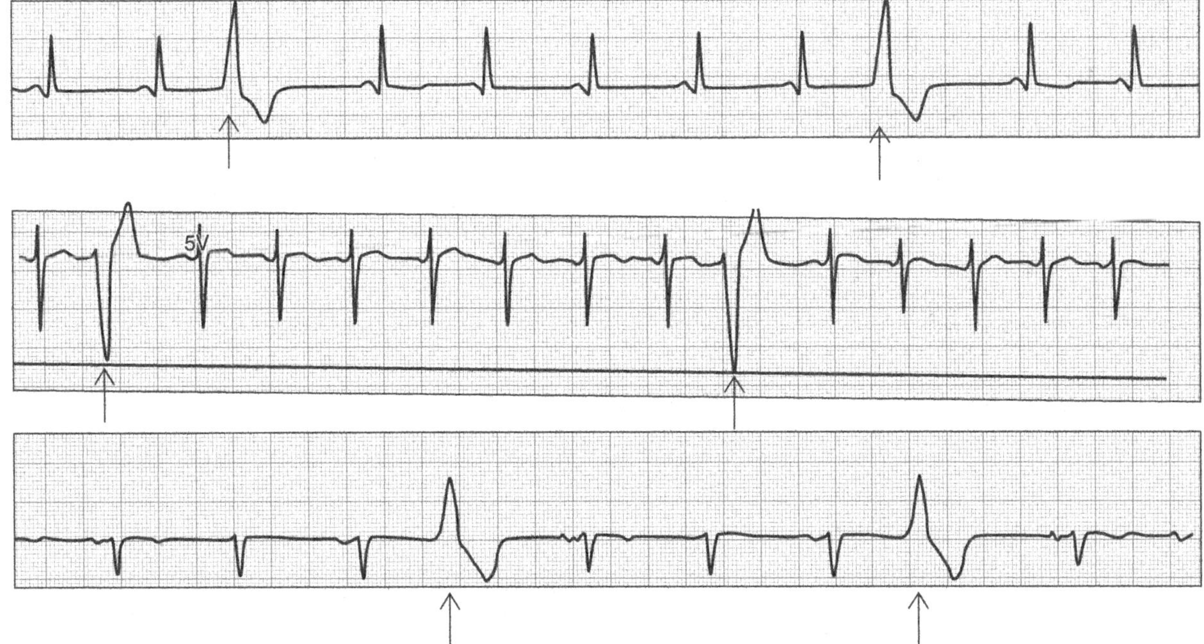

Figure 11.5 Several examples of unifocal premature ventricular contractions (arrows). Note that within each rhythm strip (i.e. within the same lead), the PVCs have identical morphology.

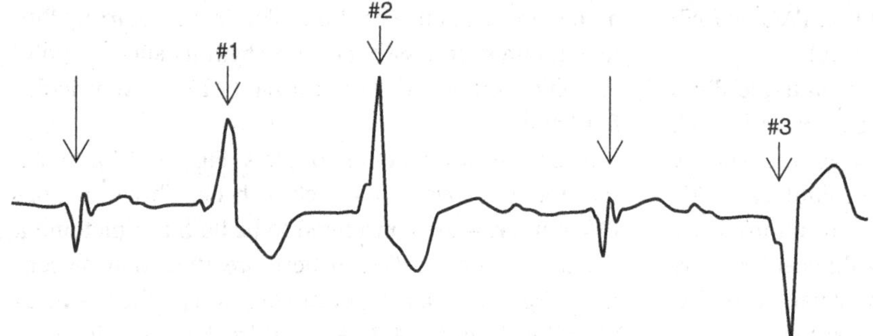

Figure 11.6 Multifocal PVCs. Note the multiple PVCs in this rhythm strip with three predominant morphologies. The primary, underlying rhythm is noted by the long arrows and the three different PVCs by the short arrows.

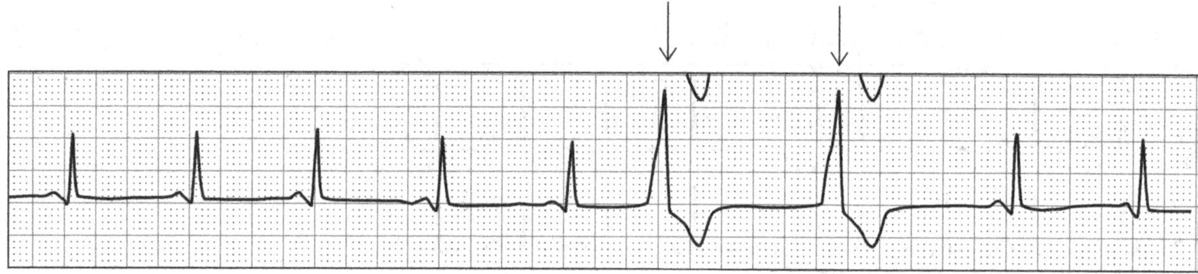

Figure 11.7 PVCs in a couplet: two consecutive PVCs (arrows), in this case, with the same morphology.

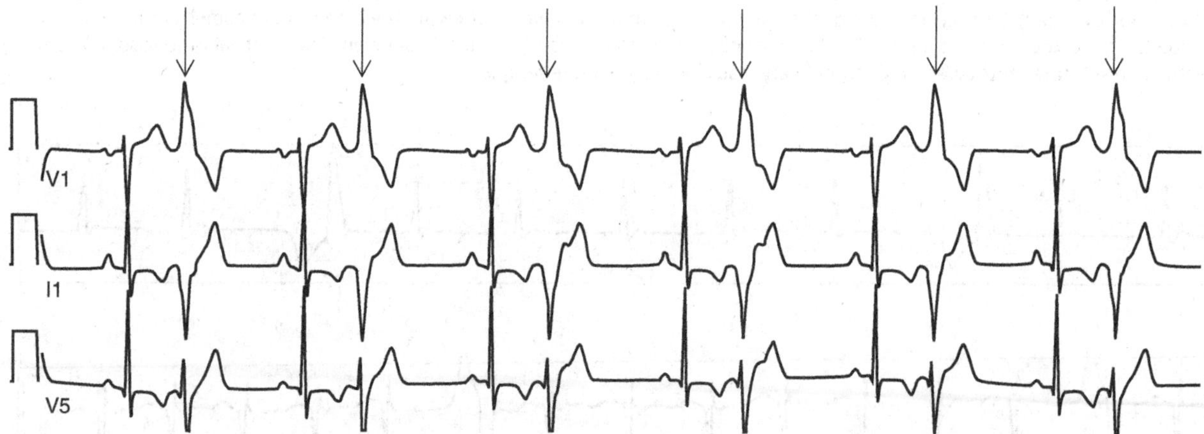

Figure 11.8 Ventricular bigeminy: every other beat is a PVC (arrows) with an underlying sinus rhythm.

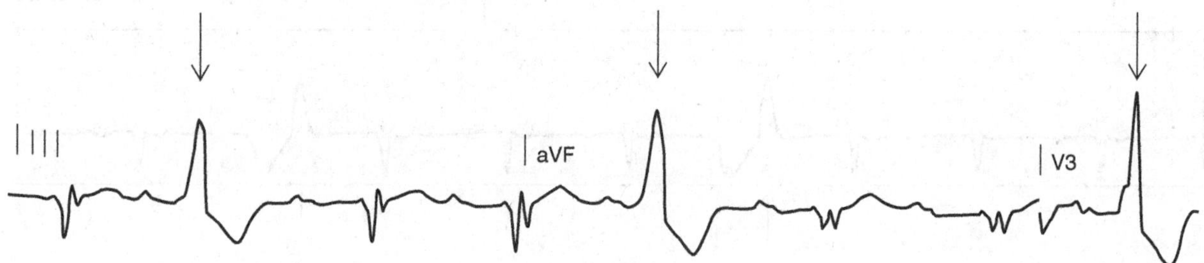

Figure 11.9 Ventricular trigeminy. In this multilead rhythm strip, the arrows indicate unifocal PVCs that occur every third beat.

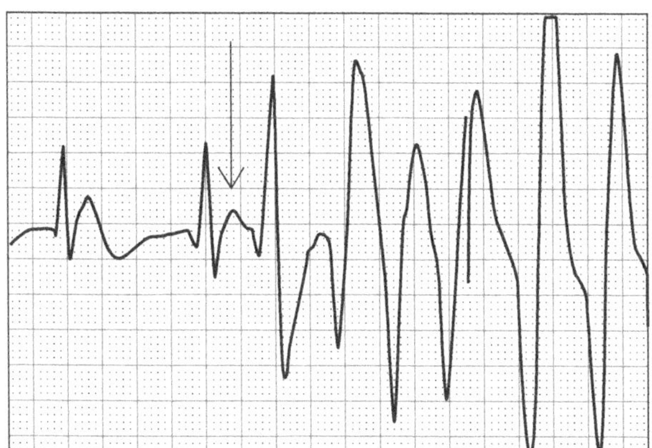

Figure 11.10 R-on-T phenomenon with PVC leading to polymorphic VT. Note how the R wave of the PVC (arrow) falls on the T wave of the preceding beat.

during the latter half of the preceding T wave and during the relative refractory period of ventricular repolarization. This event, known as an *R-on-T phenomenon* (Figure 11.10), may precipitate ventricular tachycardia or ventricular fibrillation. This form of PVC is perhaps the most significant and concerning type of ectopic electrical event.

Section III

Acute Coronary Syndrome and the 12-Lead ECG

12

Ischemic Heart Disease: Anatomic and Physiologic Considerations

Peter Pollak[1], Peter Monteleone[2], Kelly Williamson[3], David Carlberg[4], and William J. Brady[5]

[1] Mayo Clinic Specialist, Jacksonville, FL, USA
[2] Department of Internal Medicine, University of Texas at Austin Dell School of Medicine, Austin, TX, USA
[3] Department of Emergency Medicine, Northwestern University School of Medicine, Chicago, IL, USA
[4] Georgetown University School of Medicine, Washington, DC, USA
[5] Departments of Emergency Medicine and Medicine, University of Virginia School of Medicine, Charlottesville, VA, USA

The differential diagnosis of chest pain is vast, as chest pain may originate from the cardiovascular, gastrointestinal, respiratory, musculoskeletal, and nervous systems. Potentially lethal causes of chest pain, which must be considered in every patient with this complaint, include acute myocardial infarction (MI), aortic dissection, pneumothorax, pneumonia, pulmonary embolism, and esophageal perforation (Box 12.1). While many presentations of chest pain are not cardiac, the time-sensitive nature as well as dire consequences of missed cardiac chest pain make early consideration and diagnosis of this disease essential. The 12-lead electrocardiogram (ECG) plays a critical role in the evaluation of cardiac chest pain, and therefore it is important that clinicians to use the ECG early when there is a suspicion of cardiac chest pain.

Cardiac Anatomy and Basic Physiology of Depolarization

In a very basic sense, the heart is divided into two halves – the right heart and the left heart; each half of the heart is further divided into two specific chambers – atrium and ventricle. Thus, the heart is composed of four chambers, including the right atrium, right ventricle, left atrium, and left ventricle. The atria are passive receptacles for blood returning to the heart, and they, in turn, push blood into the ventricles. The ventricles are much larger and stronger than the atria because they are responsible for pumping blood to the lungs (right ventricle) and the body (left ventricle). The right heart moves deoxygenated blood from the body and pumps it to the lungs to be reoxygenated. The left heart then takes this newly oxygenated blood from the lungs and pumps it throughout the body.

When the clinician is evaluating the patient for ACS, the left ventricle is the only cardiac region that is currently considered significant and important from the perspective of the 12-lead ECG. Thus, the left ventricle is imaged by the 12-lead ECG. In fact, the 12-lead ECG primarily images the walls of the left ventricle, including the anterior, lateral, inferior, and posterior segments; the right ventricle is imaged but less completely when compared to the left ventricle.

The triggers for the atrium and the ventricle to contract come in the form of electrical impulses, and these impulses are controlled by the cardiac pacemaker and conduction system (Figures 12.1 and 12.2a). The sinus node, which is located in the right atrium, is the primary pacemaker for the heart. The electrical signal from the sinus node (Figure 12.2b) is carried through the atrium to the atrioventricular (AV node; Figure 12.2c), which is located between the atria and the ventricles. The AV node then passes the signal to the His–Purkinje system, which passes it to the ventricles, initiating repolarization (Figure 12.2d). Repolarization occurs in a reverse manner, from ventricular tissue to atrial tissue (Figure 12.2e).

The Electrocardiogram in Emergency and Acute Care, First Edition.
Edited by Korin B. Hudson, Amita Sudhir, George Glass, and William J. Brady.

Box 12.1 Causes of Non-traumatic Chest Pain

- Acute coronary syndrome (ACS, angina, unstable angina (UA), and acute myocardial infarction)
- Aortic dissection/thoracic and abdominal aortic aneurysm
- Myocarditis/pericarditis (myopericarditis)
- Pneumonia
- Pulmonary embolus
- Pneumothorax
- Esophageal perforation
- Abdominal disorders (peptic ulcer disease, gastritis, pancreatitis, cholecystitis/-lithiasis, hepatitis)
- Musculoskeletal disorders
- Herpes zoster

Coronary Anatomy and Electrocardiograhic Regional Anatomic Issues

Blood is supplied to the heart muscle, which is also called the *myocardium*, via blood vessels called the *coronary arteries*. These coronary arteries arise from the base of the aorta and run along the surface of the heart, dividing into smaller branches. Eventually, very small arteries come off of the coronary arteries and dive down into the heart tissue, providing blood directly to the myocardium. Each of the major coronary arteries follows a typical course around the heart and usually supplies a specific area of the heart muscle. The two coronary arteries that come directly off of the aorta are named the *right coronary artery* and the *left main coronary artery* (Figure 12.3). The right coronary artery wraps around the right ventricle and supplies it with blood. It is important to note that the right coronary artery supplies blood to the sinus node and the AV node. The left main coronary is short but important as it supplies nearly all of the blood flow for the left ventricle. The left main coronary artery branches into two arteries. The first is the left anterior descending (LAD) artery, which supplies the ventricular septum (the wall between the ventricles) and the anterior left ventricle. The second is the left circumflex coronary artery, which supplies the lateral wall of the left ventricle. Branches from the LAD are called *diagonals* and branches off of the left circumflex are called *obtuse marginals*.

There is important variation in the blood supply to the back of the heart. In most people (termed *right dominant*), the right coronary artery continues around the right ventricle to supply the inferior portion of the ventricular septum as well as the posterior left ventricle. When it does so, it is called the posterior descending artery (PDA). Many patients, however, have the back of their heart supplied by

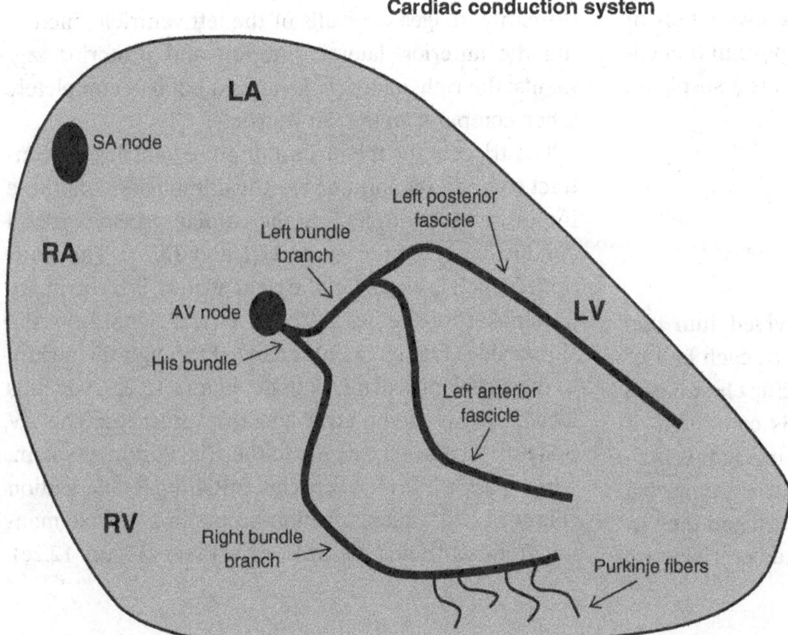

Figure 12.1 The cardiac conduction system (LA, left atrium; RA, right atrium; RV, right ventricle; LV, left ventricle; SA, sinoatrial; AV, atrioventricular).

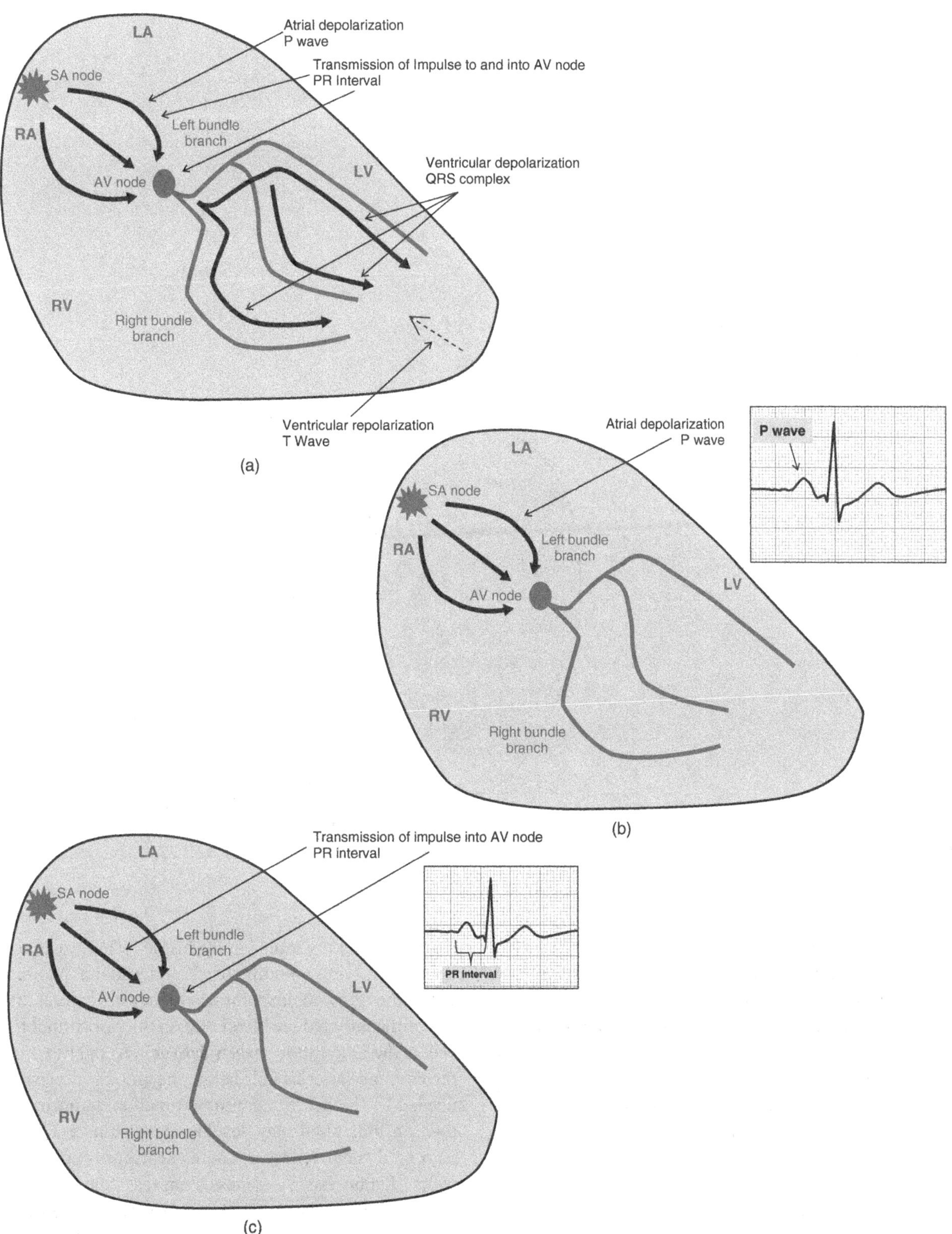

Figure 12.2 (a) The cardiac conduction system with superimposed cardiac electrical impulse with depolarization and ultimate repolarization. (b) Depolarization of the atrial tissues results in the P wave on the ECG. (c) Impulse transmission occurs through the atria and into the AV node, as described on the ECG by the PR interval. (d) The ventricle depolarizes as noted by the QRS complex. (e) The heart repolarizes in reverse manner, from ventricles to atria and is manifested on the ECG by the T wave.

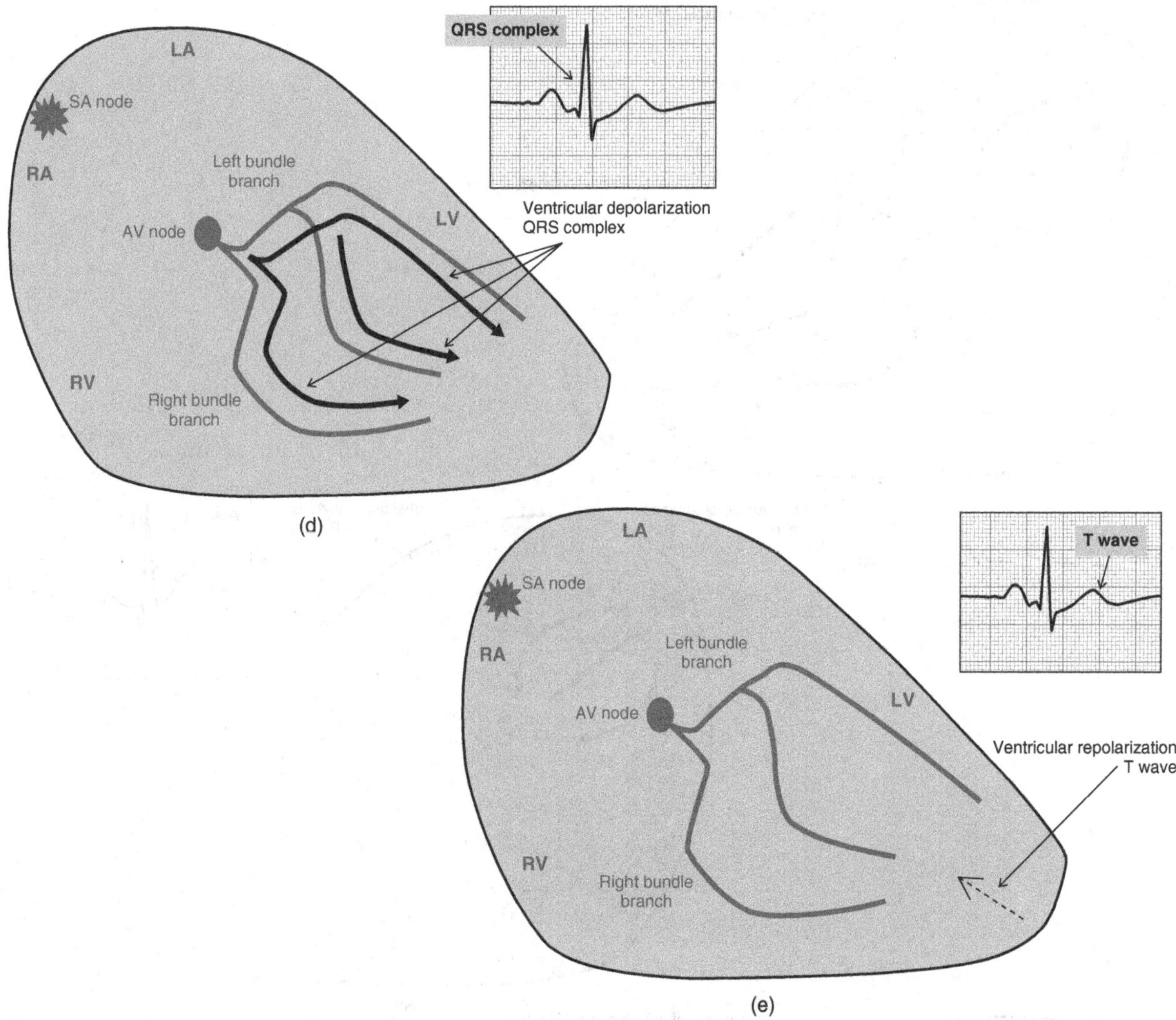

Figure 12.2 (Continued)

the left side of the coronary circulation, where the PDA arises as a continuation of the left circumflex coronary artery. A minority of people have coronary anatomy termed *codominant* where there is no specific single vessel supplying the posterior heart, but rather two smaller vessels contributed by the right and left circulations.

Figure 12.3 and Table 12.1 list the association of the anatomic cardiac wall with the related coronary artery and imaging ECG leads.

Cardiac Pathophysiology

As people age, they begin to develop atherosclerotic plaques that narrow their coronary arteries. Risk factors that accelerate the development of these plaques include hypertension, hypercholesterolemia, diabetes mellitus, cigarette smoking, and family history. These plaques, made of varying amounts of cholesterol and calcium, sometimes grow to the point where they have the ability to significantly reduce blood flow to the myocardial tissue. If the amount of oxygen delivered to the heart via the coronary arteries falls below the amount of oxygen needed by the heart to continue functioning normally, then an individual may develop chest pain or a chest pain equivalent (chest pressure, heartburn, epigastric pain, diaphoresis, dizziness, nausea, shortness of breath). This mismatch between oxygen demand and oxygen delivery and the resultant symptoms are known as *ischemia*. Ischemia is usually a reversible process, that is, reducing myocardial oxygen demand or increasing myocardial oxygen delivery leads to resolution of symptoms. Also, ischemia alone does not lead to myocardial cell death. When the myocardial oxygen and

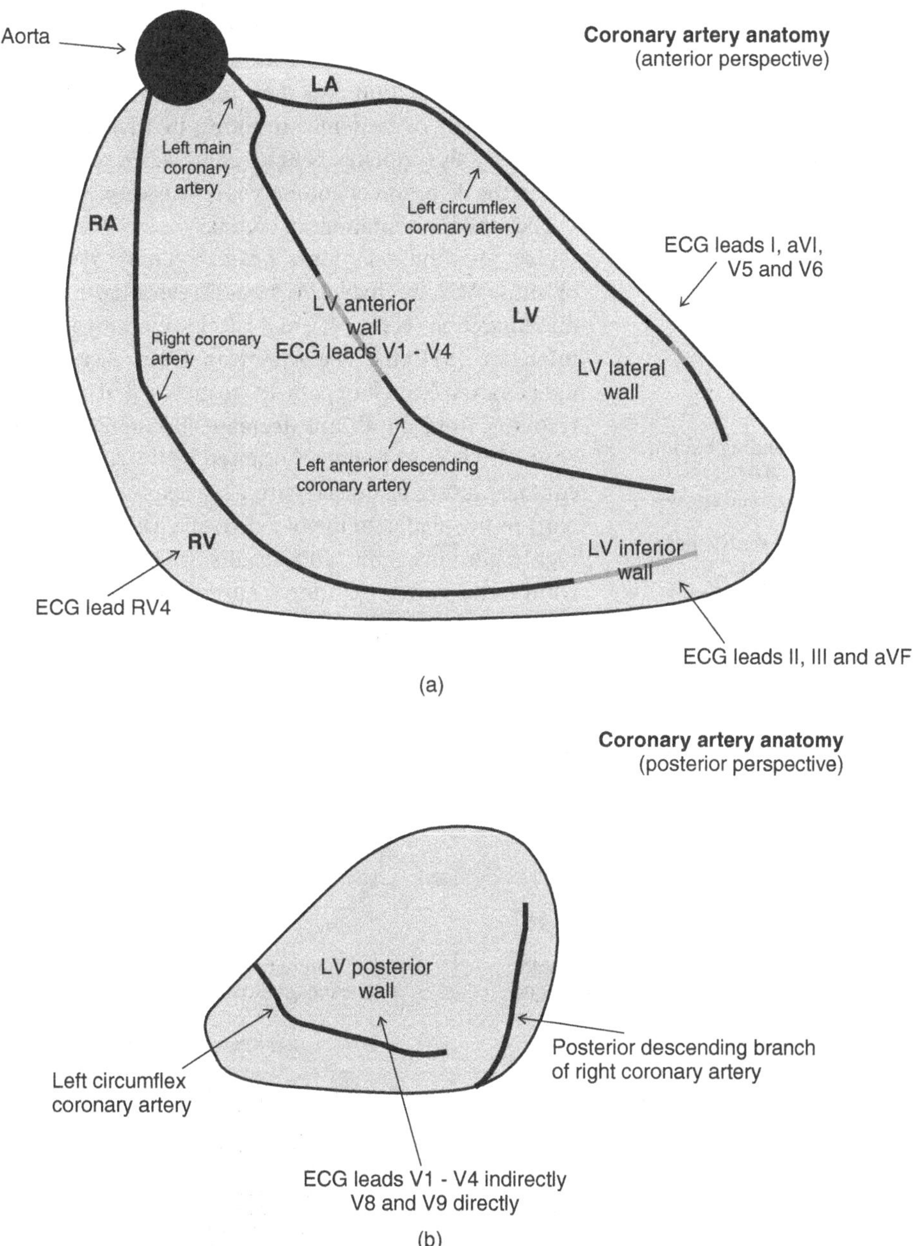

Figure 12.3 Cardiac and coronary anatomy with corresponding coronary artery, ECG lead, and cardiac segment. (a) Anterior perspective and (b) posterior perspective (LA, left atrium; RA, right atrium; RV, right ventricle; LV, left ventricle).

nutrient delivery fall so low that heart cells begin to die, this is termed a *myocardial infarction*, which is characterized by an elevation of cardiac biomarkers such as troponin into the blood.

The spectrum of coronary artery disease is broad and includes asymptomatic atherosclerotic plaques, lesions that cause ischemia, and lesions that cause MI. It can be difficult if not impossible to differentiate between these presentations solely via vital signs, history, and physical examination; thus, ECGs are vital even if suspicion for cardiac chest pain is low.

Stable angina, an indication of coronary artery disease, leads to transient, episodic chest discomfort. While stable angina is not indicative of acute infarction, its presence suggests intermittent myocardial ischemia, most often the result of a fixed atherosclerotic plaque in the coronary arteries. Since the symptoms of myocardial ischemia should be reproducible at a given level of exertion, patients who suffer from stable angina are typically familiar with their disease process. Given that stable angina is not indicative of infarction, these patients typically have relatively normal ECGs at rest. ECG changes

Table 12.1 Cardiac and coronary anatomy with corresponding coronary artery, ECG lead, and cardiac segment.

Primary chamber	Cardiac segment	ECG leads	Coronary artery
Left ventricle	Anterior wall	V1–V4	Left anterior descending artery
Left ventricle	Lateral wall	I, aVI, V5, and V6	Left circumflex artery
Left ventricle	Inferior wall	II, III, and aVF	Right coronary artery
Left ventricle	Posterior wall	V1–V4 indirectly V8–V9 directly	Posterior descending branch (RCA) or left circumflex artery
Right ventricle	Right ventricle	RV4 (RV1–RV4)	Right ventricular branch (RCA)

consistent with myocardial ischemia, including ST segment depression and T wave flattening or inversion, may appear with exertion and then resolve with rest. This phenomenon of ischemia resulting in transient ECG changes is the principle behind using the exercise stress test in the detection of coronary artery disease.

The other presentations of coronary artery disease fall under the umbrella term *acute coronary syndrome* or *ACS*. ACSs include UA, non-ST elevation myocardial infarction (NSTEMI), and ST elevation myocardial infarction (STEMI). The American Heart Association defines an ACS as chest pain due to myocardial ischemia resulting from an abrupt decrease in coronary blood flow. ACS is most frequently caused by the rupture of a coronary artery plaque (Figure 12.4), exposing the contents of the plaque to the bloodstream. This material is highly thrombogenic and results in clot formation within the coronary artery. Further, the artery can

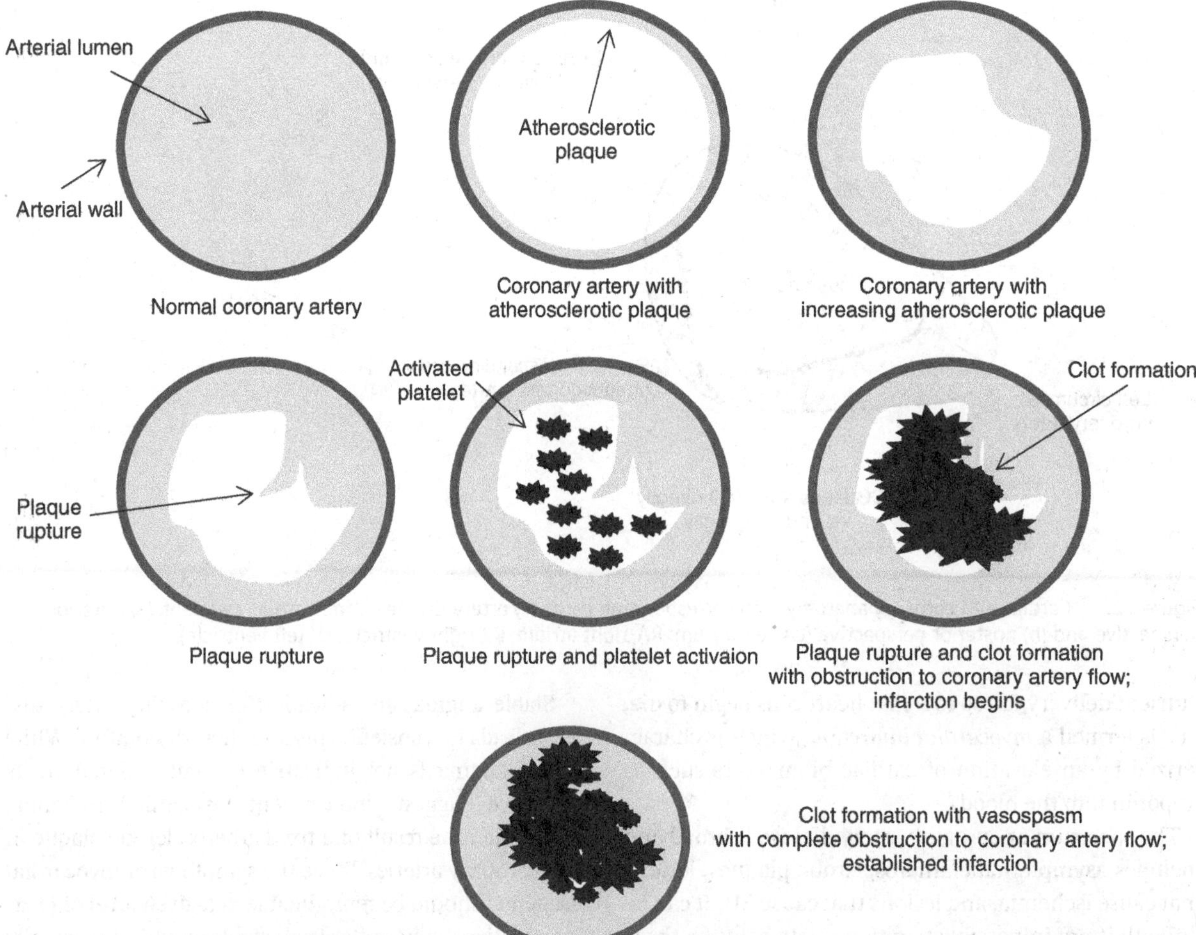

Figure 12.4 The development of atherosclerotic lesions in the coronary artery from early in life to the development of acute myocardial infarction. Note that plaque rupture initiates platelet activation, clot formation, and vasospasm, and ultimately coronary artery obstruction with myocardial infarction.

develop spasm, further reducing the lumen of the affected artery and further compromising flow. When the vessel is suddenly occluded, the heart muscle becomes starved for oxygen, resulting in pain, loss of function, and possibly ECG changes. Refer Figure 12.4 for a depiction of the progressive nature of atherosclerosis over time and development of ACS with plaque rupture, platelet activation, clot formation, and vasospasm.

UA is defined as anginal symptoms that are new, occur at rest, or those with a "crescendo" pattern of increasing duration or frequency. UA may be considered a pre-infarction state, as atherosclerotic plaque rupture may lead to thrombus formation, vasospasm, and incomplete coronary artery occlusion. Patients with UA may have a normal ECG, or the ECG may begin to reveal signs of ischemia, including T wave abnormalities and ST segment changes. Unlike the changes associated with stable angina, these signs of ischemia rarely resolve with rest alone.

Acute MIs, known by the lay public as heart attacks, occur when ischemia persists to a degree that one develops myocardial cell death. The two types of acute MI are classified on the basis of ECG abnormalities associated with each, namely, ST segment deviation. As the name suggests, NSTEMI is defined by the development of positive serum markers of infarction (troponin, CK-MB) in the absence of ST segment elevation on ECG. The ECG of an NSTEMI patient may reveal other changes corresponding to the infarction, including T wave inversion or ST segment depression. In contrast, a STEMI is defined by the presence of greater than or equal to 1 mm of ST segment elevation in two or more contiguous leads. These patients will also develop positive serum markers of infarction.

The pathophysiology of STEMI is very different from that of UA and NSTEMI. A STEMI represents the complete occlusion of a coronary artery, while UA and NSTEMI most often represent an incomplete occlusion. The total coronary occlusion that occurs with STEMI is relatively fixed in time. The heart muscle distal to the obstruction becomes progressively more hypoxic; thus, symptoms and ECG findings are generally progressive. Conversely, in the partial coronary occlusion found with UA/NSTEMI, the flow through the coronary artery changes during the dynamic process of clot formation. The affected coronary artery may also spasm and relax at the site of obstruction. Therefore, in UA and NSTEMI, flow through the affected coronary artery waxes and wanes as the infarction evolves. This leads to waxing and waning symptoms and ECG changes that do not follow a particular pattern.

The treatments of STEMI and UA/NSTEMI also vary greatly. STEMI patients benefit from the emergent opening of the blocked coronary artery via either intravenous thrombolytic drugs or cardiac catheterization with direct clot removal, angioplasty, and stenting. Thrombolytics can be given in the emergency department, while catheterization must occur in a cardiac catheterization laboratory. The use of cardiac catheterization may be limited because some hospitals do not have catheterization capabilities. Also, cardiac catheterization requires the presence of a trained cardiologist and other members of the catheterization team. UA and NSTEMI are generally treated with medical management, including antiplatelet agents and anticoagulants, as well as urgent or elective catheterization. These patients do not benefit from intravenous thrombolytic agents.

13

Electrocardiographic Findings in Acute Coronary Syndrome

Peter Monteleone[1], Peter Pollak[2], David Carlberg[3], and William J. Brady[4]

[1] *Department of Internal Medicine, University of Texas at Austin Dell School of Medicine, Austin, TX, USA*
[2] *Mayo Clinic Specialist, Jacksonville, FL, USA*
[3] *Georgetown University School of Medicine, Washington, DC, USA*
[4] *Departments of Emergency Medicine and Medicine, University of Virginia School of Medicine, Charlottesville, VA, USA*

Introduction

Ischemic and infarcted myocardium presents electrocardiographically in many different ways. Acute coronary syndrome (ACS) may present with an array of findings, ranging from the normal electrocardiogram (ECG) to obvious ST segment elevation myocardial infarction (STEMI) to a malignant dysrhythmia. In fact, ECG changes in almost any portion of the ECGs tracing can be seen with ACS and, in the appropriate setting, suggest the diagnosis. Unfortunately, these changes do not always manifest themselves in a standard, "textbook" manner. The clinician must remember that each 12-lead ECG or cardiac rhythm strip is quite literally an "electrical snapshot in time," a few seconds in the progression of the heart's ischemic state. The use of serial ECGs with or without continuous cardiac monitoring is suggested in situations where a clinical suspicion of ACS is present.

This chapter reviews and discusses the 12-lead ECG findings encountered in patients with a range of coronary syndromes, ranging from stable angina to STEMI, with or without malignant dysrhythmia.

The 12-Lead Electrocardiogram in ST Segment Elevation Myocardial Infarction Evolution of Electrocardiogram Abnormalities

Of the different types of ACS, STEMI is the most likely to demonstrate a predictable evolution of its ECG findings. The earliest ECG abnormality associated with STEMI, occurring within minutes of an interruption to myocardial blood flow, is the development of hyperacute, or prominent, T wave. In a normal ECG, the orientation of the T wave typically corresponds to the dominant direction of the associated QRS complex; in other words, if the QRS complex is largely positive, then the T wave will also be positive or upright and vice versa. The T wave is typically upright in leads I, II, and V3 through V6; inverted in leads aVR and V1; and variable in leads III, V2, aVL, and aVF. In the early stages of coronary artery occlusion, the T waves maintain their vector (i.e. do not invert) but become tall and peaked – thus the hyperacute T wave. Refer to Figure 13.1 for examples of hyperacute T waves in early STEMI.

Classically, hyperacute T waves progress directly to ST segment elevation (STE). STE itself is both an alarming and demanding ECG finding, particularly in a patient with chest pain or chest pain equivalent presentation. It is both alarming and demanding in that it can be the manifestation of STEMI, a time-sensitive myocardial infarction with significant risk for morbidity and mortality if therapy is not delivered appropriately and expeditiously. As per the American Heart Association (AHA), STE must reach at least 1 mm of magnitude in the limb leads and 2 mm in the precordial leads to meet criteria for the diagnosis of STEMI; these findings must also occur in at least two leads in the same anatomic distribution to suggest STEMI – assuming the clinical correlation is present.

While the ST segment in a normal ECG is typically at the same level as the TP segment (i.e. not elevated above the electrocardiographic baseline defined by adjacent TP segments), during STEMI the ST segment changes

The Electrocardiogram in Emergency and Acute Care, First Edition.
Edited by Korin B. Hudson, Amita Sudhir, George Glass, and William J. Brady.

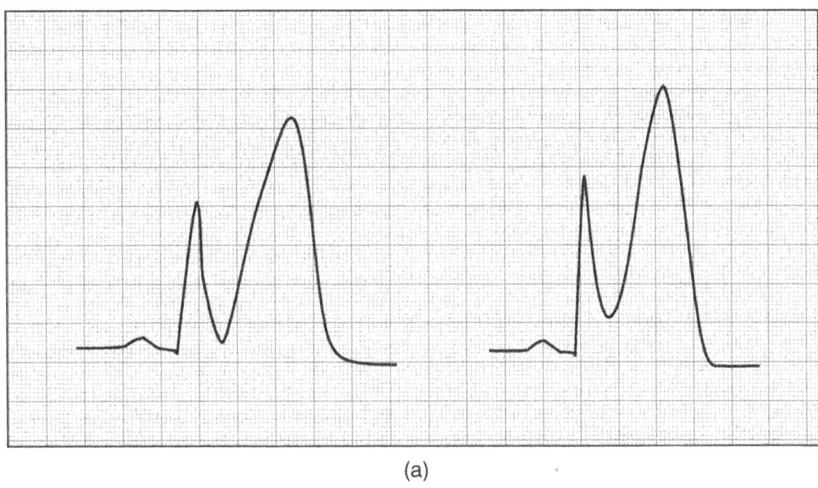

(a)

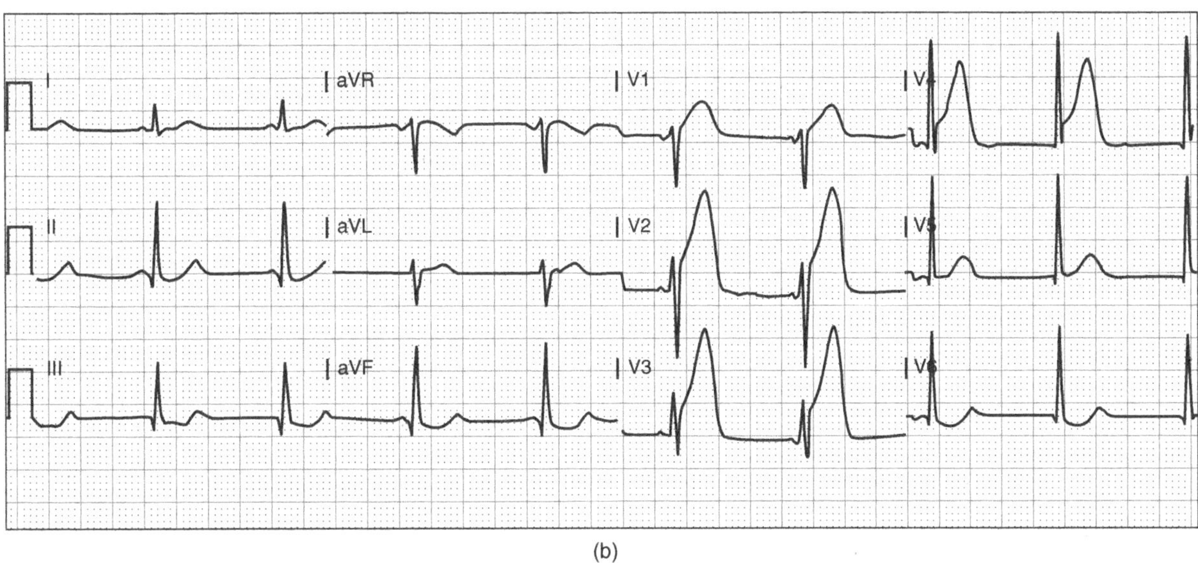

(b)

Figure 13.1 (a) Hyperacute, or prominent, T waves of early STEMI. (b) Hyperacute T wave with early ST segment elevation in the anterior region, consistent with early anterior STEMI.

from this flat and/or concave morphology to one which is elevated with either a convex or an obliquely straight morphology (Figures 13.2a, b and 13.3a, b). As the infarction progresses, the QRS complex, ST segment, and T wave fuse, leading to a single monophasic deflection on the ECG. Given its characteristic appearance and grave prognosis if left untreated, this finding has been named "the tombstone" form of STE. Refer to Figure 13.3a–e for an example of the evolution of the ECG in STEMI.

Several features of STE are important to consider. The magnitude of STE is important. As noted, expert consensus groups such as the AHA suggest that 1–2 mm of elevation is required to establish the diagnosis of STEMI. The clinician is cautioned, however, in that minimal degrees of STE, that is, subtle STE, can be encountered in certain STEMI presentations, including both inferior and lateral infarctions as well as early in the patient's course of acute myocardial infarction (AMI) (Figure 13.4). The morphology, or contour, of the elevated ST segment is also important to consider (Figure 13.2a–d). Typically, the elevated ST segment is either obliquely straight or convex in shape. Concave-shaped, elevated ST segments are less often associated with STEMI. Of course, there is an exception to every such statement – early in the course of STEMI, the elevated ST segment can be concave in appearance with evolution ultimately to either obliquely straight or convex morphologies as the infarction progresses. Regarding these electrocardiographic features of STEMI, common pitfalls in the ECG interpretation include the missed diagnosis of STEMI when the magnitude of the

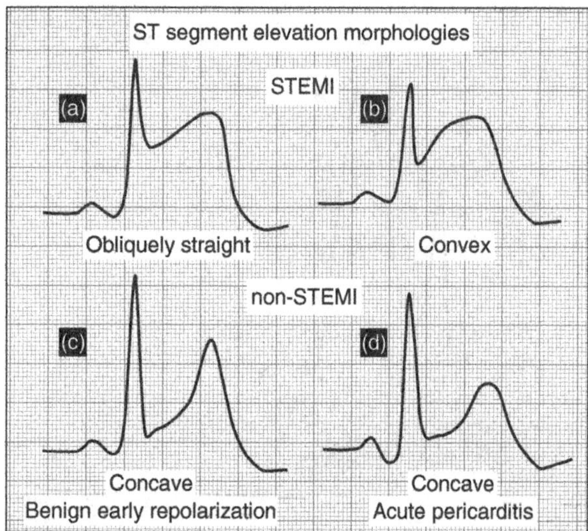

Figure 13.2 ST segment elevation subtypes in STEMI and non-STEMI presentations. (a) STEMI with obliquely straight ST segment elevation. (b) STEMI with convex ST segment elevation. (c) non-STEMI (BER) with concave ST segment elevation. (d) non-STEMI (acute pericarditis) with concave ST segment elevation.

elevation is either minimal (i.e. less than 1 mm) or atypical in contour (i.e. concave in shape). The clinician is encouraged to consider the ECG within the context of the overall patient presentation.

While pathologic Q waves, defined as the initial downsloping, or negative portion, of the QRS complex, may develop within one to two hours of symptom onset, they usually require as long as 12–24 hours after the event to fully develop (Figure 13.5a). Since nonviable cells do not conduct an electrical signal, Q waves are the ECG indication of myocardial cell death, representing an electrically inert myocardium. Clinicians must be aware, however, that the appearance of Q waves does not exclude ongoing infarction. A subset of patients with Q waves present on their ECGs in the presence of a STEMI pattern may still benefit from fibrinolytic therapy or percutaneous coronary intervention (PCI) (Figure 13.5b).

Within 48 hours after an untreated STEMI, the ST segments will usually return to their baseline and the T waves should flatten and then symmetrically invert. Within days to months, the T waves will often revert to their normal upright conformation. The Q waves may disappear over months, though they will often become a permanent feature of the patient's ECG. Refer to Figure 13.3a–e for the evolution of ECG changes with STEMI.

Reciprocal Change

Patients with STEMI frequently develop concomitant ST depression on ECG. Reciprocal change, also called reciprocal ST segment depression, is defined as at least 1 mm of ST segment depression occurring on an ECG which also demonstrates STE (Figure 13.6a, b). Further, the concept of reciprocal change cannot be used in ECG syndromes in which ST segment depression is encountered as part of that entity's normal or defined appearance. Thus, with left bundle branch block (LBBB), left ventricular hypertrophy (LVH), and ventricular paced patterns, ST segment depression is, in fact, anticipated; therefore, both the term and concept of reciprocal change cannot be used.

Reciprocal change most commonly occur in leads I and aVL, although they can occur in any lead. Reciprocal change is most commonly detected with inferior STEMI, associated with 70% of these events. Reciprocal change is only detected in 30% of anterior STEMI presentations. While not always present, reciprocal change has an important confirmatory value in STEMI diagnosis. The presence of reciprocal changes portends a 90% positive predictive value for STEMI, that is, 90% of patient with reciprocal changes are, in fact, having a STEMI. Also, the presence of reciprocal change is associated with greater cardiovascular risk as compared to STEMI patients without such abnormalities.

Left Bundle Branch Block

The conducting system of the heart is divided into two parts, the left bundle and the right bundle, just distal to the atrioventricular (AV) node. The blood supply to the left bundle comes off the left anterior descending artery (LAD); therefore the left bundle may be damaged with the occlusion of the LAD. The presence of an LBBB complicates the ACS presentation in many ways. First, from a diagnostic perspective, the presence of an LBBB pattern confounds the ability of the ECG to detect changes associated with ACS. In other words, a patient may experience AMI and demonstrate the anticipated ECG findings of a "normal" LBBB. Second, the presence of LBBB is a marker of significant increased cardiovascular risk. Patients with LBBB have higher rates of malignant dysrhythmia, cardiogenic shock, and death. Finally, the presence of a new, or "not known to be old," LBBB in the setting of acute chest pain or other anginal equivalent presentation is an indication of either fibrinolysis or PCI; of course, this last statement assumes that the clinical presentation is consistent with AMI.

Patients have an LBBB when the QRS duration exceeds 120 ms (Figure 13.7); the QRS complex is largely negative in leads V1–V3 and positive in leads I, aVl, V5, and V6. The LBBB is associated with STE with upright T waves in leads V1 through V3 and ST segment depression with inverted T waves in the lateral leads I, aVl, V5,

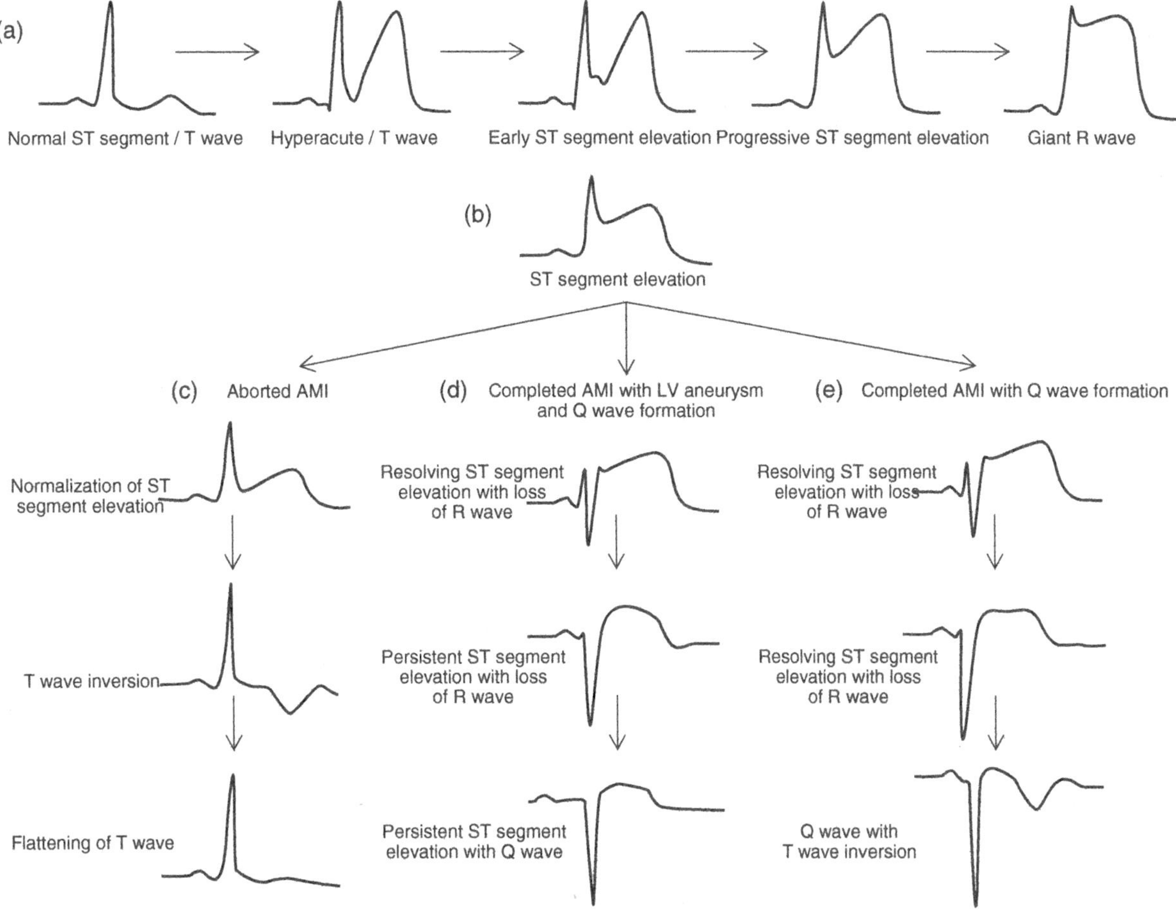

Figure 13.3 Evolution of ECG abnormalities in STEMI. The ECG structures in (a) and (b) demonstrate the typical progression of changes encountered in a STEMI. The ECG structures seen in (c–e) describe the three possible progressions of STEMI, including an aborted STEMI without significant, lasting injury, a completed STEMI with significant, lasting injury and LV aneurysm, and a completed STEMI with significant, lasting damage to the heart, respectively. (a) Progression from normal ST segment and T wave configurations to the following ECG phases of STEMI evolution: hyperacute T wave, early ST segment elevation, progressive ST segment elevation, and the giant R wave (combination of hyperacute T wave and ST segment elevation). (b) Established ST segment elevation in STEMI. (c) An aborted STEMI, either due to endogenous fibrinolysis or medical intervention, with resolving ST segment elevation, eventual T wave inversion, and ultimate T wave flattening with continued presence of the normal QRS complex (i.e. no loss of the R wave), indicating the infarction likely did not produce lasting, significant damage. (d) Completed STEMI with established infarction (indicated by the Q wave) and LV aneurysm (indicated by the persistent ST segment elevation). (e) Completed STEMI with established infarction (indicated by the Q wave and T wave inversion); note that the ST segment elevation has resolved.

and V6. The relationship of the QRS complex to the ST segment position is described by the concept of appropriate discordance; this concept states that the major, terminal portion of the QRS complex and the ST segment are located on opposite sides of the electrocardiographic baseline. Thus, primarily positive QRS complexes are usually encountered with ST segment depression and termed *discordant ST segment depression*; primarily negative QRS complexes are seen with STE and termed *discordant STE*. Refer to Figures 13.7 and 13.8 for examples of appropriate ST segment changes in LBBB.

More than 25 years ago, Sgarbossa and colleagues identified three independent electrocardiographic predictors of AMI in the presence of LBBB, including: (i) STE of at least 1 mm that is concordant with the QRS complex; (ii) ST segment depression of at least 1 mm in lead V1, V2, or V3; and (iii) STE of at least 5 mm that is discordant with the QRS; these findings were assigned weighted probability scores of 5, 3, and 2, respectively (Sgarbossa et al. 1996). To ensure the accuracy and using a specificity of 90% in AMI diagnosis, Sgarbossa and colleagues required a score of at least 3 to confirm the electrocardiographic presence of AMI. If an ECG features only discordant STE of 5 mm or more but neither of the other two criteria, further testing is recommended before one can conclude that the ECG is indicative of AMI. Stated another way, concordant ST segment changes (either elevation or depression) are

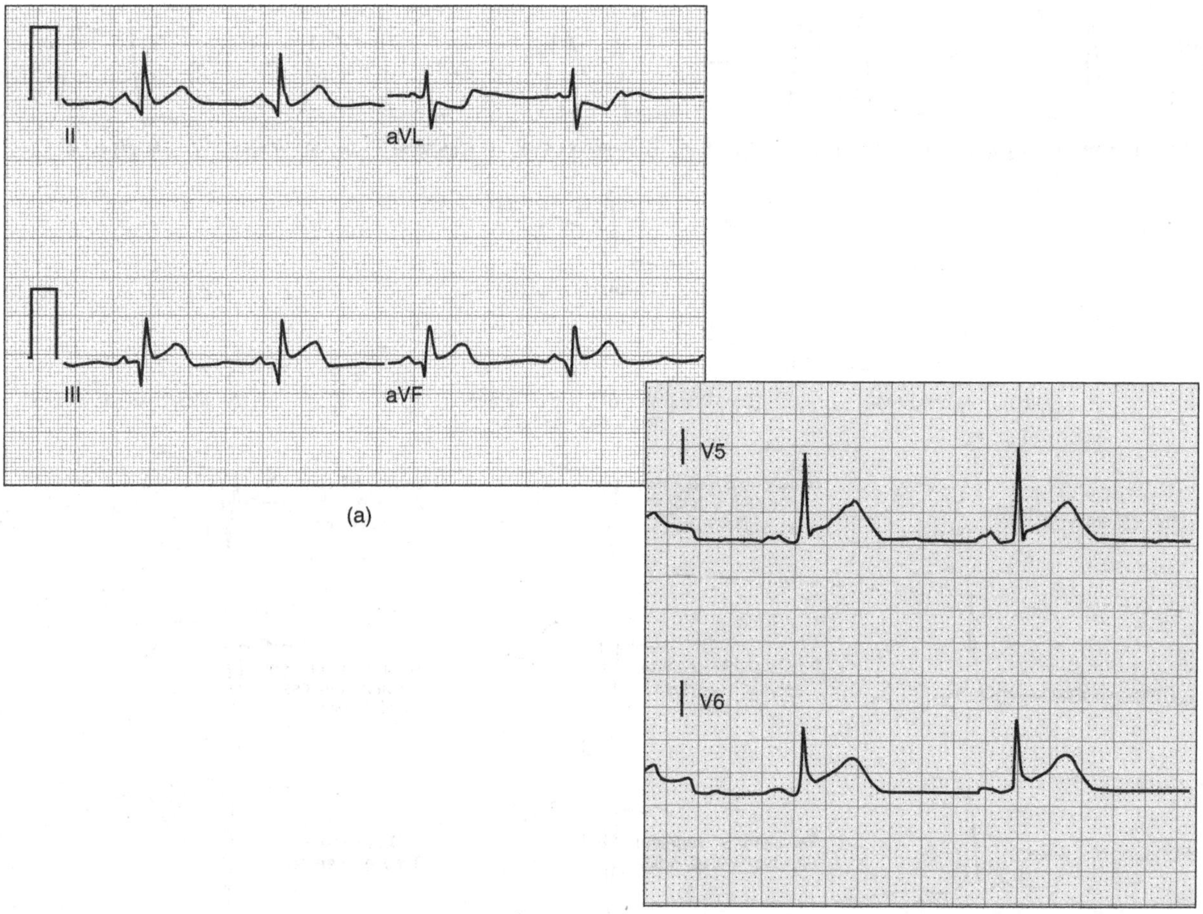

Figure 13.4 Subtle STEMI. (a) Subtle ST segment elevation in an inferior STEMI. Also note the reciprocal ST segment depression (reciprocal change) in lead aVL. (b) Subtle STEMI of the lateral wall with ST segment elevation in leads V5 and V6.

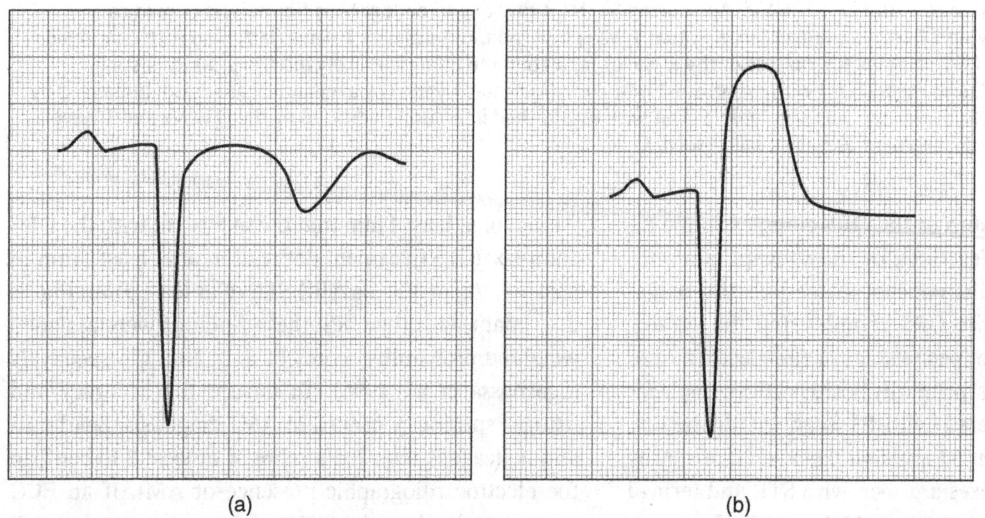

Figure 13.5 (a) Q wave likely manifesting a completed myocardial infarction. (b) Q wave with significant ST segment elevation likely representing an acute (i.e. recent) STEMI. This patient is likely still a candidate for fibrinolysis or PCI. Correlation with the patient's history is strongly encouraged in such cases to determine the onset of the STEMI.

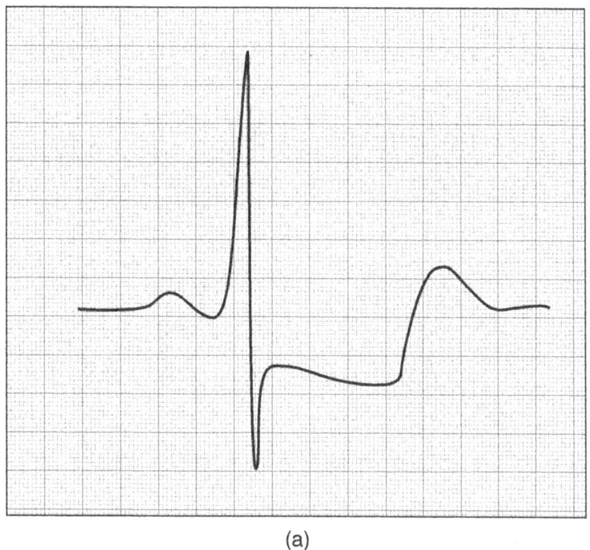

(a)

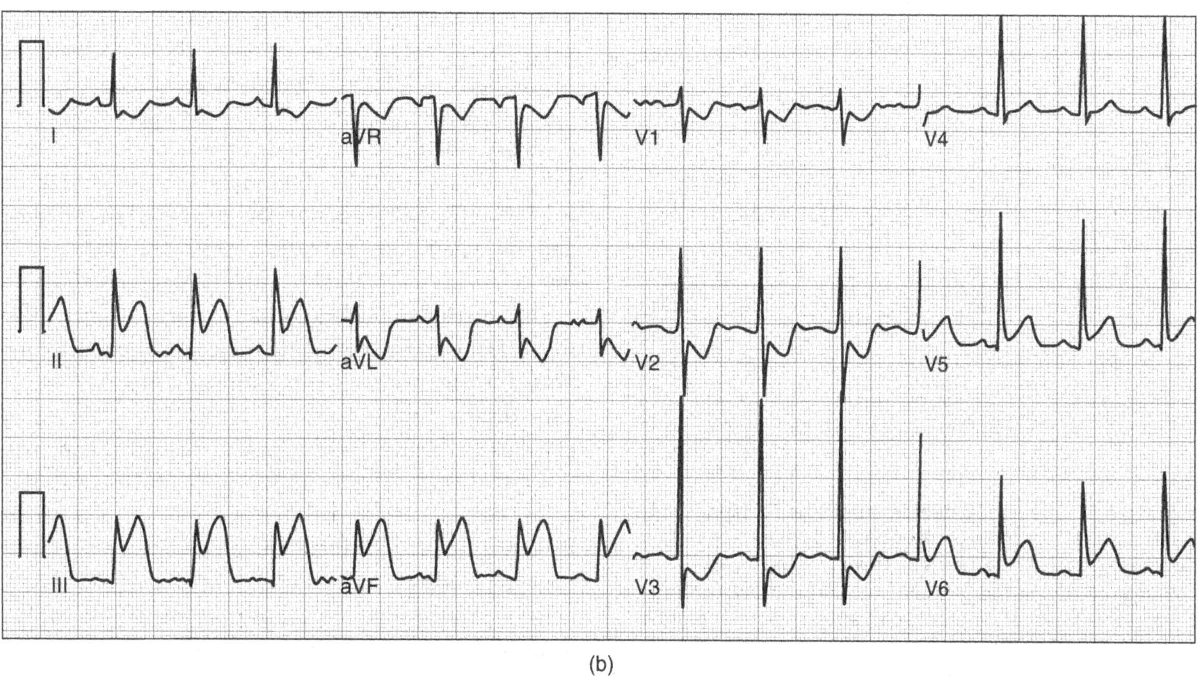

(b)

Figure 13.6 (a) Reciprocal ST segment depression, also known as reciprocal change. (b) Inferolateral STEMI along with reciprocal change in the lateral (I and aVl) and anterior leads (V1–V3).

strongly suggestive of electrocardiographic AMI; conversely, excessive discordant STE greater than 5 mm was weakly suggestive of electrocardiographic AMI. Thus, the third criterion, discordant STE greater than 5 mm, represented a significant limitation to the Sgarbossa decision rule when assessing the ECG for the electrocardiographic presence of AMI. This shortcoming was based primarily on the absolute nature of the third criterion, noting that greater than 5 mm of discordant STE was suggestive of AMI; it did not account for the proportional relationship of the ST segment to the QRS complex – basically, the magnitude of the discordant STE to the amplitude of the QRS complex.

A modified version of the Sgarbossa criteria has addressed this shortcoming of the original rule by replacing the third criterion with a proportional description of the amount, or magnitude, of discordant STE that is expected in the LBBB pattern (Meyers et al. 2015). The first two criteria remain in the modified Sgarbossa rule with the addition of the ratio of discordant STE to S (or Q) wave depth. A ratio greater than or equal to 0.25 is considered diagnostic of AMI. The modified Sgarbossa

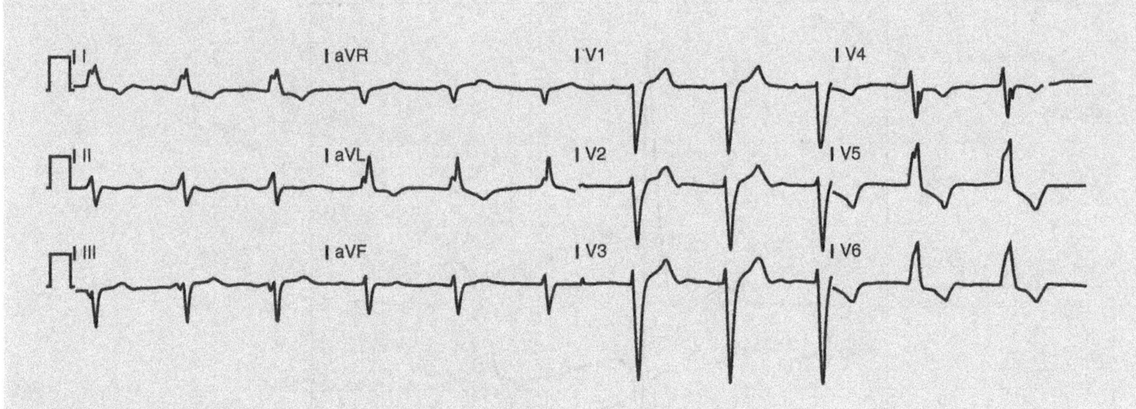

Figure 13.7 LBBB with normal, or anticipated, ST segment and T wave configurations.

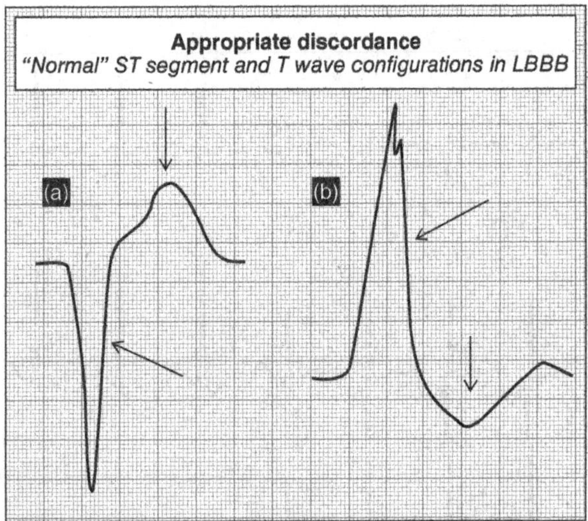

Figure 13.8 The anticipated, or "normal," ECG findings in the LBBB pattern. The common theme seen in these two ECG structures is the discordant relationship of the major, terminal portion of the QRS complex (large arrows) and the ST segment/T wave complex (small arrows). By discordant, it is meant that the QRS complex and ST segment/T wave are located on opposite sides of the electrocardiographic baseline. These relationships are described as the rule, or concept, of appropriate discordance. (a) Discordant ST segment elevation. (b) Discordant ST segment depression.

criteria reportedly yields increased sensitivity without significant loss of specificity. It is important to note that a single lead demonstrating one of the three Sgarbossa criteria abnormalities provides adequate electrocardiographic evidence of AMI. Refer to Figure 13.9 for examples of the ECG findings encountered with AMI as described by Sgarbossa.

Localization of a STEMI

ECG changes during a STEMI are found in an anatomic distribution that corresponds to the involved artery, thereby allowing the territory of a myocardial infarction to be localized by recognizing specific ECG patterns. Refer to Table 13.1 for a listing of the ECG lead and accompanying anatomic segment and involved coronary artery; refer to Figure 12.3a, b for a depiction of the coronary anatomy. Proximal arterial occlusions typically lead to more ECG abnormalities than more distal lesions; thus, recognition of the region of abnormality and its extent has both prognostic and therapeutic implications.

The anterior and inferior walls of the left ventricle are the domains most commonly subjected to acute infarction. The anterior wall is traditionally supplied by the LAD artery, and ACS in this territory is reflected by changes in leads V1 through V4, the right, and mid-precordial leads (Figure 13.10). A STEMI caused by a proximal LAD lesion is often referred to as a *widow maker* because of the high rate of death associated with these blockages. Since the LAD supplies such a large area of myocardium, it is not uncommon for cardiogenic shock and malignant dysrhythmias to occur in anterior STEMIs.

The inferior wall is most often supplied by the right coronary artery (RCA) and ACS-related changes evolve in leads II, III, and aVF. An acute infarction with STE of this segment would be termed an *inferior STEMI* (Figure 13.11). Since the RCA also supplies the AV node in 90% of the population, there is a higher incidence of conduction complications (heart block and bradycardia) when ACS involves this territory. In addition, the presence of coexisting reciprocal changes is associated with a larger infarction and increased mortality. This is especially true when there are ST depressions in leads V1 through V3.

The RCA also supplies perfusion to the right ventricle via the right ventricular (RV) branch of the RCA; thus, inferior STEMI can be complicated by RV infarction if

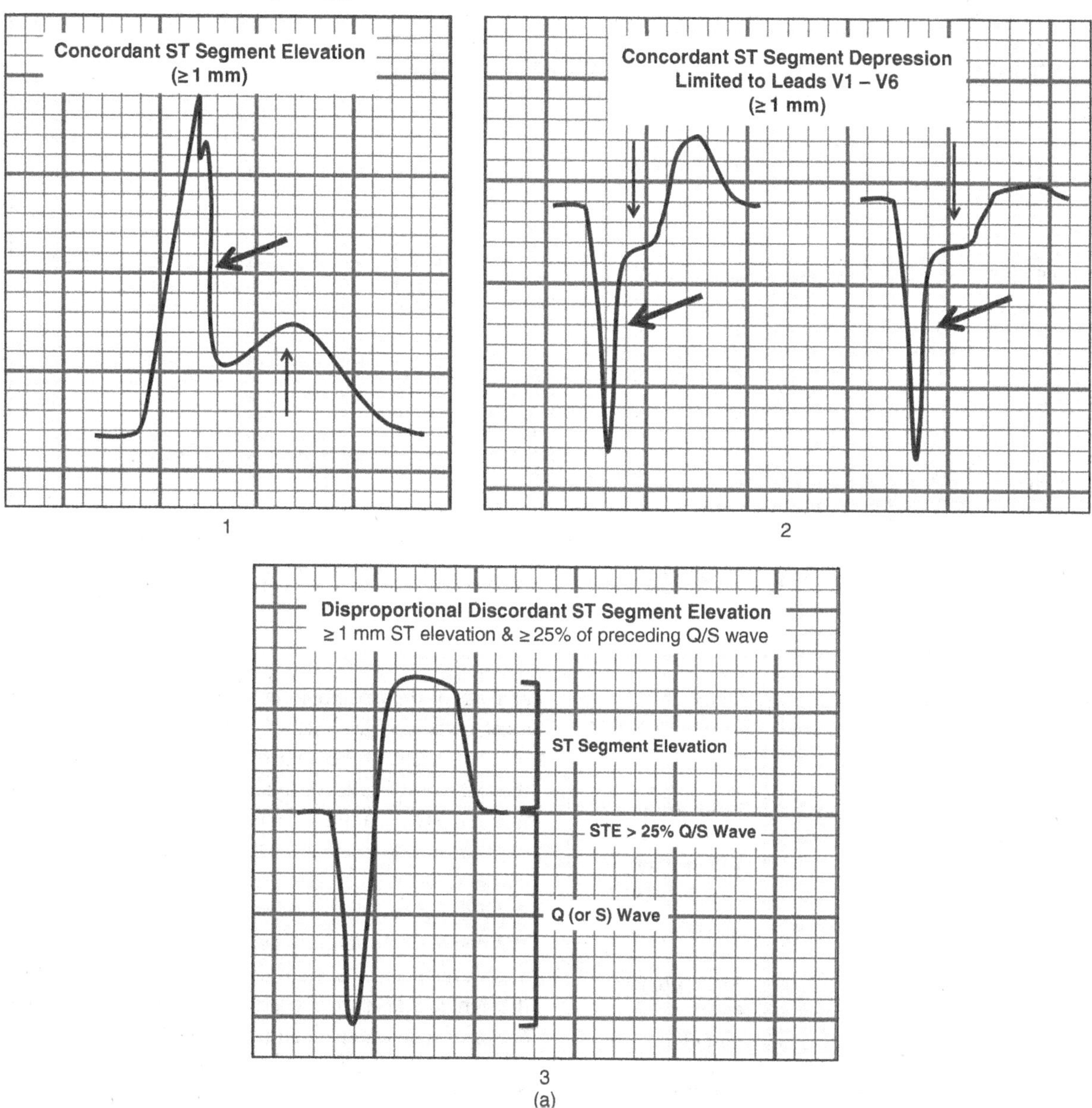

Figure 13.9 (a) The modified Sgarbossa criteria in LBBB. These three findings, if noted in a patient with a clinical presentation consistent with AMI, are suggestive of AMI and provide ECG evidence of acute infarction. (1) Concordant ST segment elevation is noted when the ST segment is elevated ≥1 mm and located on the same side of the isoelectric baseline as the major terminal portion of the QRS complex. (2) Concordant ST segment depression is noted when the ST segment is depressed ≥1 mm and located on the same side of the isoelectric baseline as the major terminal portion of the QRS complex. This finding validated only in leads V1–V6. (3) Disproportionate, or excessive, discordant ST segment elevation is noted when the ST segment is elevated ≥1 mm and, when compared to the magnitude of the negative portion of the QRS complex, is ≥25% the accompanying negative QRS complex. (b) 12-lead ECG of a patient with the LBBB pattern (widened QRS complex ≥0.12 seconds) with negatively oriented QRS complexes in leads V1–V3 and positively oriented QRS complexes in leads I, aVL, and V6. Concordant ST segment elevation is noted here in leads V5 and V6; disproportionate ST segment elevation is also seen in leads V2, V3, and V4. In leads V2–V4, the ST segment is elevated and discordant relative to the QRS complex; yet, the magnitude of the ST segment elevation is disproportionate relative to the magnitude of the negative portion of the QRS complex. These ECG findings are suggestive of AMI. Importantly, while this ECG demonstrates 5 leads with modified Sgarbossa-defined abnormality, the criteria only requires one lead with such an abnormality to electrocardiographically suggest the presence of AMI.

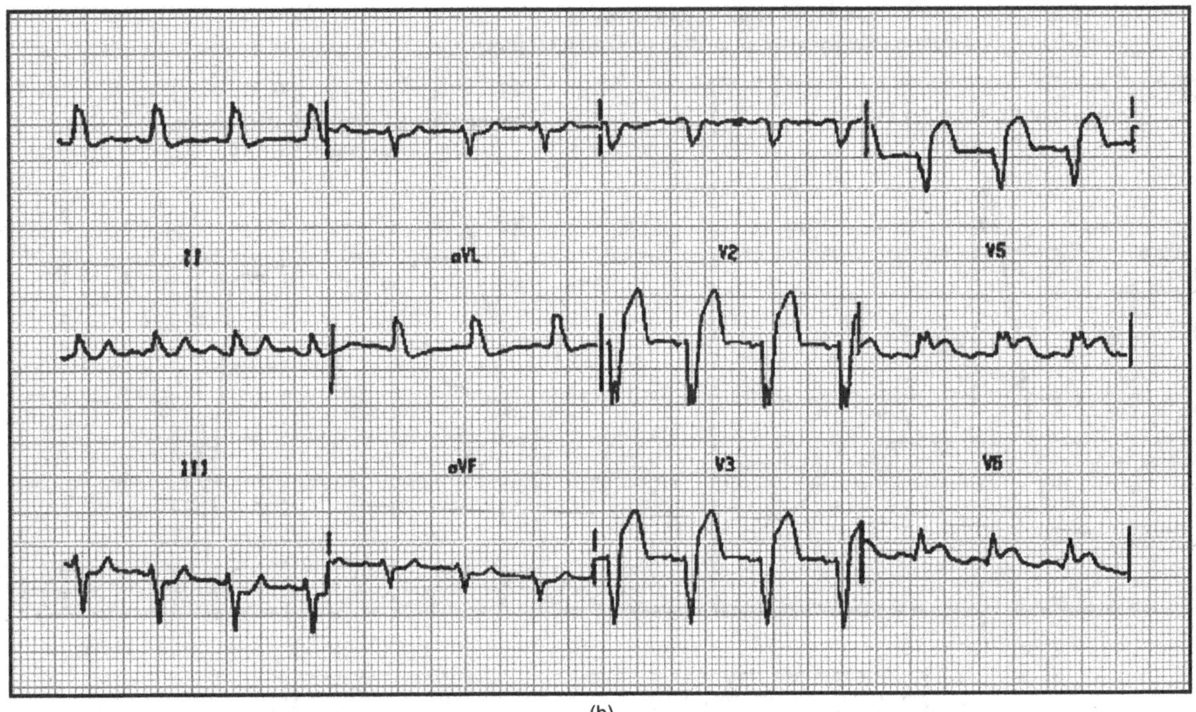

(b)

Figure 13.9 (Continued)

Table 13.1 The association of cardiac chamber and anatomic segment with ECG leads and coronary anatomy.

Primary chamber	Cardiac segment	ECG leads	Coronary artery
Left ventricle	Anterior wall	V1–V4	Left anterior descending artery
Left ventricle	Lateral wall	I, aVl, V5, and V6	Left circumflex artery
Left ventricle	Inferior wall	II, III, and aVf	Right coronary artery
Left ventricle	Posterior wall	V1–V4 indirectly V8 and V9 directly	Posterior descending branch (RCA) or left circumflex artery
Right ventricle	Right ventricle	RV4 (RV1–RV4)	Right ventricular branch (RCA)

the occlusion occurs proximal to the RV branch. RV infarction (Figure 13.12) is another area that is often overlooked, as the standard 12 lead is not a sensitive indicator of myocardial damage in this area. Acute infarction of the right ventricle is rarely an isolated event; however, it is associated with 40% of inferior infarctions and complicates some anterior infarcts. STE in lead V1 in the setting of inferior STEMI is concerning for concomitant RV infarction and should prompt analysis of the placement of right-sided ECG leads – in most instances, lead RV4 is adequate to evaluate the right ventricle. Given that the smaller muscle mass of the right ventricle leads to a corresponding decrease in size of the QRS complex, changes may appear more subtly than they do in other leads. Lead RV4 (Figure 13.13), placed in the right fifth intercostal space at the midclavicular line is the most sensitive lead to detect RV damage.

When the right ventricle becomes ischemic, the patient may develop an acute right heart syndrome. In this case, the right heart becomes a passive conduit and circulation becomes preload dependent, meaning that venous return to the right heart is the only force moving blood through the right heart. These patients are frequently hypotensive and may be bradycardic. Therapy with nitrates can be troublesome, as such therapy reduces ventricular preload, compromising filling pressures to the left ventricle. Treatment requires normal saline volume loading to maintain blood pressure and reperfusion therapy as soon as possible. As previously mentioned, RV infarctions are not always clinically obvious; thus a greater than expected drop in blood pressure in response to nitrates could be a clue to an RV infarction. Patients with RV infarctions experience more in-hospital complications and increased mortality rates when compared to patients with isolated inferior wall MIs.

The lateral wall of the left ventricle, reflected by leads I, aVL, V5, and V6, is variably supplied by either the

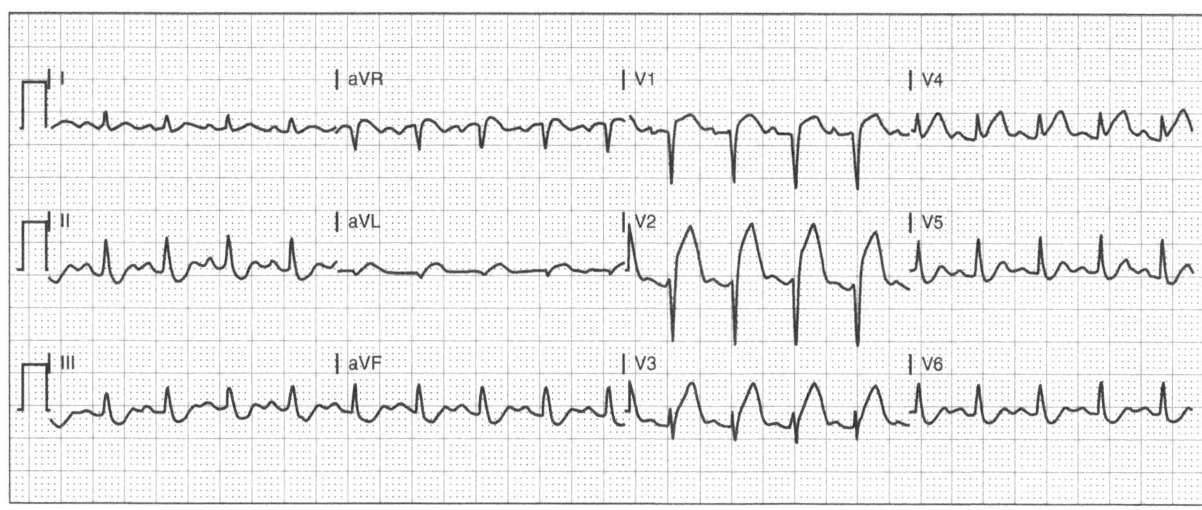

Figure 13.10 Anterior wall STEMI with ST segment elevation in leads V1–V4. Also, reciprocal change is noted in the inferior leads.

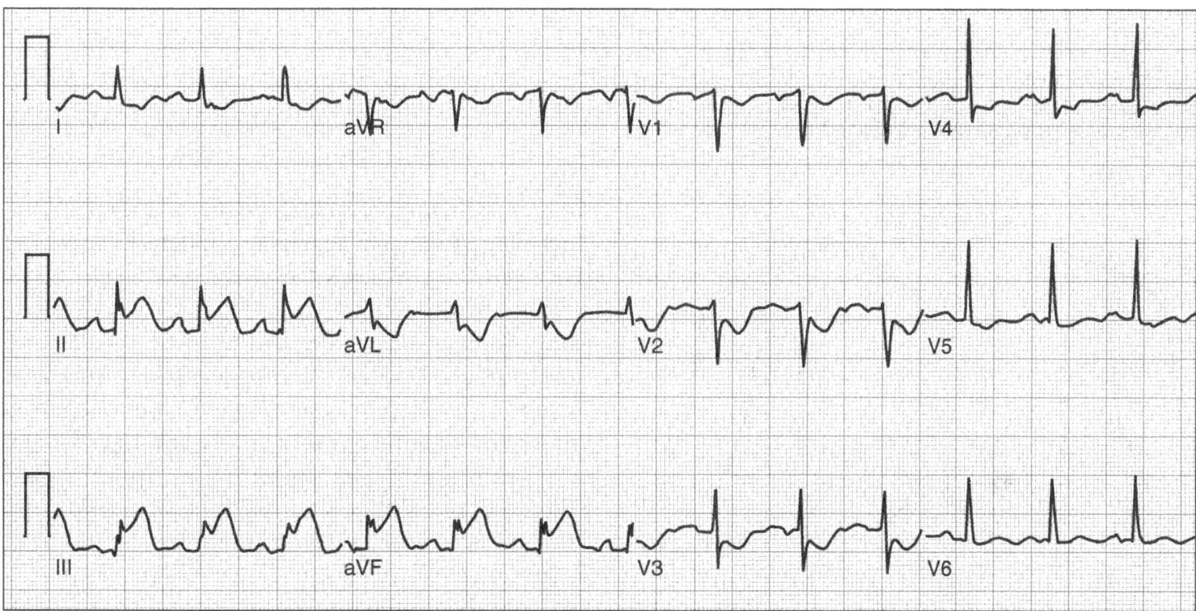

Figure 13.11 Inferior STEMI with reciprocal change in the anterior and lateral leads.

LAD, the RCA, or the left circumflex artery (LCX). While lateral wall infarctions rarely develop as isolated events, extension into this segment may occur with involvement of each of the above-mentioned arteries. Refer to Figure 13.14 for an example of a lateral wall STEMI.

The posterior wall of the left ventricle is a segment of the heart that is less easily and less accurately imaged by the 12-lead ECG. There is an important variation in the blood supply to the back of the heart. In the majority of people, the RCA continues around the right ventricle to supply the inferior portion of the ventricular septum as well as the posterior wall of the left ventricle – the so-called right dominant pattern. In this situation, the arterial continuation is called the *posterior descending artery* (PDA). Many patients, however, have the back of their heart supplied by the left side of the coronary circulation, where the PDA arises as a continuation of the left circumflex coronary artery – a "left dominant" pattern. A minority of people have coronary anatomy termed *codominant* where there is no specific single vessel supplying the posterior wall, but rather two smaller vessels

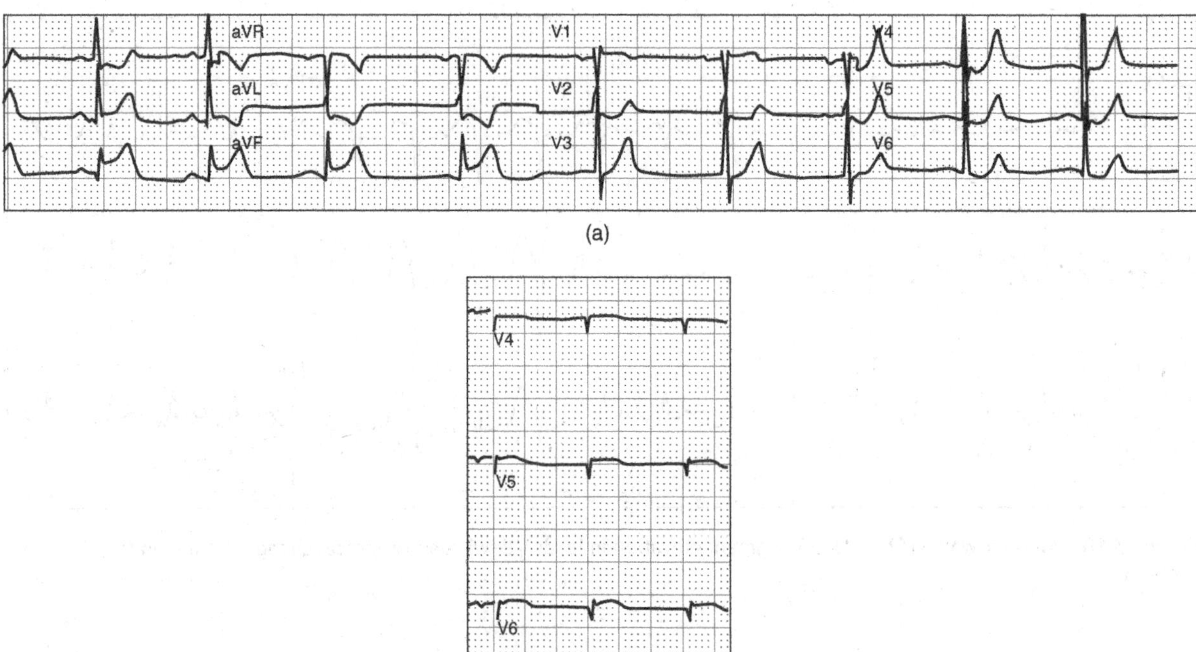

Figure 13.12 Inferior STEMI. RV infarction is also suspected for the following reasons: excessive ST segment elevation in lead III compared to either leads II or aVf in (a); ST segment elevation in lead V1 in (a); and additional ECG leads RV4 to RV6 demonstrating ST segment elevation in (b).

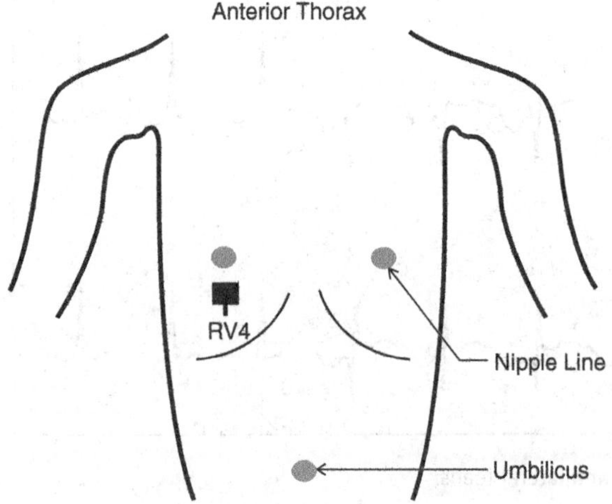

Figure 13.13 Additional ECG lead imagining the right ventricle, lead RV4. This lead is placed on the right side of the patient's chest, in the similar position of left-sided lead V4.

contributed by the right and left circulations. Thus, the most typical posterior wall infarction presentation is the inferior STEMI with posterior wall; lateral STEMI with posterior infarction is also seen. The "isolated" posterior infarction, that is, no inferior or lateral STEMI is present, can occur.

Acute infarction can involve the posterior wall of the left ventricle. From the anterior perspective, reciprocal or reverse findings of STEMI are noted in leads V1–V4, including ST segment depression, upright T waves, and positive QRS complexes (i.e. R waves) (Figure 13.15); these leads are indirectly imaged by leads V1–V4. These three findings, when reversed, produce STE, T wave inversion, and Q waves – findings classically associated with STEMI. Direct imaging of the posterior wall can be performed with the posterior ECG leads, leads V8 and V9, which are placed directly on the patient's back (Figure 13.16). STE in these two leads, frequently subtle, can indicate acute infarction of the posterior wall (Figure 13.15).

While ACS is primarily thought of as a discrete event in a single "culprit" artery, this observation is not always the case. Autopsy studies have documented the rate of multiple culprit lesions to range from 10% to 50% of fatal AMIs. These multiple culprit cases are relatively infrequent in clinical practice because of their high mortality – that is, the patient frequently expires either before calling for assistance or soon thereafter, before the delivery of any significant amount of medical care or the performance of diagnostic study. These patients are more likely to suffer cardiogenic shock and life-threatening arrhythmias. Nevertheless, major academic centers report multiple culprit lesions in about 5% of patients who survive to the cardiac catheterization laboratory.

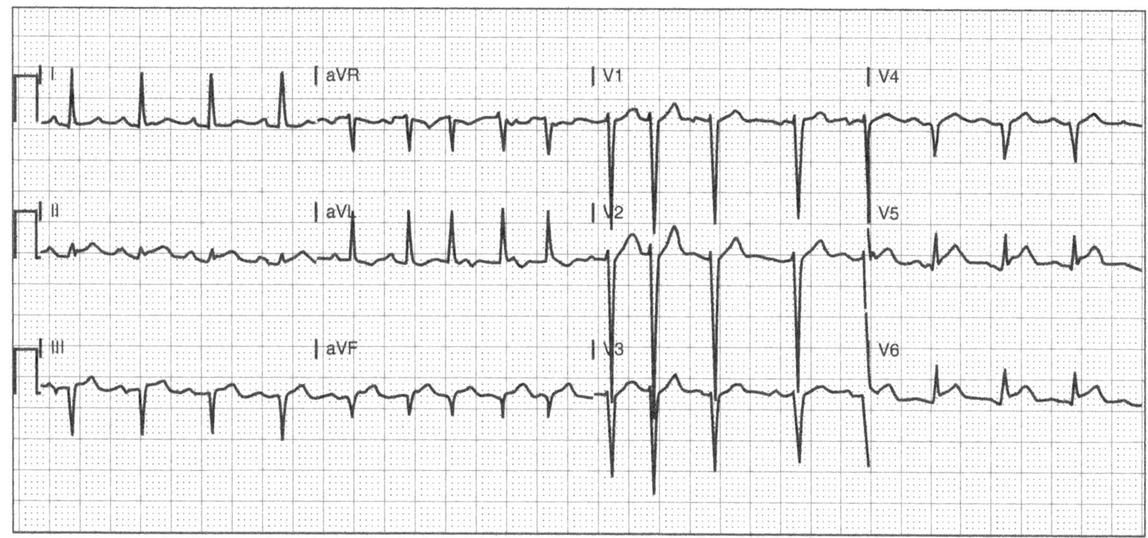

Figure 13.14 Lateral STEMI with ST segment elevation in leads V5 and V6.

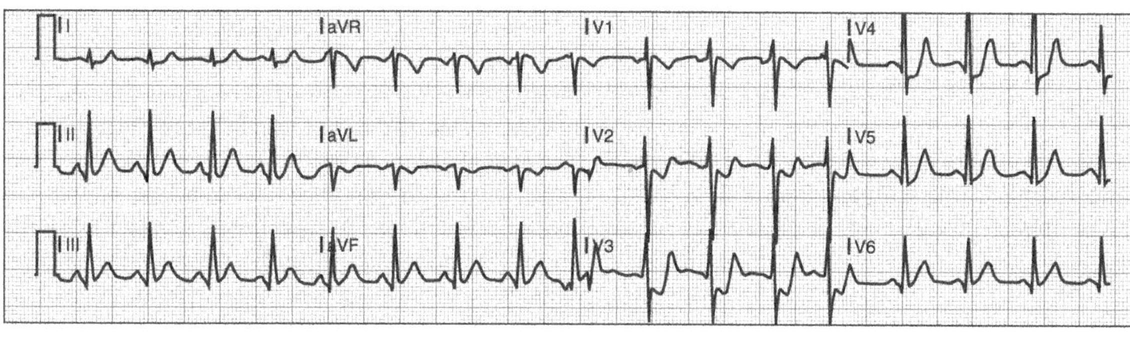

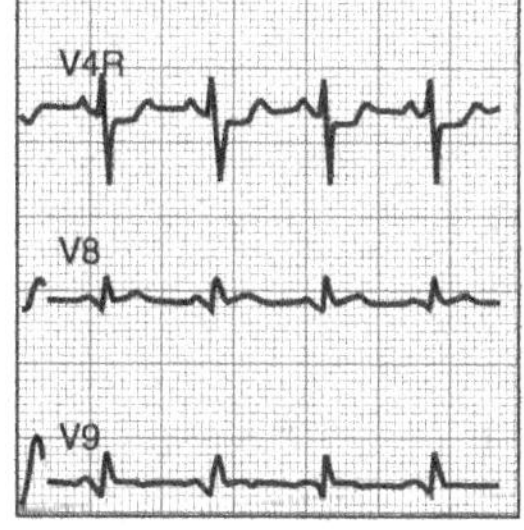

Figure 13.15 "Isolated" posterior wall acute myocardial infarction. Note the ST segment depression in leads V2–V4 with prominent R waves and upright T waves in the same distribution. The insert, the additional ECG leads V4R (right ventricle) and V8/V9 (posterior wall of LV) are performed to further evaluate the ST segment depression in the anterior leads. Leads V8 and V9 demonstrated ST segment elevation, consistent with a posterior STEMI.

The 12-Lead Electrocardiogram in non-ST Segment Elevation Myocardial Infarction Presentations

ST Segment Depression

ST segment depression (Figure 13.17) may be captured on the ECG in both ischemia and infarction. ST depression may have a morphology that is downsloping or horizontal, though a horizontal depression is more indicative of ischemia than a downsloping shape. ST segment depression may precede STE in a STEMI as ischemia progresses to infarction. Conversely, ST segment depression may be the primary ECG abnormality associated with a non-ST segment elevation myocardial infarction (NSTEMI). In fact, ST depression greater than or equal to 2 mm in two or more leads is indicative of widespread ischemia. Finally, ST depression in the

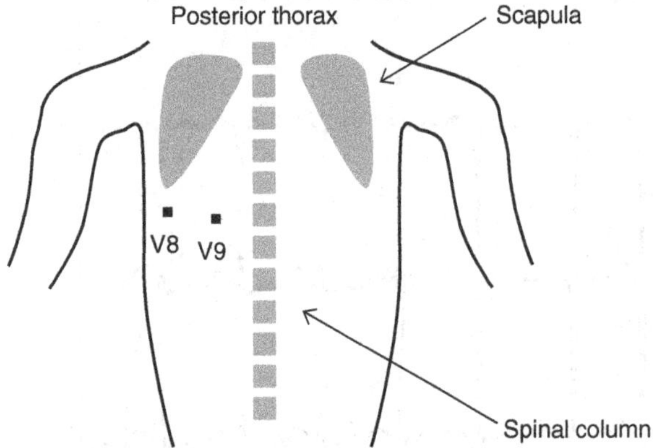

Figure 13.16 Additional posterior leads, V8 and V9. Lead V8 is placed on the patient's left back at the tip of the scapula, while lead V9 is placed halfway between lead V8 and the spinal column. These leads imagine the posterior wall of the left ventricle.

right to midprecordial leads may indicate a STEMI of the posterior wall.

T Wave Inversion

As previously mentioned, the orientation of the T wave normally corresponds with the orientation of the associated QRS complex. While isolated T wave inversion is a non-specific finding, T wave inversion in contiguous leads is highly suggestive of myocardial ischemia. In addition, T wave inversion may persist indefinitely following infarction. T wave inversions associated with ACS tend to be symmetrical in morphology with similar downsloping and upsloping limbs (Figure 13.18).

Pseudonormalization of the T wave refers to chronically inverted T waves undergoing T wave inversion and becoming upright again. This pseudonormalization may be a sign of acute myocardial ischemia; however, this phenomenon can only be recognized by comparing a current ECG to prior study. In addition, the predictive value of T wave pseudonormalization for significant coronary blockage is poor.

A specific syndrome involving T wave inversions in ACS is worthy of additional review. This syndrome, termed *Wellens' syndrome* (Figure 13.19), is a pattern of electrocardiographic T wave changes associated with critical, proximal LAD artery obstruction. Syndrome criteria include T wave changes plus a history of anginal chest pain without serum marker abnormalities; patients lack Q waves and significant STE; such patients demonstrate normal precordial R wave progression. The T wave inversion can assume one of two presentations: the deeply inverted, "Wellenoid" T waves and biphasic T waves (both upright and inverted within a single T wave) (Figure 13.19). The natural history of Wellens' syndrome is anterior wall AMI. The T wave abnormalities are persistent and may remain in place for hours to weeks; the clinician will likely encounter these changes in the sensation-free patient. With definitive management of the stenosis, the changes resolve with normalization of the ECG.

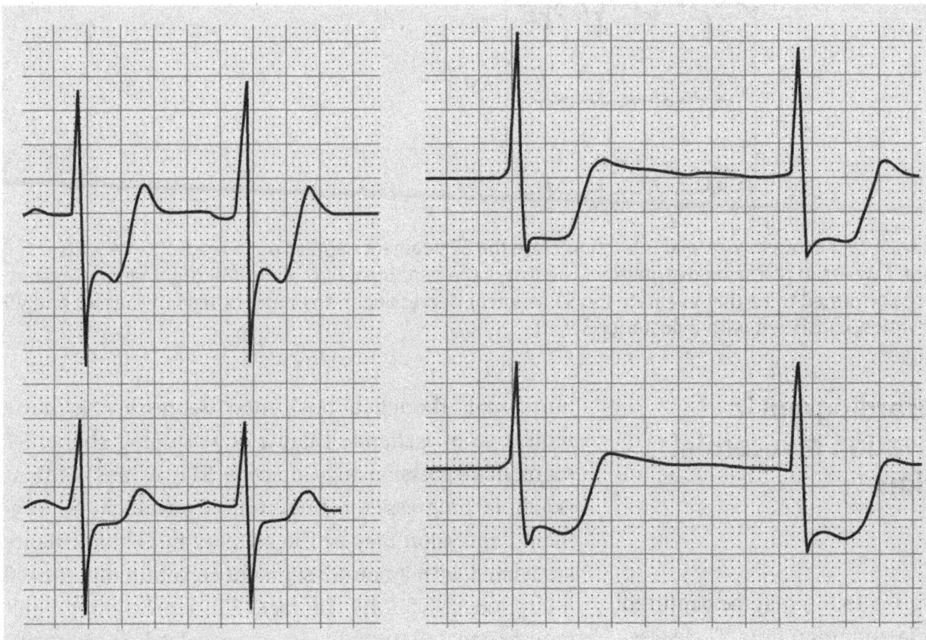

Figure 13.17 ST segment depression.

De Winter Syndrome

The de Winter ECG pattern, also referred to as the de Winter Syndrome, represents another electrocardiographic presentation which is suggestive of ACS. The electrocardiographic findings associated with this presentation include very prominent T waves with J point depression producing ST segment depression seen in the precordial leads, coupled with STE in lead aVR (Figure 13.20). The de Winter Syndrome is associated with proximal LAD artery LAD lesions. These patients are usually ill-appearing with ongoing chest discomfort. ECG findings may progress to classic anterior STEMI over a very short period of time; lack of progression, however, has also been associated with significant LAD artery occlusion and subsequent large myocardial infarction. Some clinicians consider the de Winter Syndrome a STEI-equivalent presentation while others approach this entity as a pre-infarction ECG pattern; in either case, the de Winter ECG presentation is a high-risk finding that warrants urgent care and careful observation (de Winter et al. 2016).

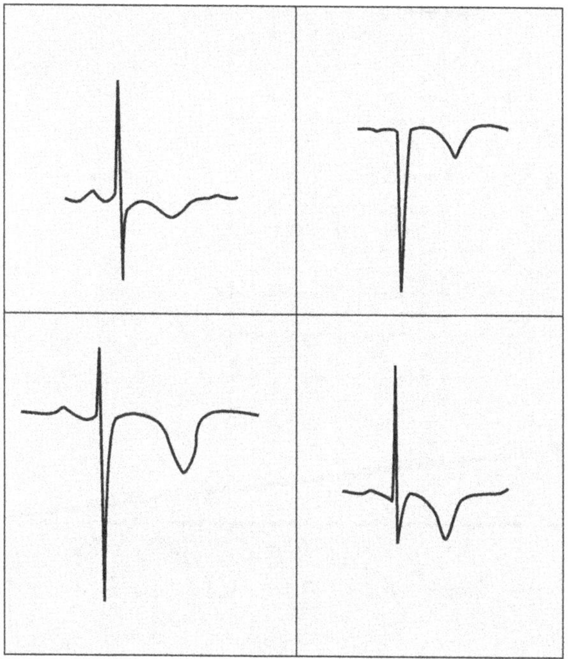

Figure 13.18 T wave inversions associated with ACS.

R-Wave Progression

R-wave progression refers to the increase in the size of the R wave across the precordium. In normal patients (i.e. those patients without current or past ACS), the R wave is absent in lead V1, present but much smaller than the S wave in lead V2, and increases in size relative to the S wave until it is larger than the S wave in lead V4. When there is a loss of R wave progression, the R wave remains small in leads V1–V3. It is a non-specific marker of ischemia, yet can indicate past myocardial infarction.

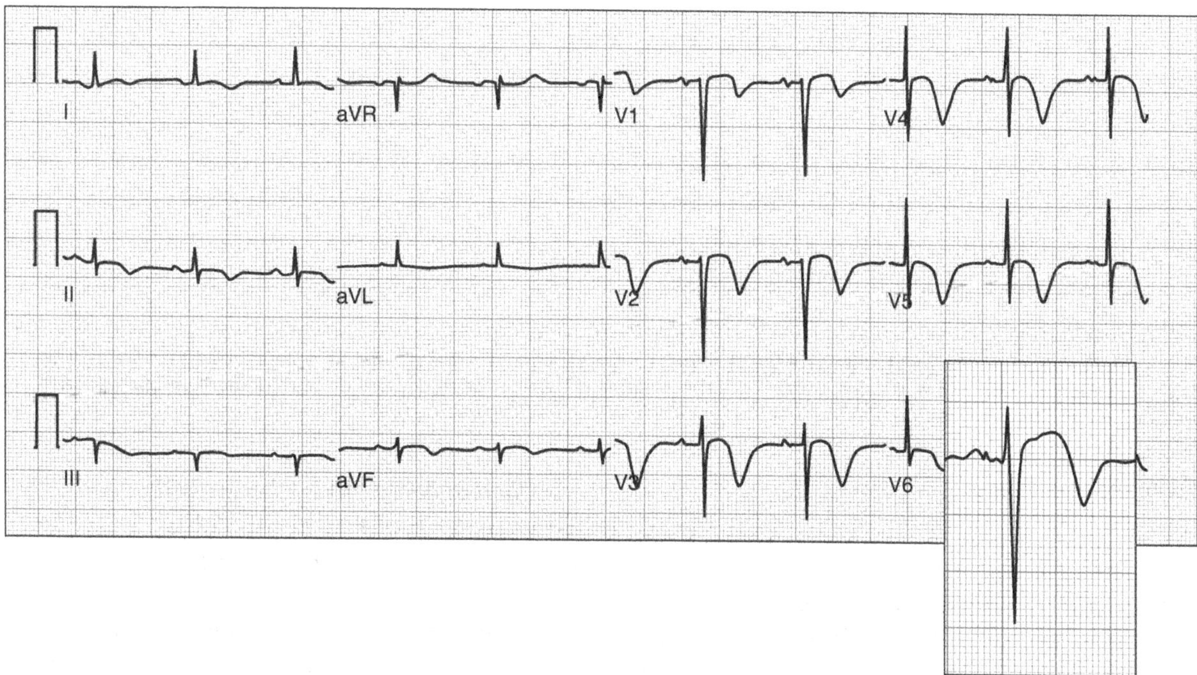

Figure 13.19 Wellens' syndrome with deeply inverted T waves in the anterolateral distribution. The insert shows the other T wave abnormality seen in Wellens' syndrome, the biphasic T wave.

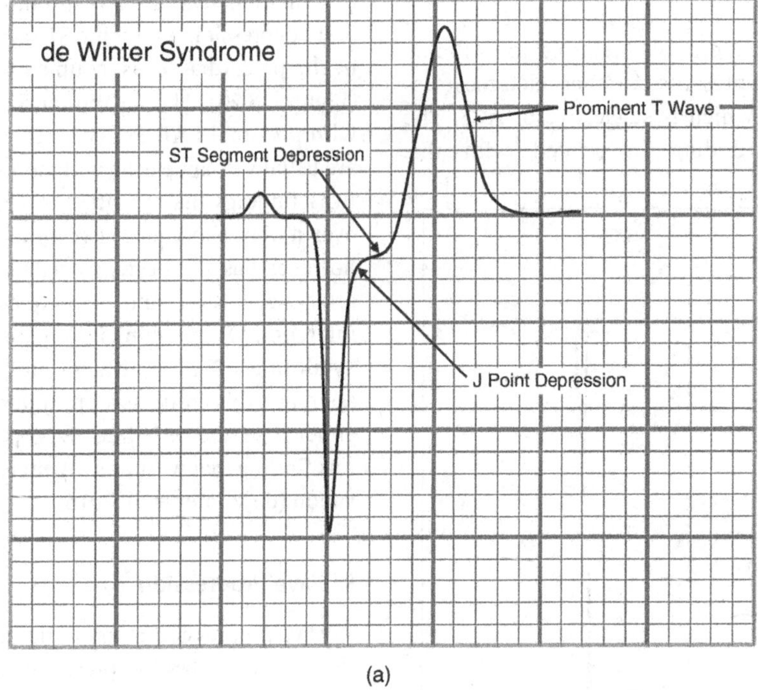

(a)

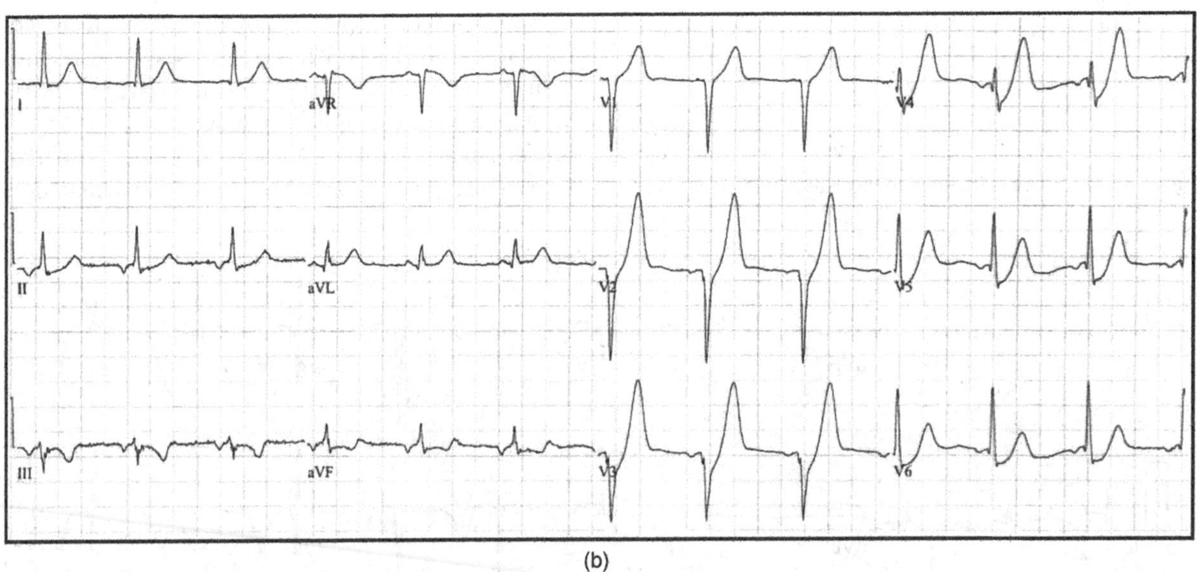

(b)

Figure 13.20 (a) de Winter Syndrome: note the prominent T wave, J point depression, and ST segment depression. (b) 12-lead ECG of a patient with the de Winter Syndrome: note the prominent T wave, J point depression, and ST segment depression in leads V2, V3, and V4.

Complete Heart Block

Heart block can be a feature in the presentation of myocardial ischemia. The AV node is supplied by the RCA and may cease to function when ischemic. This association is most common with RCA infarctions – inferior STEMI – and may require transcutaneous pacing. In fact, the association of unstable complete heart block and chest pain has been noted to be strongly predictive of STEMI.

Electrocardiogram ST Segment Elevation Myocardial Infarction Mimickers and Confounders

Several electrocardiographic entities beyond STEMI cause STE as well as other findings typically associated with ACS. While making a diagnosis of STEMI is crucial in the acute setting, there are many ECG patterns that can both mimic changes seen with AMI and confound, or hide, the findings seen in STEMI. The mimicking patterns include benign early repolarization (BER), acute pericarditis, and left ventricular aneurysm, while the ECG confounders include LVH, LBBB, and ventricular paced patterns; the confounding patterns also mimic changes seen with STEMI and other ACS presentations.

Benign Early Repolarization

BER is an ECG syndrome producing STE that occurs in 1% of the general population and is seen frequently in emergency department (ED) chest pain patients. This entity is a benign ECG finding that neither suggests nor rules out an ACS. It is characterized (Figure 13.21) by widespread STE, upward concavity of the initial portion of the ST segment, notching or slurring of the terminal QRS complex at the J point (the juncture of the QRS complex with the ST segment), and concordant T waves of large amplitude. It is important to note that the J point elevation in BER is usually less than 3.5 mm and that the STE is generally maximum in the precordial leads. BER rarely presents with "isolated" limb lead STE; most often, STE related to BER is seen in the right to midprecordial leads, at times accompanied by STE in the inferior leads; it is usual to observe BER-related ST >segment elevation noted only in the inferior leads – thus, if this occurs, STEMI should be carefully considered.

Pericarditis

Pericarditis is characterized by inflammation of the pericardium, the sac surrounding the heart. While the pericardium is electrically silent, the superficial epicardium (the outermost layer of the myocardium), if irritated, can cause ST segment changes associated with acute pericarditis, or more appropriately termed, *acute myopericarditis*. In fact, STE (Figure 13.21) is generally present in multiple leads with the exception of lead aVr. Pericarditis may be associated with diffuse PR segment depression as well, which can best be seen in the inferior leads and lead V6; lead aVr can demonstrate "reciprocal" PR segment elevation, which is easily seen. Refer to Figure 13.22 for ECG findings of acute myopericarditis (acute pericarditis).

Left Ventricular Aneurysm

Left ventricular aneurysm is defined as a localized area of infarcted myocardium, which bulges outward during both systole and diastole. Left ventricular aneurysms most often are noted after large anterior wall infarctions, but may also be encountered status post inferior and posterior wall MIs. In most cases, left ventricular aneurysm is manifested electrocardiographically by varying degrees of STE, which may be difficult to distinguish from ST segment changes due to STEMI. STE is generally associated with well developed, completed Q waves in the anterior precordial leads; also, the T waves will either be upright and of a small amplitude or inverted.

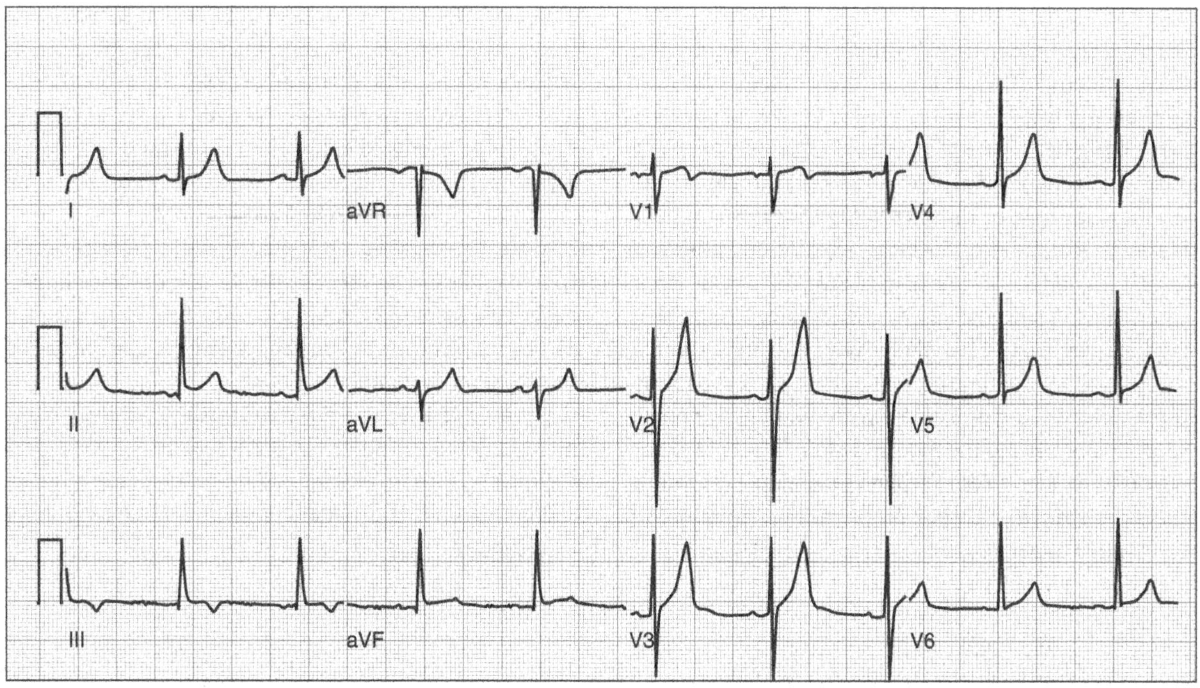

Figure 13.21 Benign early repolarization with concave ST segment elevation in leads V1–V5 as well as lead II.

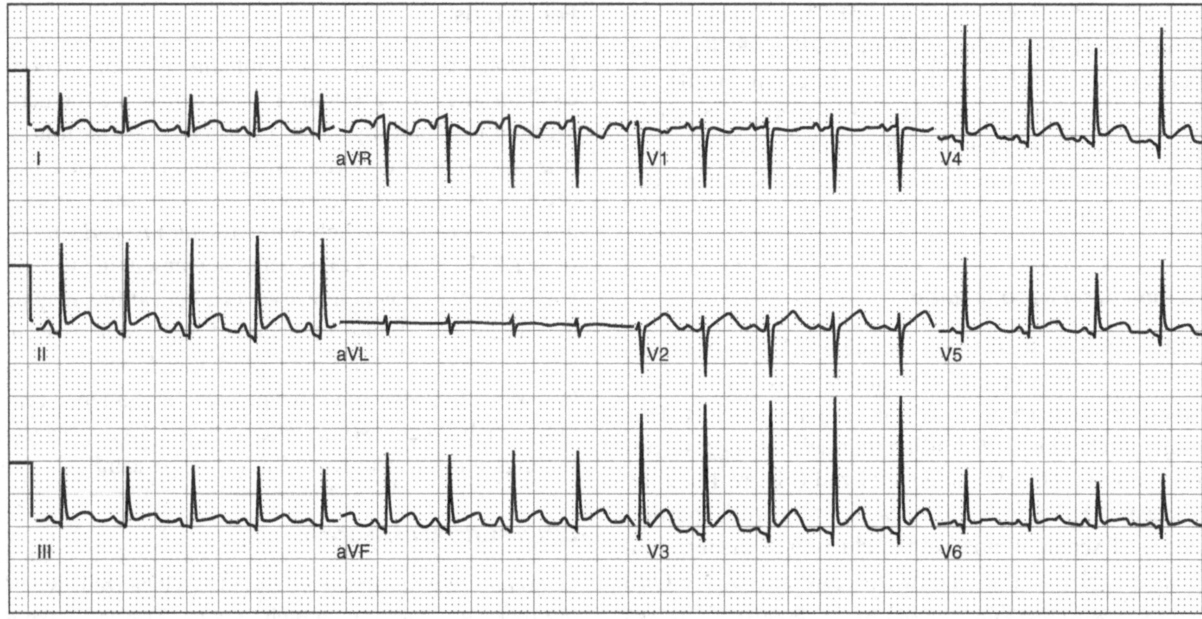

Figure 13.22 Acute myopericarditis, also commonly referred to as acute pericarditis, with diffuse ST segment elevation in the anterior and inferior leads. PR segment changes are best seen in the inferior leads (PR segment depression) and lead aVr (PR segment elevation).

Left Bundle Branch Block and Ventricular Paced Pattern

LBBB and the ventricular paced pattern are both a confounding and mimicking pattern. They have been discussed earlier in this chapter.

Left Ventricular Hypertrophy

The LVH pattern, such as LBBB, is both a confounding and mimicking ECG syndrome. Many models, with varying specificity and sensitivity, exist for the diagnosis of LVH by the ECG. One of the most accurate and easiest to use models is the Sokolow–Lyon criteria. This model considers the size of the QRS complexes in the precordial leads. If the size of the largest Q wave in either lead V1 or V2 is added to the size of the largest R wave in either V5 or V6 and the total is greater than 35 mm, then the diagnosis of LVH is likely. Why is it important to consider the diagnosis of the LVH pattern? Approximately 75% of patients with the LVH by voltage pattern demonstrate the "strain pattern"; the strain pattern includes significant ST segment changes (elevation and depression) and T wave abnormalities (prominent T waves and T wave inversion).

The LVH with strain pattern is associated with poor R wave progression, most commonly producing a QS pattern; these complexes are located in leads V1, V2, and V3. STE is encountered in this distribution along with prominent T waves and can be greater than 5 mm in height, mimicking acute anterior wall STEMI. The initial, upsloping portion of the ST segment–T wave complex is frequently concave in LVH. The lateral leads, leads I, aVL, V5, and V6, demonstrate large, prominent, positively oriented QRS complexes with marked ST segment depression and T wave inversion – again, consistent with ACS-related change. In a general sense, the ST segment–T wave abnormalities can be predicted based on the direction of the QRS complex. The ST segment–T waves are directed opposite from the polarity of the QRS complex. The anterior leads demonstrate largely negatively oriented QRS complexes; in these leads, the ST segment is elevated and the T wave is upright and at times rather prominent. The lateral leads display positively oriented QRS complexes; in these leads, ST segment depression and inverted T waves are seen. Refer to Figure 13.23 for an example of the ST segment changes encountered in the patient with the LVH by voltage ECG pattern.

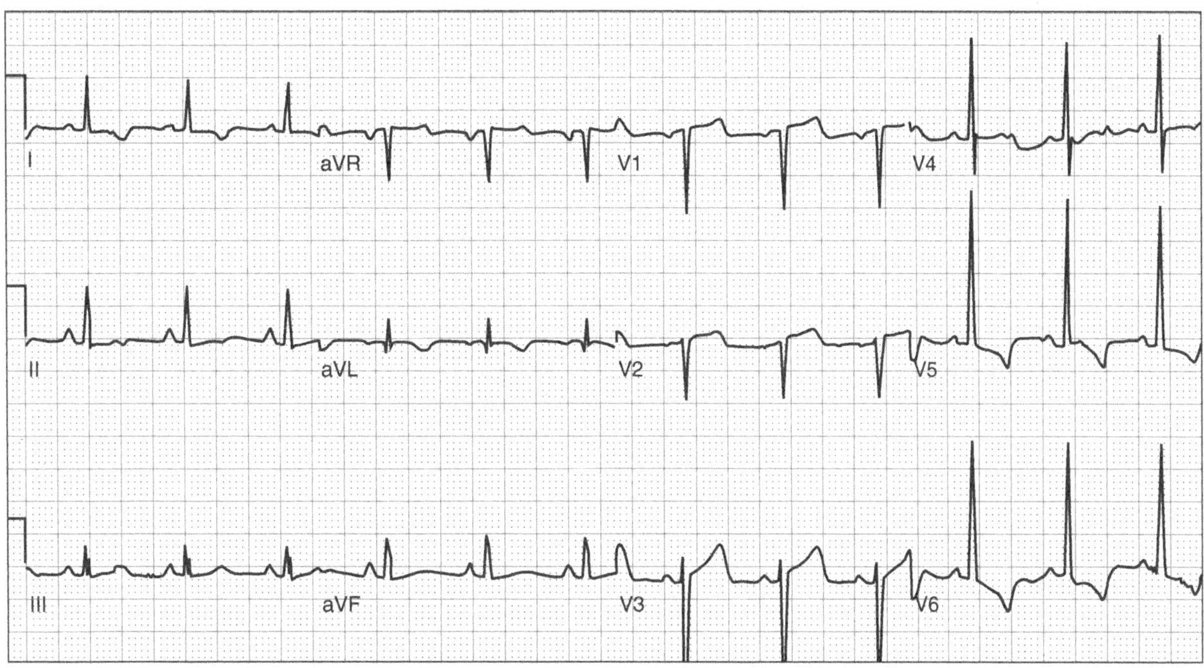

Figure 13.23 Left ventricular hypertrophy by voltage pattern with strain. Note the large QRS complexes in the precordial leads. Also note the strain pattern, the ST segment and T wave abnormalities, seen in the precordial leads. ST segment elevation is seen in leads V1–V3 along with ST segment depression with T wave inversion in leads V5 and V6.

Further Reading

Brady, W.J. and Chan, T.C. (1999). Electrocardiographic manifestations: benign early repolarization. *J. Emerg. Med.* 17: 473–478.

Brady, W.J., Harrigan, R.A., and Chan, T.C. (2006). Acute coronary syndromes. In: *Rosen's Emergency Medicine: Concepts and Clinical Practice*, 6e (ed. J.A. Marx, R.S. Hockberger, R. Walls, et al.), 1154–1199. Mosby Elsevier.

Bauml, M.A. and Underwood, D.A. (2010). Left ventricular hypertrophy: an overlooked cardiovascular risk factor. *Cleve Clin. J. Med.* 77: 381–387.

Khandaker, M.H., Espinosa, R.E., Nishimura, R.A. et al. (2010). Pericardial disease: diagnosis and management. *Mayo Clin Proc.* 85: 572–593.

References

Meyers, H.P., Limkakeng, A.T., Jaffa, E.J. et al. (2015). Validation of the modified Sgarbossa criteria for acute coronary occlusion in the setting of left bundle branch block: A retrospective case-control study. *Am. Heart. J.* 170: 1255–1264.

Sgarbossa, E.B., Pinski, S.L., Barbagelata, A. et al. (1996). Electrocardiographic diagnosis of evolving acute myocardial infarction in the presence of left bundle branch block. *N. Engl. J. Med.* 334: 481–487.

de Winter, R.W., Adams, R., Verouden, N.J.W. et al. (2016). Precordial junctional ST-segment depression with tall symmetric T-waves signifying proximal LAD occlusion, case reports of STEMI equivalence. *J. Electrocardiol.* 49: 76–80.

Section IV

Special Populations, High-Risk Presentation Scenarios, and Advanced Electrocardiographic Techniques

14

The Electrocardiogram in the Pediatric Patient

Robert Rutherford[1], *Robin Naples*[2], *and William J. Brady*[3]

[1] Swedish Medical Center-Edmonds Campus, Edmonds, WA, USA
[2] Thomas Jefferson University, Philadelphia, PA, USA
[3] Departments of Emergency Medicine and Medicine, University of Virginia School of Medicine, Charlottesville, VA, USA

The approach to the pediatric electrocardiogram (ECG) is similar to that of the adult ECG with the notable exception of an awareness of age-related norms regarding rate, interval length, complex width, and so on; in addition, certain findings, both normal and abnormal, are particular to the pediatric ECG. It is important to remember that pediatric ECGs, especially in the neonate and infant, have significant, age-related differences from their adult counterparts. Nonetheless, a systematic evaluation of rate, rhythm, axis, and evaluation of PR, QRS, and QT intervals will identify the majority of clinically relevant pediatric ECG abnormalities.

For most clinicians, understanding the age-related findings and trends in the ECG are more important than remembering specific, age-dependent values. The recognition of normal morphologic findings with respect to age is also important. A brief understanding of fetal circulation, and its transition to adult physiology, is important in the understanding of the pediatric ECG. In fetal circulation, the pulmonary circuit is a high-pressure system because of the hypoxic vasoconstriction of the pulmonary vessels. Blood is preferentially shunted from the right side to the left side of the heart because of the pressure gradient produced. These factors all contribute to the fetus being right-heart dominant. In the neonatal period, pulmonary vascular resistance falls, leading to the adult circulatory pattern over the first several years of life. Over time, these changes cause the left ventricle to mature. Thus, early in life, the ECG will demonstrate a right-sided pattern of morphologic findings; as the heart grows and circulation becomes "more left-sided," the adult ECG patterns will predominate and become the age-related normal. By early to mid-adolescence, the pediatric and adult heart – and ECGs – become nearly indistinguishable.

Rate and Rhythm

Pediatric heart rates vary as a function of age (Table 14.1). Peaking near the second month of life, the heart rate trends down to adult levels in the adolescent years as the increasingly mature left ventricle is able to contribute to cardiac output by increasing the stroke volume as opposed to increasing its rate. The accepted normal values for pediatric heart rates cover a broader range than those for adults, such that the patient's clinical status must be taken into account even if the heart rate is within normal ranges for that age.

As with the adult, the normal pediatric rhythm is sinus rhythm with the P wave originating from the sinoatrial (SA) node, a consistent PR interval, and a P wave associated with each QRS complex (Figure 14.1a, b); in the 12-lead ECG, the T waves are upright in leads I, II, and III (Figure 14.1b). Sinus arrhythmia (Figure 14.1c) is a normal variant rhythm, not indicative of underlying pathology of any sort; it is seen when all aspects of normal sinus rhythm are satisfied with the exception of a regular rhythm – slight irregularity is seen in this rhythm. An analysis of these structures and their relationship to one another will aid in rhythm assessment and will enable the clinician to determine most cardiac rhythms.

The Electrocardiogram in Emergency and Acute Care, First Edition.
Edited by Korin B. Hudson, Amita Sudhir, George Glass, and William J. Brady.

Table 14.1 Pediatric ECG normal values by age.

Age	Pulse (bpm)	QRS complex axis (degrees)	PR interval (s)	QRS complex (s)
First week	90–160	60–180	0.08–0.15	0.03–0.08
1–3 wk	100–180	45–160	0.08–0.15	0.03–0.08
1–2 mo	120–180	30–135	0.08–0.15	0.03–0.08
3–5 mo	105–185	0–135	0.08–0.15	0.03–0.08
6–11 mo	110–170	0–135	0.07–0.16	0.03–0.08
1–2 yr	90–165	0–110	0.08–0.16	0.03–0.08
3–4 yr	70–140	0–120	0.09–0.17	0.04–0.08
5–7 yr	65–140	0–110	0.09–0.17	0.04–0.08
8–11 yr	60–130	−15 to 110	0.09–0.17	0.04–0.09
12–15 yr	65–130	−15 to 110	0.09–0.18	0.04–0.09

QRS Axis

The axis of the pediatric ECG is distinct from that of the adult in that it is predictably dynamic over periods of time. This dynamic nature is primarily the result of changes in right versus left heart forces that occur with the change from fetal to neonatal to adult circulatory patterns. The most pronounced changes occur over the first year of life, when the axis goes from an age-appropriate right axis to a pattern more consistent with a normal adult axis. Most obvious of these is a prominent R wave in leads V1 and V2, reflecting the dominant right ventricle and diminutive R waves in leads V5 and V6, indicative of the relatively thin-walled left ventricle (Figures 14.1b and 14.2). As the left ventricle matures under its increased workload, the R wave progression approaches the adult norm, with minimal to no R wave in the right precordial leads (V1–V3) to prominent R wave in the left precordial leads (V4–V6).

T Waves

The T wave on the pediatric ECG is most often upright in the limb leads. In the precordial leads (predominantly lead V1–V4), however, the T wave is frequently inverted and is, in fact, considered normal when inverted, creating an important area of "interpretation disparity" between the adult and pediatric ECG (Figures 14.1b and 14.2). This distribution of T wave inversion is termed the *juvenile* T wave pattern. This juvenile T wave pattern can persist into adolescence. In fact, in the pediatric population, upright T waves in the right to midprecordial leads can be evidence of cardiac pathology, namely, right ventricular hypertrophy (RVH).

Intervals

As with heart rate, the pediatric PR interval and QRS complex duration vary as a function of age (Table 14.1). Neonates have shorter PR intervals and more narrow QRS complex widths that increase as the cardiac muscle and conduction system mature. In evaluating the ECG, the age-appropriate intervals must be used to determine the presence of atrioventricular (AV) block and QRS complex widening. For example, a neonate with a PR interval of 0.2 is clearly outside of the normal range, and thus has a first-degree block, whereas an older child or adult with the same PR interval would be considered normal.

The evaluation of the QT interval is more straightforward in the infant, child, and adolescent. The QT interval is corrected for the heart rate and is expressed as the corrected QT interval, or QTc interval. The calculation of QTc is the same in children as in adults ($QTc = QT/\sqrt{RR}$). A normal QTc is under 0.450 s.

Common Dysrhythmias

Paroxysmal Supraventricular Tachycardia

Paroxysmal supraventricular tachycardia (PSVT) is the most common pediatric dysrhythmia (Boxes 14.1 and 14.2). It can occur at any age but it most often occurs during infancy. The two common mechanisms by which PSVT occurs are either an accessory pathway (i.e. Wolff–Parkinson–White syndrome) that conducts the electrical impulse (more likely in children) or an AV nodal reentry (more likely in adolescents). Differentiating between these two causes is difficult and largely unnecessary for the emergency clinician.

The clinical presentation of a patient with PSVT often is fussiness, lethargy, or poor feeding in infants, and palpitations, dyspnea, or lightheadedness in older children. The ECG will reveal a regular, narrow QRS complex tachycardia with a heart rate around 220 bpm (range 180–300 bpm) without obvious P waves and little R-R variability (Figure 14.3a [neonate] and Figure 14.3b [adolescent]). With extremely rapid ventricular rates, the QRS complex can widen as a result of the bundle branch system's inability to repolarize at a

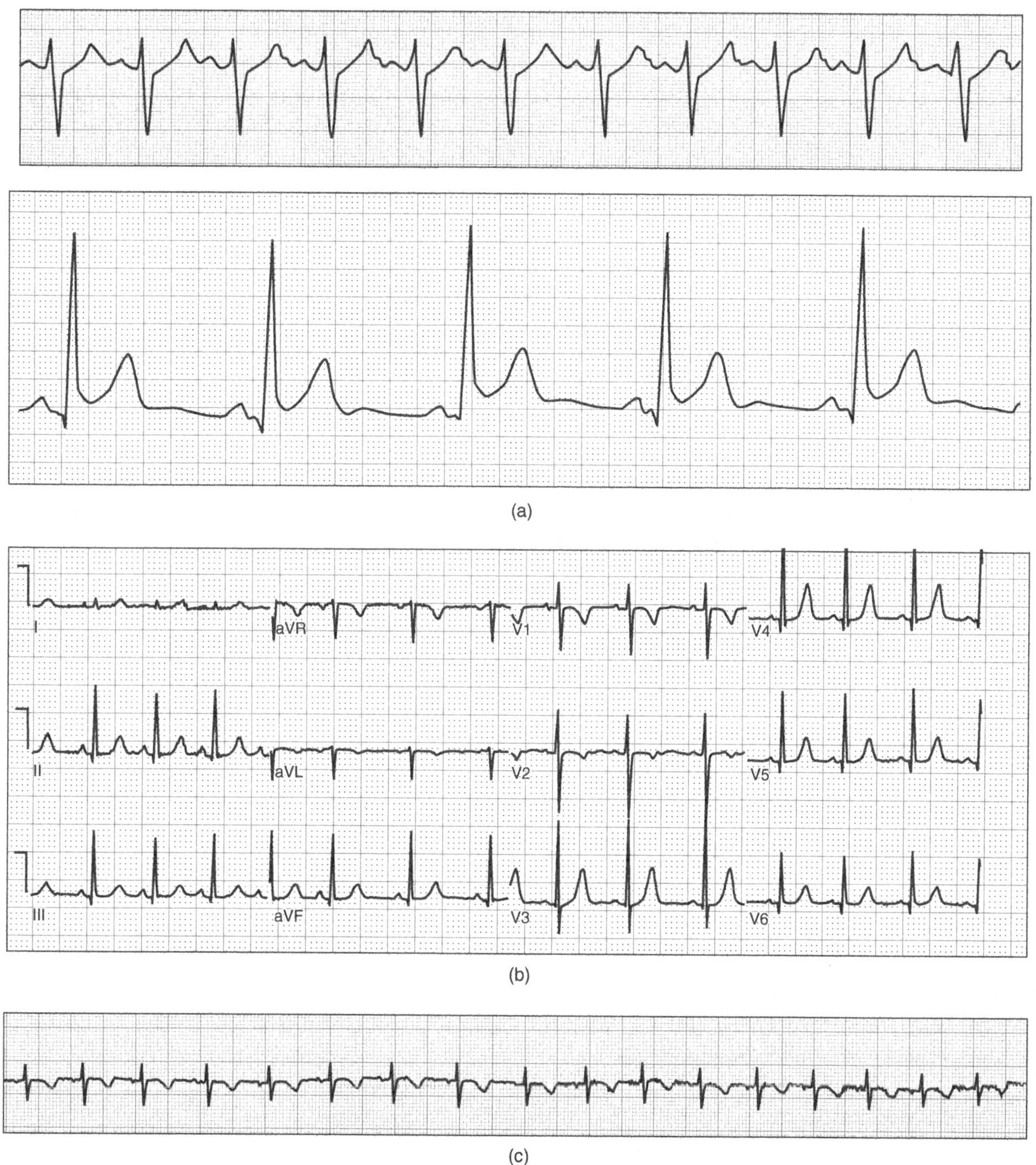

Figure 14.1 (a) Normal sinus rhythm in two pediatric patients. The upper panel in a 2-month-old infant and the lower panel in a 16-year-old male. (b) Normal sinus rhythm in an older infant with upright P waves in the limb leads. Also note the T wave inversions in the right precordial leads (juvenile T wave pattern) as well as the positive QRS complex across the precordial leads. (c) Sinus arrhythmia, a normal variant.

sufficiently rapid rate, thus producing bundle fatigue and a widened QRS complex (Figure 14.3c [six month-old infant]).

P waves can occur in certain individuals, the so-called retrograde P wave (Figure 14.3d). This type of P wave has nothing to do with rhythm genesis; rather, as the impulse is generated in the supraventricular focus, it moves distally into the ventricle, producing a ventricular depolarization (and QRS complex) and simultaneously, in retrograde manner, back into the atrial tissues,

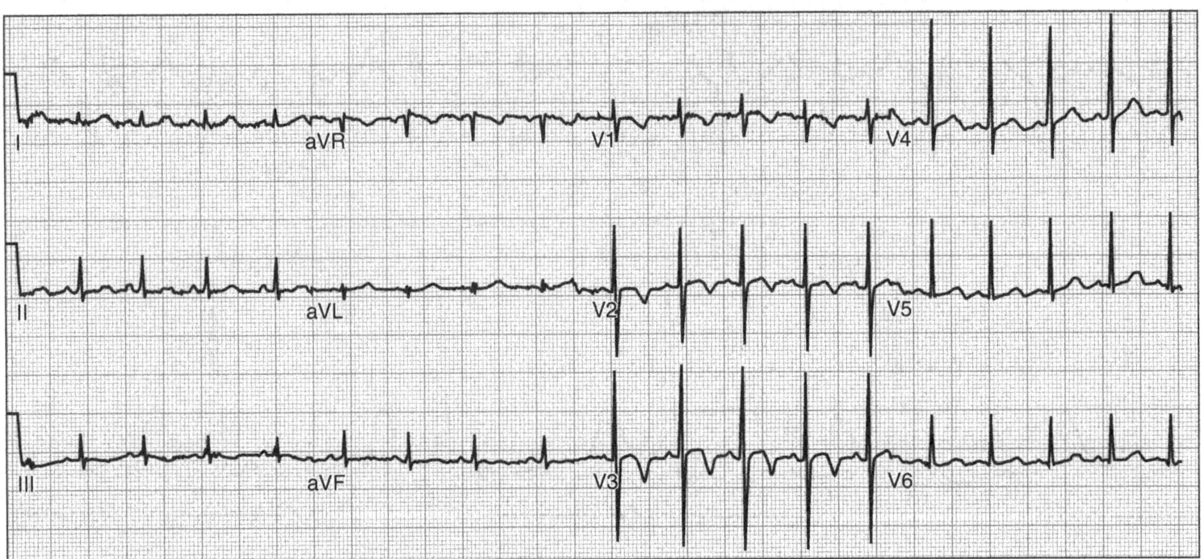

Figure 14.2 Normal sinus rhythm in an infant with the T wave inversions in the right to midprecordial leads (juvenile T wave pattern) as well as the positive QRS complex across the precordial leads.

Box 14.1 Clinical Considerations – Pediatric Dysrhythmias

Sinus arrhythmia

- Irregular R–R intervals.
- Pulse rate increases during inspiration and decreases during expiration.
- Normal finding, no treatment is indicated.

Sinus tachycardia

- Consider age-appropriate range.
- Can be precipitated by agitation, fever, hypovolemia, hypoxia, or pain.
- Look for cause.

Wolff–Parkinson White syndrome

- In normal sinus rhythm, demonstrates shortened PR interval, slurred QRS complex upslope (delta wave), and minimal widening of QRS complex.
- Associated with PSVT-like narrow complex tachycardia.
- Can also present with two other tachycardias: (i) atrial fibrillation with rapid ventricular response and wide QRS complex and (ii) wide complex tachycardia.

Atrial fibrillation/flutter

- Rare in children.
- Usually associated with congenital or acquired heart disease.

Long QT syndrome with or without polymorphic VT

- Several congenital forms.
- Can also be associated with electrolyte abnormalities and medication adverse effect.
- May have family history of syncope or sudden death.
- Presents as palpitations, syncope, or sudden cardiac death as a result of VT or torsades de pointe.

Accelerated idioventricular rhythm (AIVR)

- Benign pediatric rhythm often confused with VT.
- Rarely faster than 150 bpm.
- May be present many years after congenital heart repair.

Ventricular tachycardia (VT)
- Rare in children.
- Consider age-appropriate QRS complex duration.
- Inappropriately wide complexes should be assumed VT until proven otherwise.
- Identify any potential reversible cause and treat to the extent possible.

Ventricular fibrillation
- May be presenting rhythm in pediatric arrest patients.
- Initiate advanced life support therapy including electrical defibrillation.

Box 14.2 Treatment Considerations – General Management of Pediatric Dysrhythmias

Paroxysmal supraventricular tachycardia
- Vagal maneuvers (mammalian diving reflex, Valsalva maneuvers, unilateral carotid massage)
- Adenosine 0.1 mg/kg IV (max dose of 0.25 mg/kg)
- Cardioversion 0.5–2 J/kg if unstable

Bradycardia
- Supplemental oxygen
- Epinephrine (1 : 10 000) 0.01 mg/kg IV
- Atropine 0.02 mg/kg IV

Long QT syndrome/Torsade de pointes
- Magnesium sulfate 3–12 mg/kg IV
- Defibrillation 1–2 J/kg if compromising ventricular dysrhythmia

Ventricular tachycardia (stable)
- Amiodarone 5 mg/kg IV

Ventricular tachycardia (unstable) or VF
- Cardioversion/defibrillation 1–2 J/kg
- Epinephrine (1 : 10000) 0.01 mg/kg IV

causing depolarization and resultant P wave – the retrograde P wave. These P waves are frequently located immediately adjacent to the QRS complex, before or after, and are usually inverted.

Bradycardia

Bradycardia (Figure 14.4) in the pediatric patient is often a sign of a more significant, acute underlying disorder. It is important to consider the age appropriate ranges for the pediatric patient and recognize the bradycardic rhythm. Frequently, bradycardia is a result of acute respiratory failure with hypoxemia, although it can also manifest from increased intracranial pressure, hypothyroidism, and medication overdose (e.g. clonidine, digoxin, β-adrenergic blockers, calcium channel blockers). Identifying and treating to the extent possible any reversible causes of bradycardia can be a life-saving measure. Bradycardia can be sinus in origin with all the feature of sinus rhythm (upright P wave with P wave – QRS complex relationship); the obvious exception is a rate less than the lower limit of normal for sinus rhythm (Figure 14.4(a)). Junctional (or nodal, Figure 14.4(b)) and idioventricular (Figure 14.4(c)) bradycardias are also encountered, yet usually in more extreme cardiorespiratory situations. Junctional bradycardia is seen when the QRS complex is normal in width and occurring regularly without evidence of a P wave; idioventricular bradycardia is seen with a widened and regularly occurring QRS complex that also does not demonstrate an associated P wave.

Heart Block

When determining the degree of AV block in a pediatric patient, it is important to remember the age-appropriate ranges. In all such cases, the same criteria is used to diagnose the AV blocks in the pediatric patient as applied to the adult; the key issues are the nature of the PR interval and the relationship of the P wave to the QRS complex. First-degree AV block is usually a benign condition in the pediatric patient unless it is a manifestation of an underlying disease process such as a toxic ingestion. Second-degree AV blocks are also seen in the pediatric patient. Mobitz type I blocks are generally considered to be a normal variant in the pediatric patient – unless, of course, acute pathology such as an ingestion is being managed; a Mobitz type II AV block is always abnormal and is suggestive of significant underlying cardiac pathology. Third-degree, or complete, AV blocks can

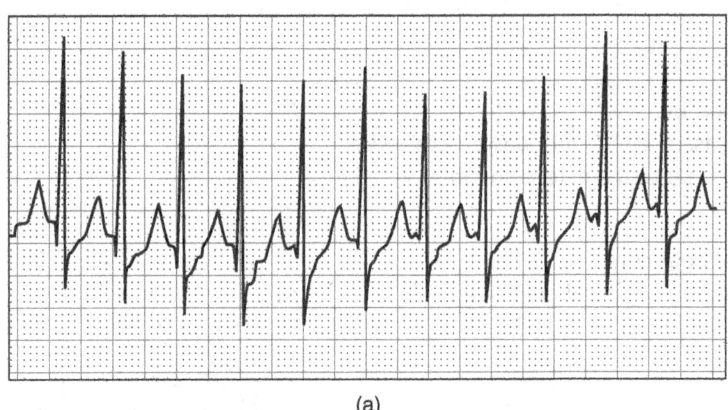

(a)

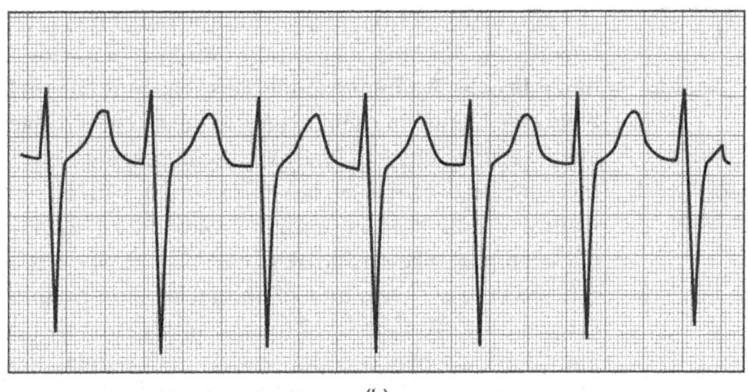

(b)

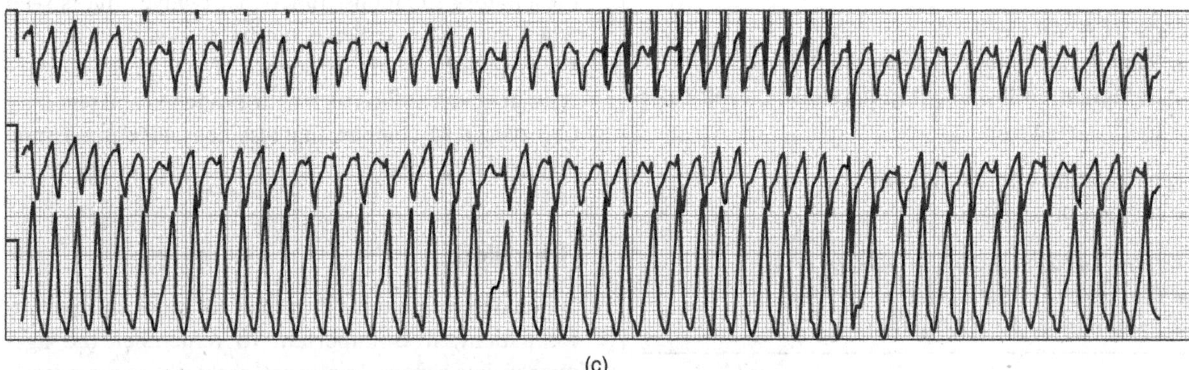

(c)

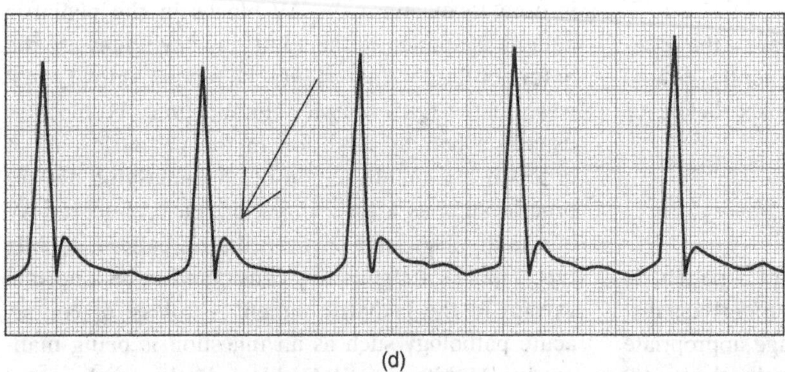

(d)

Figure 14.3 Paroxysmal supraventricular tachycardia. (a) Rapid, narrow complex tachycardia in a neonate. This rhythm is consistent with PSVT. (b) Rapid, narrow complex tachycardia in an adolescent, consistent with PSVT. (c) Extremely rapid tachycardia with intervening periods of narrow and wide QRS complexes. This rhythm is PSVT with intermittent widened QRS complexes due to bundle fatigue (rate-related bundle branch block) resulting from the extremely rapid ventricular rate. (d) Retrograde P wave (arrow) in PSVT.

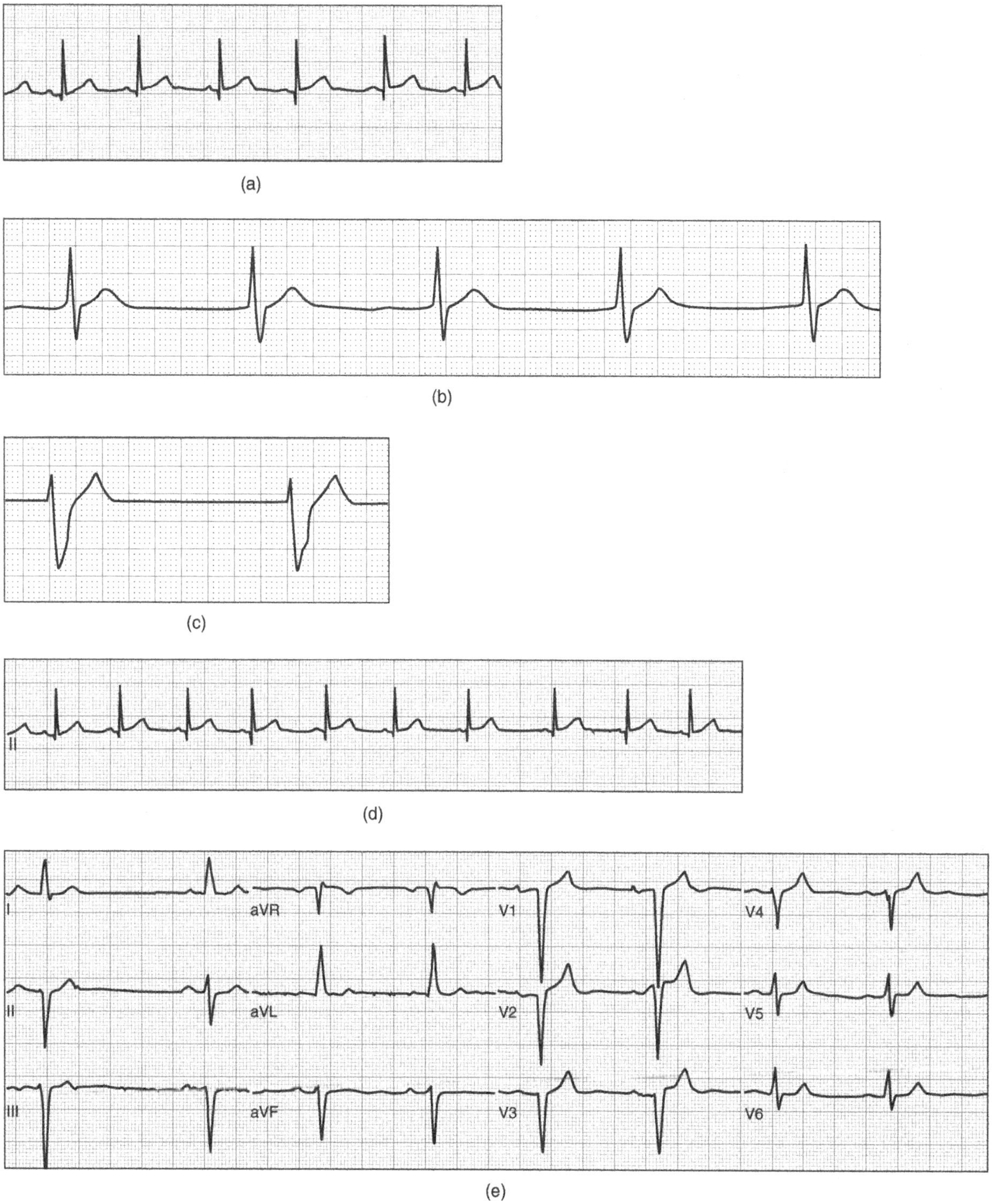

(a)

(b)

(c)

(d)

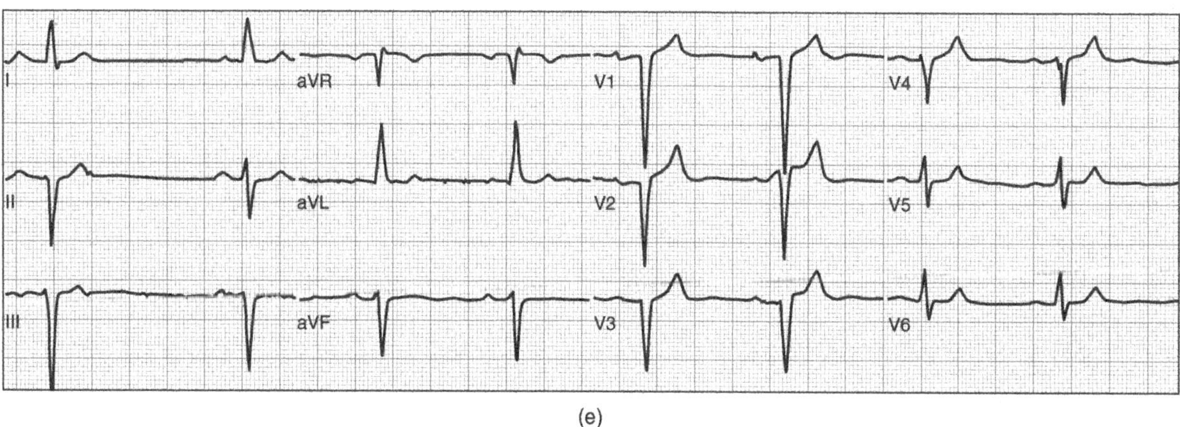

(e)

Figure 14.4 Bradycardia. (a) Sinus bradycardia. (b) Junctional bradycardia. (c) Idioventricular bradycardia. (d) Sinus bradycardia in a neonate with congenital hydrocephalus and increasing intracranial pressure. (e) Marked sinus bradycardia with a first-degree AV block and widened QRS complex in a one-day old with congenital heart disease.

be either congenital or acquired – and are always abnormal. Congenital third-degree AV blocks not related to structural heart disease are usually detected in utero by the presence of persistent fetal bradycardia. Complete congenital blocks associated with structural heart disease carry a poor prognosis. Congenital forms of third-degree heart block tend to have a narrow QRS complex, while the QRS complex in acquired forms of complete AV block seen in older children tend to be wide.

15

The Electrocardiogram in the Poisoned Patient

Steven H. Mitchell[1], Christopher P. Holstege[2], and William J. Brady[3]

[1] *Department of Emergency Medicine, University of Washington School of Medicine, Seattle, WA, USA*
[2] *Division of Medical Toxicology, Department of Emergency Medicine, University of Virginia School of Medicine, Charlottesville, VA, USA*
[3] *Departments of Emergency Medicine and Medicine, University of Virginia School of Medicine, Charlottesville, VA, USA*

The proliferation and wide spread usage of medications that result in cardiotoxicity in overdose is a reality of prehospital medicine today. Toxicity can result in a variety of electrocardiographic changes that pose life-threatening risks to the patient. Clinicians managing the overdose patient should be aware of the various electrocardiographic changes that can potentially occur in the acutely poisoned patient. ECG abnormalities including the PR interval prolongation, widening of the QRS complex, alterations in the T wave and the ST segment, and lengthening of the QT interval can all be seen (Figure 15.1).

Potential toxins can be placed into broad classes based on their cardiac effects (Box 15.1). Recognizing changes consistent with each class will assist the clinician in determining the severity of toxicity and its associated risks; also, recognizing these changes can suggest the most appropriate therapy in overdose situations (Box 15.2). The primary medication toxicity classes are discussed in detail below.

Potassium Efflux Blocking Agents

Myocardial repolarization, which is represented electrocardiographically by the T wave, is predominantly created by potassium moving out of cardiac cells. Blockade of the outward potassium movement prolongs the action potential and subsequently prolongs the QT interval of the ECG (Figure 15.1). In these situations, patients can experience ventricular dysrhythmias, including torsades de pointes. Commonly encountered medication classes include antibiotics, antiemetics, and antihistamines (Table 15.1).

Electrocardiographic Manifestations of the Potassium Efflux Blocking Agents

A prolonged QT interval (Figure 15.2a) is the hallmark of potassium efflux blocking agents and may result in vulnerability to reentry rhythms such as polymorphic ventricular tachycardia, most often in the form of torsades de pointes (Figure 15.2b). The QT interval is measured from the beginning of the QRS complex to the end of the T wave and is influenced by the patient's heart rate. Several formulas have been developed to correct the QT interval for the effect of heart rate using the RR interval. When evaluating a rhythm strip for a patient in sinus rhythm, a QT interval that is greater than half the RR interval may indicate QT interval prolongation (Figure 15.2c). Computerized ECG interpretations report the corrected interval as the QTc, using the formula $QTc = QT/\sqrt{RR}$. In general, the QTc is considered prolonged when it exceeds 450 ms; specifically, the QT interval is considered long when the QTc interval is greater than 440 ms in men and is greater than 460 ms in women. Arrhythmias are most common with values greater than 500 ms.

Sodium Channel Blocking Agents

The cardiac sodium channels are located in the cell membrane and open rapidly in response to an action potential. This rapid opening of sodium channels leads to cell depolarization, which in turn propagates the action potential throughout the ventricles. The QRS complex represents depolarization of cardiac myocytes located in the right and left ventricles. Blockade of

The Electrocardiogram in Emergency and Acute Care, First Edition.
Edited by Korin B. Hudson, Amita Sudhir, George Glass, and William J. Brady.

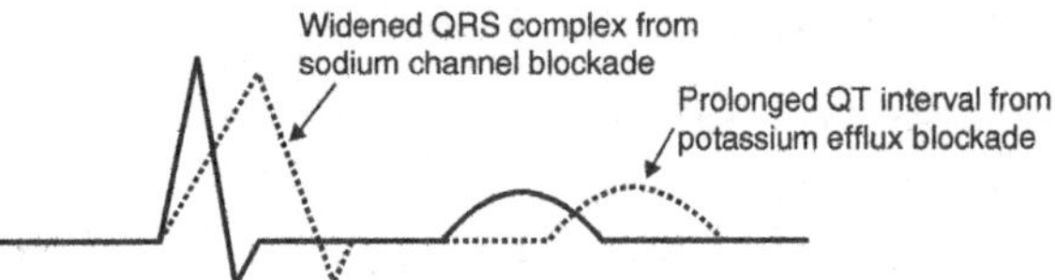

Figure 15.1 Impact of sodium channel and potassium efflux blocking drugs on the ECG with QRS complex widening and QT interval prolongation.

Box 15.1 Clinical Considerations – Toxic Ingestions with a Mixed Picture Presentation

Cocaine	Sodium channels blockade and sympathomimetic toxidrome
Diphenhydramine	Sodium channel blockade and anticholinergic toxidrome
Propoxyphene	Sodium channel blockade and opioid toxidrome
Tricyclic antidepressants	Sodium channel blockade and potassium efflux blockade
Digitalis	Cardiac glycoside toxicity and hyperkalemia
Verapamil and diltiazem	Calcium channel blockade and sodium channel blockade
Propranolol	β-Adrenergic blockade and sodium channel blockade
Sotalol	β-Adrenergic blockade and potassium efflux blockade

sodium influx causes a widening of the QRS complex (Figure 15.1). Common medications that are sodium channel blocking agents include antidepressants, antiarrythmics, and diphenhydramine (Table 15.2).

Electrocardiographic manifestations of the sodium channel blocking agents: Sodium channel blockage manifests electrocardiographically as a widened QRS complex, usually greater than 120 ms. Early stages of toxicity affect the first phase of depolarization (phase 0) and as a result, the upslope of depolarization is slowed. As toxicity increases and fewer sodium channels are available for depolarization, the QRS complex continues to widen (Figure 15.3a, b), ultimately resulting in a sine wave pattern. Eventually the rhythm will degrade to asystole. Sodium channel blockers may also slow intraventricular conduction, which can lead to a reentrant circuit that results in ventricular tachycardia (Figure 15.3c). Thus, wide complex tachycardia can be seen in this setting, resulting from either supraventricular tachycardia with aberrant intraventricular conduction or ventricular tachycardia.

Cardiac Glycoside Toxicity

Cardiac glycosides work to inhibit the sodium-potassium-adenosine triphosphatase pump in cardiac cells that moves sodium out of the cell and potassium into the cell. The increased potassium outside the cell

Box 15.2 Treatment Considerations of Specific Cardiotoxic Effects

Potassium efflux blockade	Torsade de pointes	IV Magnesium sulfate (1–2 g/adult); overdrive pacing
Sodium channel blockade	Wide QRS Complex	IV Sodium bicarbonate (1–2 mEq/kg) bolus every 1–2 min until QRS complex narrows
Cardiac glycoside toxicity	Bradycardia	For bradycardia: • IV Atropine (0.5–2 mg)
	Hyperkalemia	For hyperkalemia: • IV Sodium bicarbonate (1 meq/kg), IV insulin, and dextrose • AVOID calcium which may potentiate asystole
	Ventricular tachydysrhythmias	For ventricular dysrhythmias: • IV Lidocaine (50–100 mg for adult, 1 mg/kg for child)
Calcium channel blockade	Hypotension	For hypotension: • IV Calcium chloride or gluconate every 5–10 min
	Bradycardia	For bradycardia: • IV glucagon (3–5 mg over 1–2 min, repeat every 5 min to max dose of 10 mg) • IV epinephrine (1 mcg/min infusion, titrate as necessary)
β-Adrenergic blockade	Bradycardia hypotension	For both bradycardia and hypotension: • IV glucagon (5–10 mg bolus, repeat as necessary) • IV epinephrine (1 mcg/min infusion, titrate as necessary)

Table 15.1 Potassium efflux channel blocking drugs.

Antihistamines	Bepridil	Class III antiarrhythmics	Erythromycin
• Astemizole	Chloroquine	• Amiodarone	Fluoroquinolones
• Clarithromycin	Citalopram	• Dofetilide	• Ciproßoxacin
• Diphenhydramine	Clarithromycin	• Ibutilide	• Gatißoxacin
• Loratidine		• Sotalol	• Levoßoxacin
• Terfenadine			• Moxißoxacin
			• Sparßoxacin
Antipsychotics	Class IA antiarrhythmics	Cyclic antidepressants	
• Chlorpromazine	• Disopyramide	• Amitriptyline	
• Droperidol	• Quinidine	• Amoxapine	
• Mesoridazine	• Procainamide	• Desipramine	
• Pimozide	Class IC antiarrhythmics	• Doxepin	
• Quetiapine	• Encainide	• Imipramine	
• Risperidone	• Flecainide	• Nortriptyline	
• Thioridazine	• Propafenone	• Maprotiline	
• Ziprasidone			

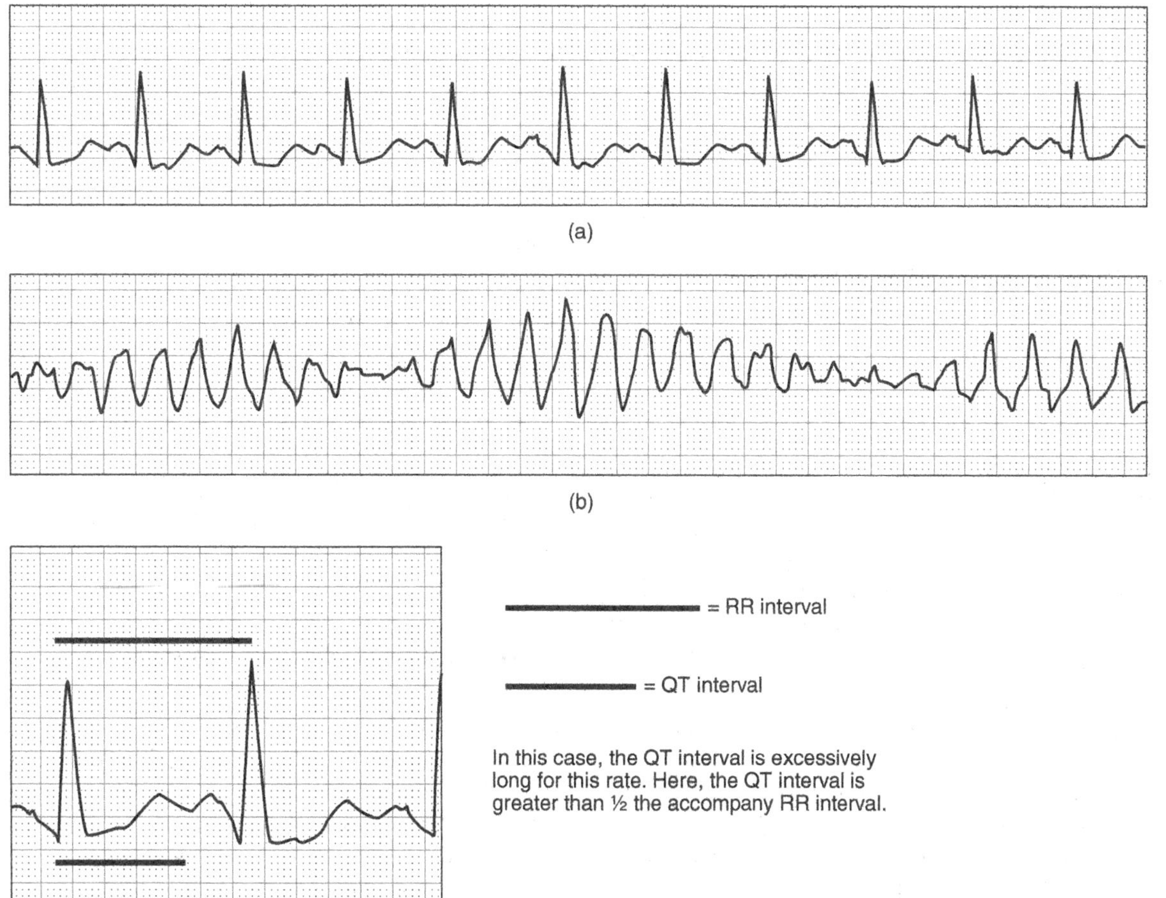
(a)
(b)
= RR interval
= QT interval
In this case, the QT interval is excessively long for this rate. Here, the QT interval is greater than ½ the accompany RR interval.
(c)

Figure 15.2 (a) Sinus tachycardia at 104 with prolonged QT interval. (b) Polymorphic VT (torsades de pointes) associated with QT interval prolongation. (c) Determination of the prolonged QT interval – if the QT interval is longer than half the accompanying RR interval, then that QT interval is prolonged.

Table 15.2 Sodium channel blocking drugs.

Amantadine Carbamazepine Chloroquine Citalopram Cocaine Diltiazem Diphenhydramine	Class IA antiarrhythmics • Disopyramide • Quinidine • Procainamide Class IC antiarrhythmics • Encainide • Flecainide • Propafenone	Cyclic antidepressants • Amitriptyline • Amoxapine • Desipramine • Doxepin • Imipramine • Nortriptyline • Maprotiline	Hydroxychloroquine Phenothiazines • Medoridazine • Thioridazine Propranolol Propoxyphene Quinine Verapamil

and increased sodium inside the cell, together with increased vagal tone that may lead to direct atrioventricular (AV) nodal depression, can result in significant cardiac disturbances and ECG abnormalities in the setting of toxicity.

Cardiac glycosides are used therapeutically to increase myocardial contractility and to slow AV conduction. Cardiac glycosides, such as digoxin and other digitalis derivatives, are encountered widely in daily life. Digoxin historically has been used to treat atrial fibrillation and congestive heart failure. Cardiac glycosides are also found in non-prescription and plant forms and have been associated with toxicity (Table 15.3).

Electrocardiographic Manifestations of the Cardiac Glycosides

The *digitalis effect* is a term used for several electrocardiographic changes that are associated with digoxin therapy. These changes include a sagging or scooped ST segment and T wave complex that takes the appearance of a hockey stick (Figure 15.4a). The T wave may be flattened or abnormally inverted and the ST segment depressed. These findings are most pronounced in leads with tall R waves. The increased vagal tone may result in lengthening of the PR interval and the QT interval may be shortened. These changes do not indicate toxicity but are rather seen at therapeutic levels of the drug – and are strictly considered the "digitalis effect."

The effects of toxic levels of cardiac glycosides result in a mixture of excitatory and suppressant activity that can produce a variety of electrocardiographic abnormalities and a wide assortment of dysrhythmias (Figure 15.4a, b). In practice, it is reasonable to assume that patients who are toxic from cardiac glycosides may have any or all of the following rhythm abnormalities related to these mechanisms:

Augmented automaticity (heightened ability of pacemakers to depolarize)

- Increased calcium inside the cells leads to premature beats within the atria, AV node, or ventricles. The most common dysrhythmia associated with toxicity is frequent premature ventricular beats (Figure 15.4c) in the setting of either sinus rhythm or atrial fibrillation.

Increased vagal tone

- Slowed conduction through the AV node leads to sinus bradycardia, junctional bradycardia (Figure 15.4b), bundle branch blocks, or all grades of AV nodal block (first-, second-, and third-degree).

Combination of excitant and suppressant activity

- This combination may result in a mixed picture of atrial tachycardia with AV block or second-degree AV block with junctional premature beats. Dysrhythmias, which are highly suggestive of glycoside toxicity as a result of the combination of excitatory and suppressive effects, include paroxysmal atrial tachycardia with variable block, an accelerated junctional rhythm, and atrial fibrillation with significant slowing of the ventricular response.

Calcium Channel Blocker Toxicity

The number of toxic exposures to calcium channel blockers (CCBs) has increased significantly as the use of this family of medications has increased dramatically. There are three classes of CCB medications that have varying cardiovascular effects (Table 15.4).

All CCBs inhibit the calcium channel within the cell membrane of cardiac and smooth muscle cells. In cardiac cells, the inhibition of calcium channels prevents movement of calcium from outside the cell to sites within. Decreased calcium within the myocardial cells

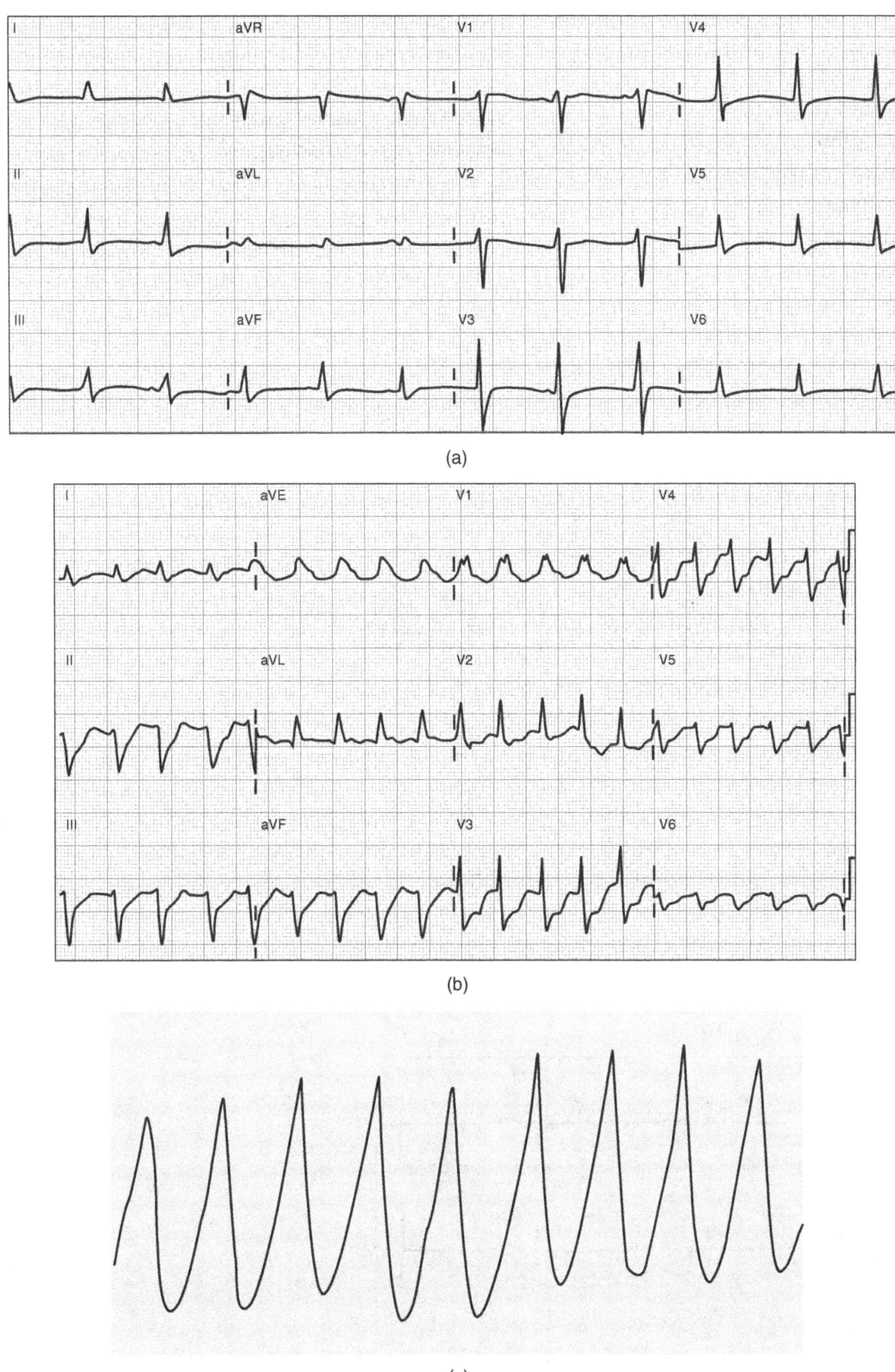

Figure 15.3 (a) Minimally widened QRS complex in the setting of a cardiotoxic ingestion with sodium channel blocking ability. (b) Tricyclic antidepressant overdose with characteristic changes on ECG, including sinus tachycardia, deep S wave in lead I, R wave in lead aVr, and widened QRS complex. (c) Ventricular tachycardia related to sodium channel blockade.

Table 15.3 Plants associated with cardiac glycoside toxicity.

Digitalis purpurea, D. lanata (foxglove)
Nerium oleander (oleander)
Strophanthus gratus (oubain)
Thevetia peruviana spp. (yellow oleander)
Convallaria majalis (lily of the valley)
Urginea maritima (squill)

results in slowing of conduction, decreased contractility, and decreased cardiac output.

Electrocardiographic Manifestations of the Calcium Channel Blockers

Following significant exposure with CCBs, the initial rhythm is typically a sinus bradycardia that may or may not be symptomatic. As levels of CCB increase, the

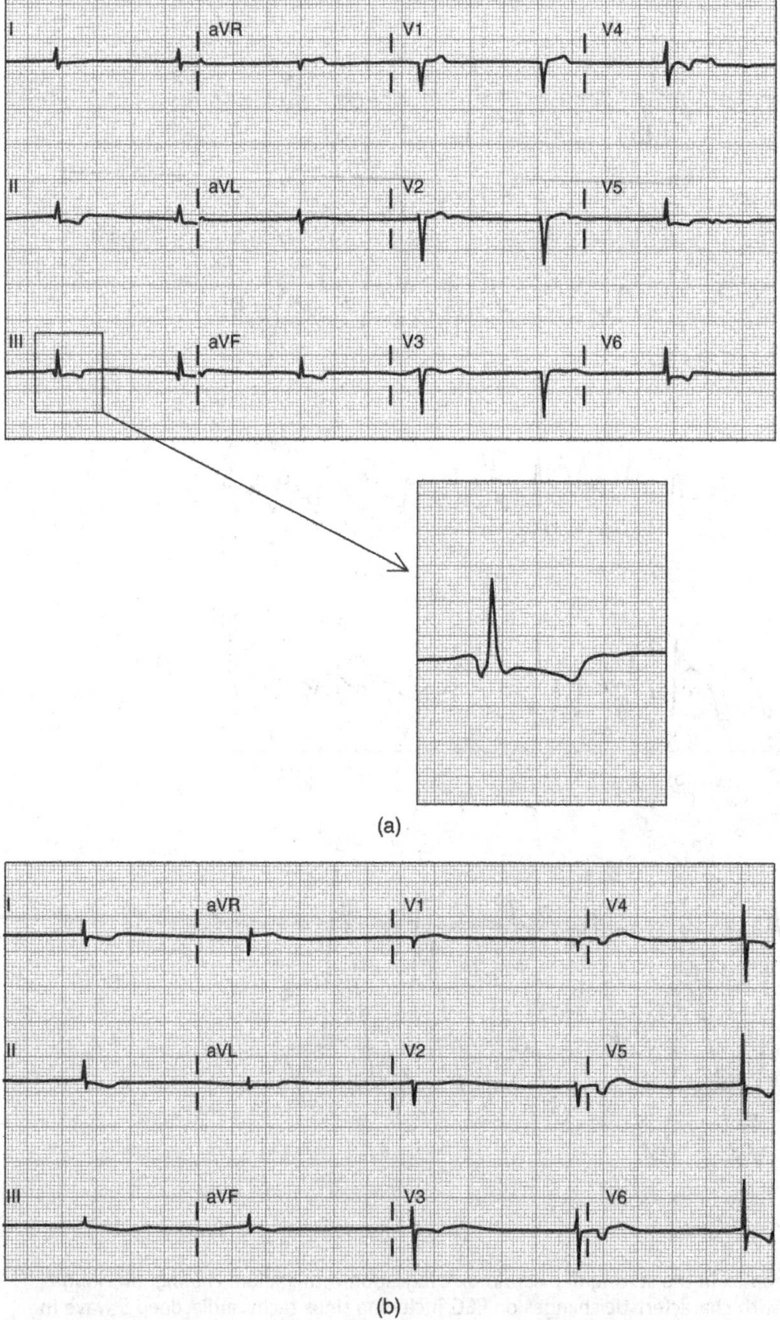

Figure 15.4 (a) ECG with characteristic changes of "digitalis effect," a nontoxic manifestation of digoxin's presence in the body; the rhythm in this case, however, is a junctional rhythm, a potential indication of toxicity. (b) Electrocardiogram in the setting of digitalis toxicity with a junctional bradycardia. (c) Frequent ventricular ectopy with bradycardia seen in a digoxin overdose.

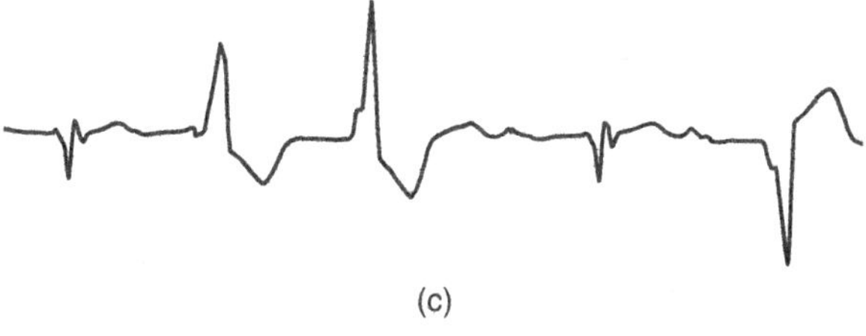

Figure 15.4 (Continued)

patient may develop rhythms that correspond to greater inhibition of the conduction system. All types of AV block (first-, second-, and third-degree) may be encountered as well as junctional and ventricular bradydysrhythmias (Figure 15.5a). There is also strong evidence that the CCBs also have a cross affinity for cardiac sodium channels that results in widening of the QRS complex. This subsequent QRS complex widening increases the potential for ventricular dysrhythmias (Figure 15.5b).

Table 15.4 Subtype classification of calcium channel blockers, channel affinity, and cardiac effects.

Subtype name	Peripheral vascular smooth muscle channels	Myocardial channels	Cardiac effects
Dihydropyridine (identified by the suffix "-dipine") • Nifedipine • Nicardipine • Nimodipine • Amlodipine	High	Low	Hypotension and reflex tachycardia; not useful in terminating tachydysrhythmias
Phenylalklamine • Verapamil	Low	High	Strong AV nodal blockade, useful in terminating tachydysrhythmias
Benzothiazepine • Diltiazem	Mixed	Mixed	Causes both hypotension and bradycardia

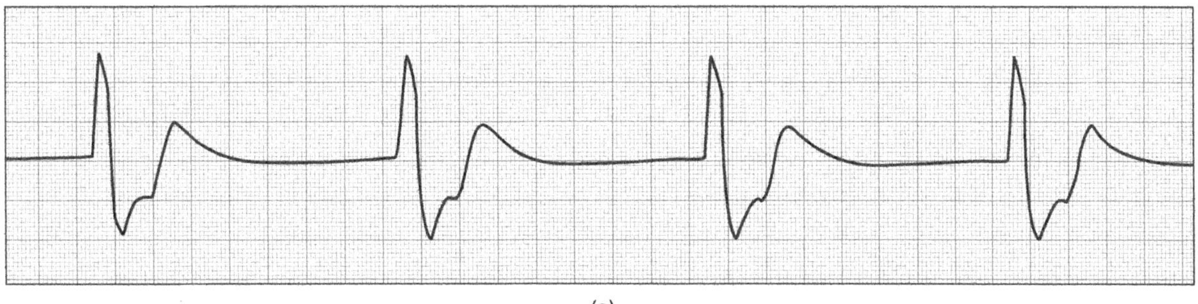

(a)

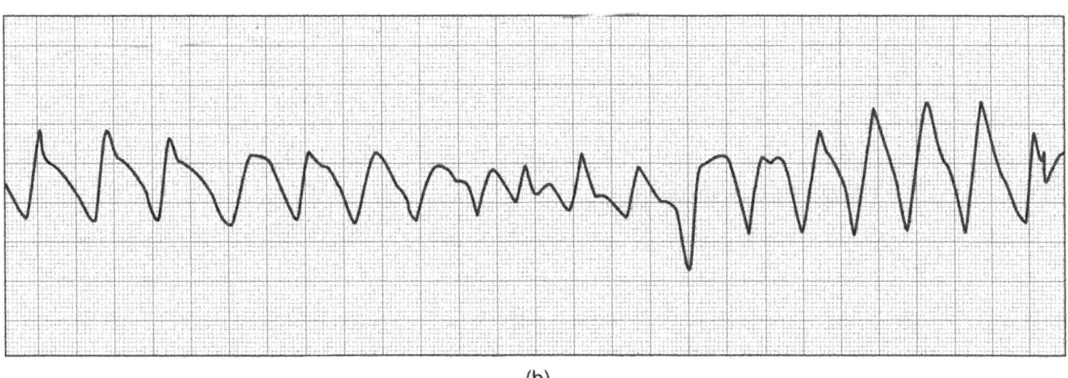

(b)

Figure 15.5 (a) Bradydysrhythmia (idioventricular rhythm) with heart rate of 35 and QRS complex widening in calcium channel toxicity. (b) Ventricular dysrhythmia consistent with torsades de pointes-type of polymorphic ventricular tachycardia due to calcium channel blocker toxicity.

β-Adrenergic Blocker Toxicity

β-Blockers (BBs) are widely used because of their efficacy in the treatment of hypertension, ischemic heart disease, and dysrhythmias, among other medical conditions. There are currently numerous BBs available (Table 15.5). BBs competitively inhibit β receptors throughout the body. β-1 receptor inhibition results in a decrease in heart rate and contractility along with decreased AV nodal conduction. β-2 receptor inhibition results in relaxation of the smooth muscles located in blood vessels, bronchi, and the gastrointestinal tract. Each type of BB has varying affinity for the β-1 and β-2 receptors. Some agents block other receptor types concurrent with their β receptor activity. Examples include the α-adrenergic receptors (e.g. labetalol), cardiac sodium channels (e.g. propranolol), and cardiac potassium channels (e.g. sotalol).

Table 15.5 β-Adrenergic blocking drugs.

Acebutolol	Nebivolol	Pindolol	Nadolol
Atenolol	Metoprolol	Carvedilol	Propranolol
Betaxolol	Acebutolol	Labetalol	Sotalol
Bisoprolol	Carteolol	Levobunolol	Timolol
Esmolol	Penbutolol	Metipranolol	

Electrocardiographic Manifestations of the β-Adrenergic Blockers

In acute overdose, the most pronounced effects of BBs are on the cardiovascular system. Similar to CCBs, augmented β-1 blockade results initially in sinus bradycardia (Figure 15.6) and diminished AV nodal conduction, which may lead to varying degrees of AV block. Impaired contractility may also result in hypotension.

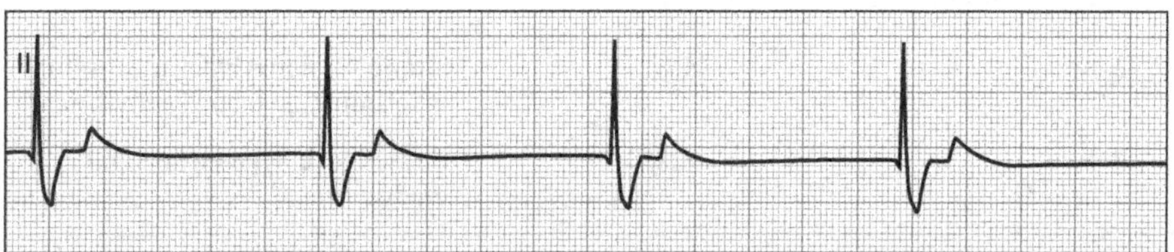

Figure 15.6 Junctional bradydysrhythmia with heart rate of 30 in the setting of β blocker toxicity.

16

The Electrocardiogram in Hyperkalemia

Steven H. Mitchell[1] *and William J. Brady*[2]

[1] *Department of Emergency Medicine, University of Washington School of Medicine, Seattle, WA, USA*
[2] *Departments of Emergency Medicine and Medicine, University of Virginia School of Medicine, Charlottesville, VA, USA*

Hyperkalemia, the elevation of serum potassium, is a common electrolyte disturbance that can be seen in many clinical situations (Box 16.1). Hyperkalemia can be considered a true "silent killer" as elevated serum levels may produce few symptoms despite ECG changes that may rapidly lead to terminal events. Recognition of ECG changes from toxic potassium levels can lead to early, life-saving interventions (Box 16.2).

Potassium (K^+) is the most abundant cation in the body, with most being stored intracellularly. It is this large potassium gradient across the cell's membrane that contributes to the excitability of cardiac cells as well as other cells throughout the body. The body's internal potassium management is primarily managed by the kidney. Most daily potassium loss (90%) is through renal excretion. Patients with renal failure, therefore, have impaired ability to regulate serum potassium and become prone to hyperkalemia. In addition, there are a number of medications and clinical conditions that may contribute to or cause hyperkalemia. In a basic sense, elevated serum potassium disrupts electrical function in the heart. This disruption not only affects the pacemaking foci of the heart but also the conduction tissues, resulting in bradycardia and conduction abnormalities.

Electrocardiographic Manifestations

Serum potassium concentration is tightly regulated in the normal range. It is important to note that the relation between ECG changes and serum potassium will vary between people. Patients with frequent past exposures or slowly progressive elevations tend to tolerate higher serum levels before the development of significant ECG abnormality. Conversely, the sudden increase in serum potassium, such as with a toxin ingestion or rapid development of acute kidney injury (renal failure), will likely produce ECG abnormality at lower total levels of elevation. In a general sense, Table 16.1 lists the association between serum potassium level and ECG manifestation; this association should be used as a guide and is most often seen with sudden, acute elevations as opposed to chronic, recurrent hyperkalemia.

The ECG changes of hyperkalemia progress in a relatively predictable manner and are outlined below.

T Wave

The peaked, or "tented" T wave, as a result of increased membrane repolarization, is the earliest ECG manifestation of hyperkalemia (Figure 16.2). It is also perhaps the most easily observed finding. Peaked T waves are best seen in the inferior (leads II and III) and precordial (leads V2–V4) leads (Figure 16.3). The peaked T wave is typically tall and narrow. It has the appearance of a "church steeple"; the T wave will broaden as further increases in serum potassium occur (Figure 16.3). Whether the T wave is narrow or wide, however, the morphology remains symmetric, which helps differentiate it from the asymmetric appearance of the ischemic, hyperacute T wave of early ST segment elevation myocardial infarction (STEMI). T waves that are typically inverted such as in left ventricular hypertrophy may become upright or "pseudonormalized."

The Electrocardiogram in Emergency and Acute Care, First Edition.
Edited by Korin B. Hudson, Amita Sudhir, George Glass, and William J. Brady.

Box 16.1 Clinical Considerations – Causes of Hyperkalemia

- Renal failure (acute and chronic)[a]
- Liver disease (severe/end-stage)[a]
- Heart failure (severe/end-stage)[a]
- Medications (partial list)[a]
  - Angiotensin-converting-enzyme (ACE) inhibitors (e.g. lisinopril)
  - Angiotensin receptor blockers (e.g. losartan)
  - Non-steroidal anti-inflammatory agents (e.g. ibuprofen)
  - Exogenous (excessive potassium supplementation)
  - Potassium-sparing diuretics (e.g. spironolactone)
  - Immunosuppressants (cyclosporine, tacrolimus)
  - β-blockers (e.g. metoprolol)
  - Trimethoprim (antibiotic)
  - Succinylcholine (burns, neuromuscular disease patients)
- Excessive use of dietary salt substitutes (potassium chloride)[a]
- Hemolysis (increased release with cell death after trauma, burns, chemotherapy)
- Metabolic acidosis
- Diabetic ketoacidosis
- Addison's disease
- Hyperkalemic periodic paralysis

[a]Denote the most commonly encountered causes of hyperkalemia.

P Wave and PR Interval

Early in the rise of potassium, the PR interval will become prolonged. With further increases in the serum potassium, the P wave is impacted. The amplitude of the P waves diminishes in hyperkalemia and may eventually disappear entirely as the condition worsens. This diminution of the P wave is likely secondary to increased sensitivity of atrial tissue to hyperkalemia and depression of sinoatrial (SA) and atrioventricular (AV) node conduction.

QRS Complex

In the intermediate stage of potassium elevation, the QRS complex is minimally, or subtly, widened (Figure 16.3). As the potassium levels increase, the QRS complex structure widens further (Figure 16.4) and can masquerade as a bundle branch block. Ultimately, the QRS complex will widen and assume a "sine wave" configuration (Figure 16.5).

Sinoventricular Rhythm

As the potassium levels rise, the QRS complex widens further, fusing with the T wave and forming a sine wave pattern; the P wave is not detectable. At this stage of ECG abnormality, the sinoventricular rhythm of severe hyperkalemia is noted (Figure 16.6). It is characterized most often by a relatively slow rate, ranging from 50 to 70 bpm, with sine wave QRS complex and no P wave. This rhythm is a preterminal rhythm, meaning that this rhythm is a true medical emergency, requiring emergent treatment.

Consider significant hyperkalemia when bradycardia with widened QRS complexes is noted; this diagnosis is rather challenging.

Cardiac Arrest

Cardiac arrest from hyperkalemia presents initially with either ventricular fibrillation or asystole.

The progression of electrocardiographic changes noted above account for the typical abnormalities related to hyperkalemia. The impaired conduction resulting from hyperkalemia, however, may also result in more atypical conduction abnormalities. These include AV block, right and left bundle branch blocks, bifascicular block, and trifascicular block.

Box 16.2 Management Considerations

Three management goals:

- Stabilization of cardiac cell membrane
- Transient shifting of potassium intracellularly
- Removal of potassium from the body permanently

Treatment usually produces rapid results with lessening of ECG abnormalities.

Impact and effect of treatment is transient/repeat therapy is indicated in many situations.

Management is guided by patient condition and ECG manifestations (Figure 16.1).

Stabilization of cardiac cell membrane

- Calcium chloride/gluconate 1 g IV

Transient shifting of potassium intracellularly

- Sodium bicarbonate 1 ampule IV
- Magnesium sulfate 1–2 g IV
- Dextrose (50%) 1 ampule IV
- Insulin (regular) 2–10 units IV
- Albuterol nebulized administration
- Epinephrine (1:10 000) IV – portions of 1 mg dose/titrated/only with impending cardiac arrest

Removal of potassium from the body permanently

- GI tract via binding resins and cation exchange polymers
- Renal excretion through the use of loop diuretics
- Hemodialysis

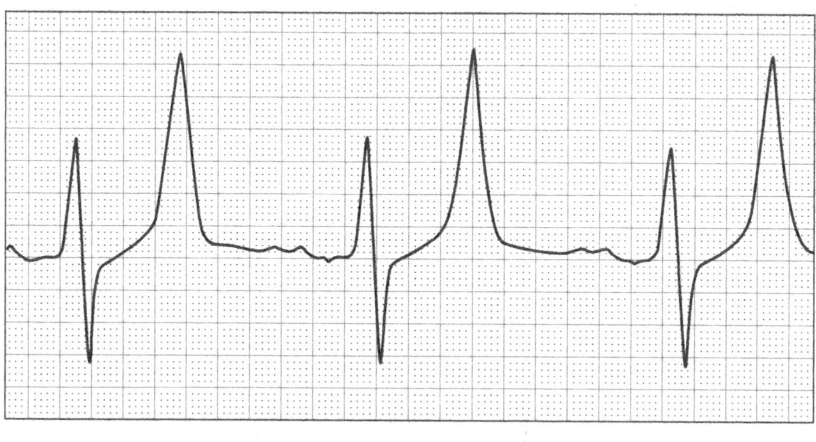

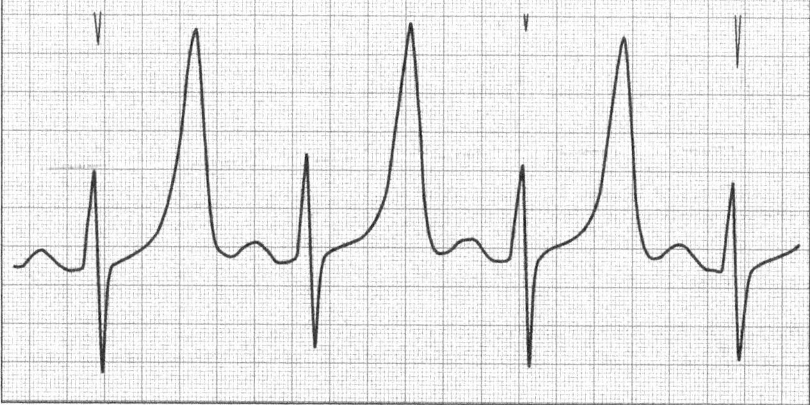

Figure 16.1 Peaked, or prominent, T waves. Note the tall, narrow, symmetric T waves, associated with hyperkalemia. Peaked T waves are best seen in the inferior (leads II and III) and precordial (leads V2–V4) leads (Figure 16.2).

Table 16.1 Serum potassium concentration and ECG manifestations.

Serum potassium[a]	ECG manifestation
Mild elevation (5.5–6.5 mEq/l)	Peaked T waves
Moderate elevation (6.5–8.0 mEq/l)	Decreased P wave amplitude
	Lengthening of PR interval
	Widening of QRS complex
Severe elevation (>8.0 mEq/l)	Absent P wave
	Conduction delays (atrioventricular/intraventricular)
	QRS complex widens with slurring into T wave creating "sine wave"
	Sinoventricular rhythm
	Ventricular fibrillation/asystole

[a]Significant variation is found with respect to serum potassium level and ECG manifestation; the currently listed association should be used as a guide and is most often seen with sudden, acute elevations.

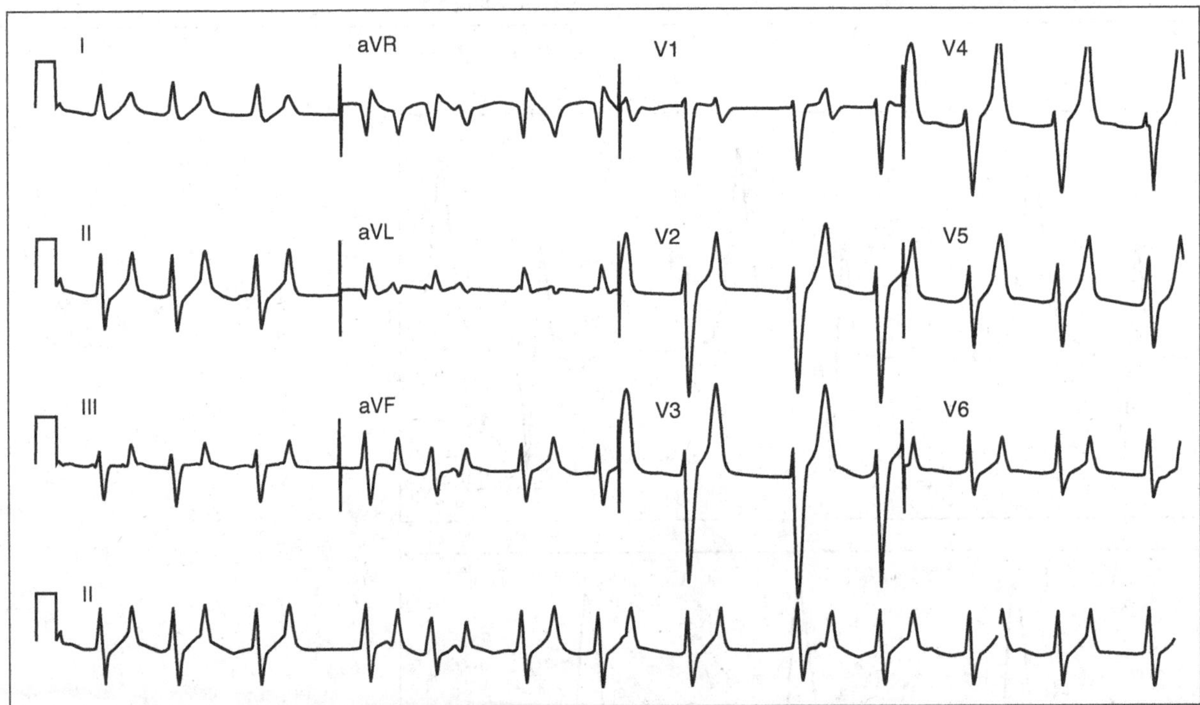

Figure 16.2 QRS complex widening in hyperkalemia: The 12-lead ECG with prominent T waves, best seen in leads V2–V5. Also note the widening of the QRS complex and the absence of easily identified P waves.

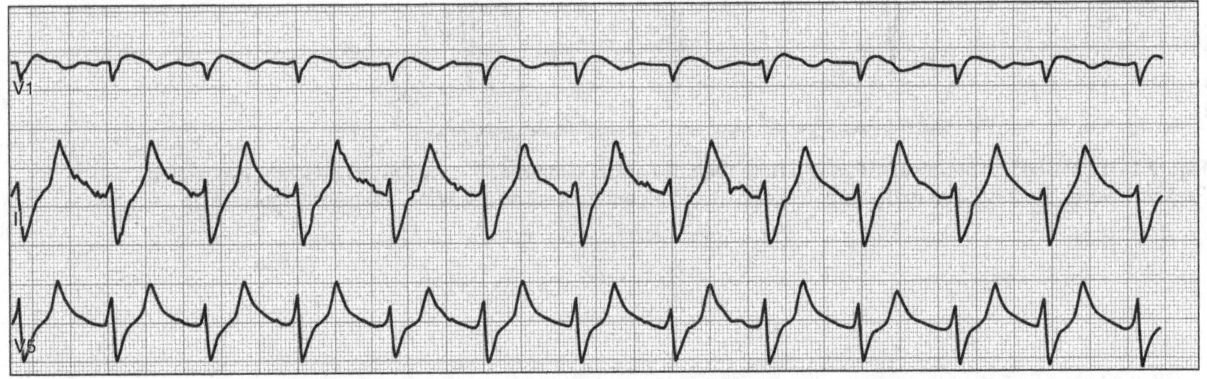

Figure 16.3 Severe hyperkalemia with widened QRS complex and symmetric peaked T waves.

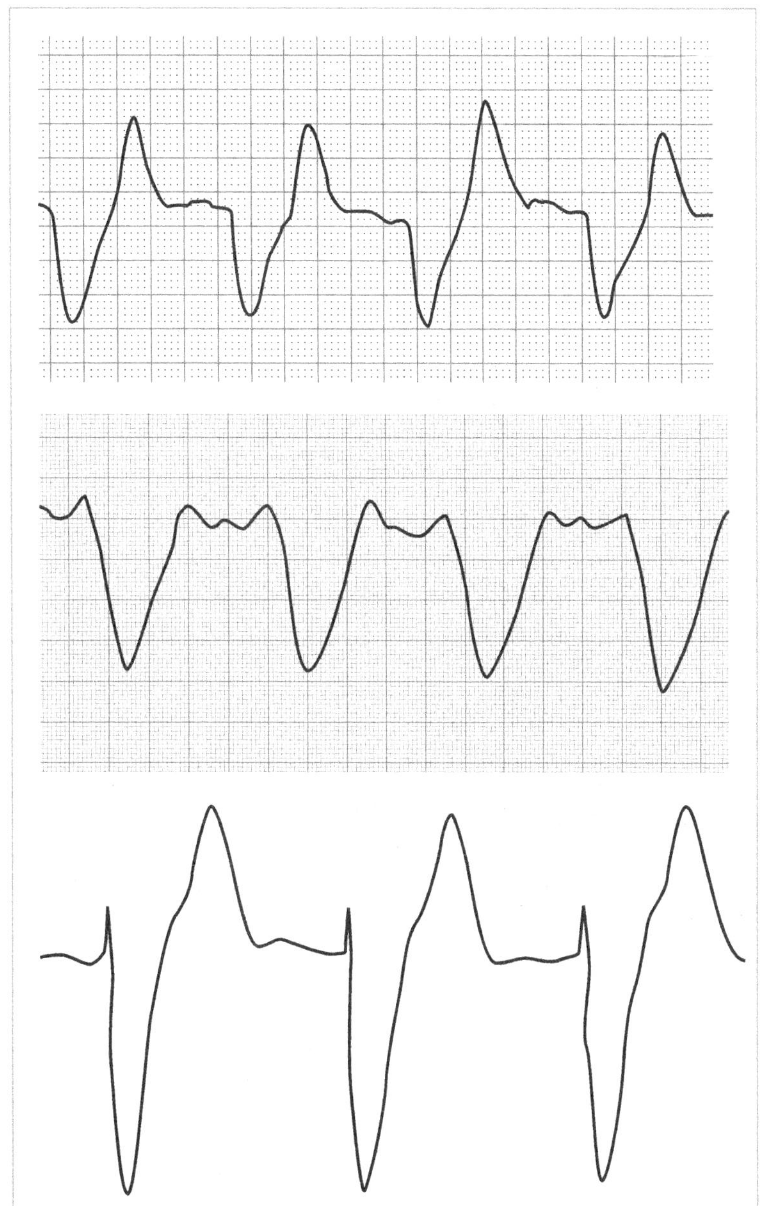

Figure 16.4 Widened QRS complex in severe hyperkalemia.

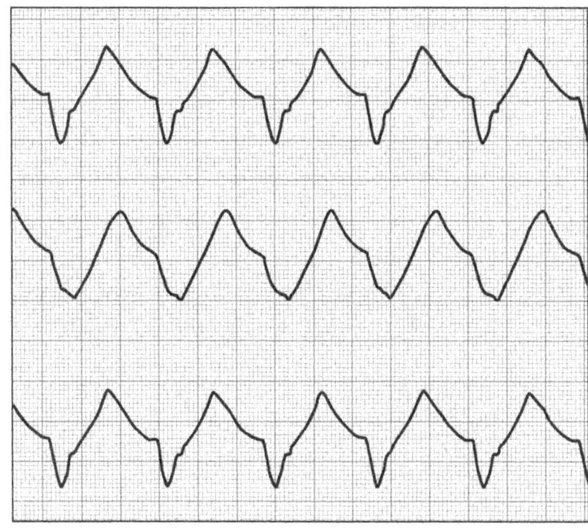

Figure 16.5 Significantly widened QRS complexes in three separate patients with severe hyperkalemia.

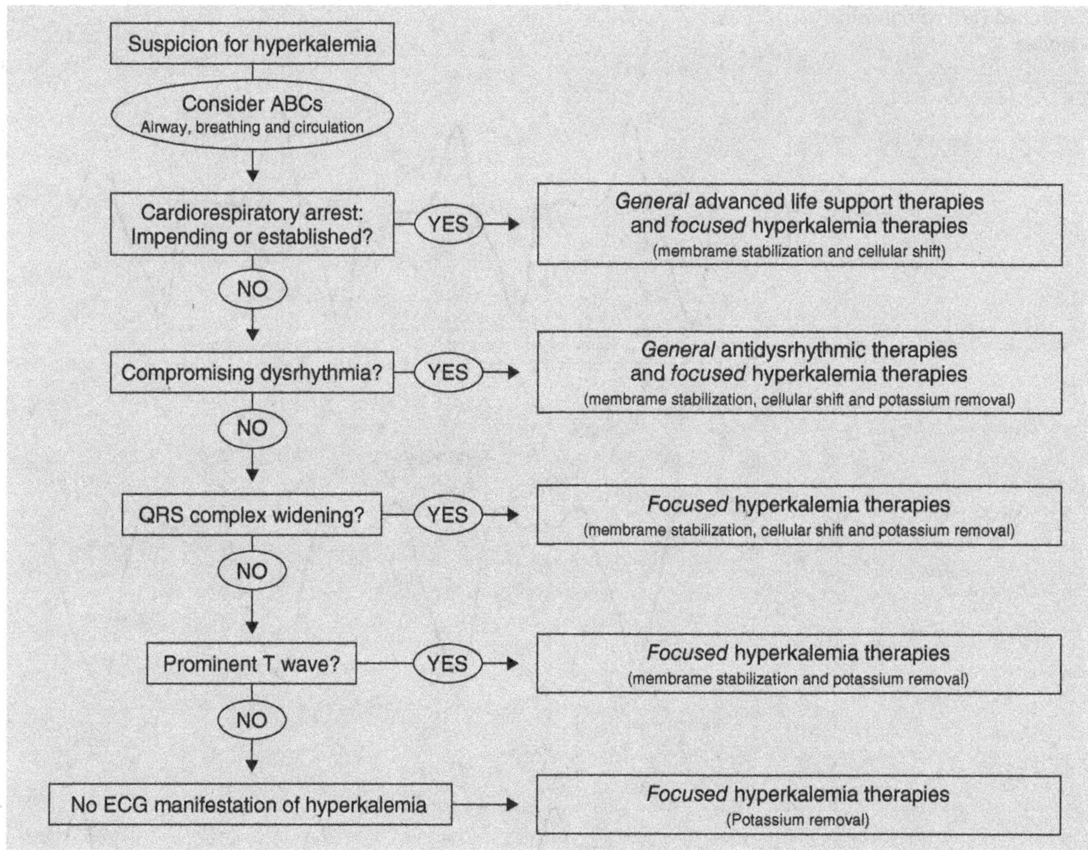

Figure 16.6 ECG-directed guideline for the treatment of hyperkalemia. Of course, the clinician managing the patient is in the best position to determine specific therapy in an individual patient situation.

17

Life-Threatening Electrocardiographic Patterns

Steven H. Mitchell[1], Richard B. Utarnachitt[2], and William J. Brady[3]

[1] Department of Emergency Medicine, University of Washington School of Medicine, Seattle, WA, USA
[2] Airlift Northwest, Harborview Medical Center, University of Washington School of Medicine, Seattle, WA, USA
[3] Departments of Emergency Medicine and Medicine, University of Virginia School of Medicine, Charlottesville, VA, USA

There are several distinct ECG patterns that deserve special mention because they can represent potentially lethal underlying pathology. Each of the ECG patterns discussed below, when recognized in the appropriate clinical situation, should prompt further investigation. Though not an exhaustive list, Table 17.1 summarizes the patterns discussed in this chapter.

Wellens' Syndrome

Wellens' syndrome is a pre-infarct pattern seen on the 12-lead electrocardiogram (ECG). It occurs in the patient with acute coronary syndrome (ACS), who may or may not be experiencing chest discomfort but in whom there is no other evidence of acute myocardial infarction. The natural history of the associated lesion is catastrophic anterior wall myocardial infarction or death within 60–90 days in up to 75% of such patients (Box 17.1).

Electrocardiographic Manifestations

Wellens' syndrome is a characteristic ECG pattern of changes to the T wave in the right to midprecordial leads (leads V1–V4; Figure 17.1). Two patterns of changes to the T waves have been described as follows:

Deeply inverted T wave pattern

- It occurs predominantly across the right and mid-precordial leads (leads V1–V4) but may involve all anterior leads (leads V1–V6) (Figure 17.1a). The pattern typically results in inverted T waves that are symmetric in contour but deeper than "typical" ischemic T waves. This pattern occurs in 75% of cases.

Biphasic T wave pattern

- It is more subtle than the inverted T wave and most commonly occurs in leads V2–V3 (Figure 17.1b). The biphasic T wave morphology is an initial positive, or upright, component of the T wave followed by a secondary inverted, or negative, T wave. This pattern occurs in 25% of cases.

Brugada Syndrome

In 1992, Pedro and Joseph Brugada described a syndrome that is associated with sudden cardiac death in patients with no atherosclerosis and a structurally normal heart. The abnormality found in these patients involves a mutation of the ion channels in the cardiac cell membrane. The mutation leads to a predisposition toward malignant dysrhythmias (Figure 17.2) that terminate in ventricular fibrillation. Patients with this syndrome were noted to have characteristic changes on their ECGs that can lead the informed clinician to diagnose a potentially fatal condition.

Electrocardiographic Manifestations

Characteristic electrocardiographic changes of Brugada syndrome include a complete or incomplete right

The Electrocardiogram in Emergency and Acute Care, First Edition.
Edited by Korin B. Hudson, Amita Sudhir, George Glass, and William J. Brady.

Table 17.1 Etiology and clinical manifestations of life-threatening ECG patterns.

ECG pattern	Etiology	Clinical manifestations
Wellens' syndrome	• High-grade stenosis of the proximal LAD artery	• Anterior wall STEMI • Malignant ventricular dysrhythmia • Death
Brugada syndrome	• Genetic mutation of cardiac sodium channels	• Syncope/"seizure"[a] • Malignant ventricular dysrhythmia • Sudden death
Hypertrophic cardiomyopathy (HCM)	• Genetic mutation of cardiac sarcomere	• Syncope (exertional) Malignant ventricular dysrhythmia Sudden death
Long QT syndrome (LQTS) – congenital	• Genetic mutations of transmembrane ion channels	• Syncope/"seizure"[a] Torsades de pointes Sudden death
Long QT syndrome – acquired	• Medications/toxins, Electrolyte abnormality, CNS event	• Syncope/"seizure"[a] Torsades de pointes Sudden death

[a] Primary seizure disorder is not infrequently misdiagnosed when, in fact, the patient has experienced convulsive syncope as a result of a malignant ventricular dysrhythmia.

Box 17.1 Clinical Consideration – Wellens' Syndrome

Syndrome criteria

- History of recent chest pain
- No ECG evidence of evolving or established AMI
  - No Q waves
  - No loss of R wave progression
  - Normal or minimally elevated (<1 mm) ST segments
- T wave changes: deep symmetric inversion or biphasic morphology
- Normal to minimally elevated cardiac markers

Natural history

- Anterior wall ACS event, frequently STEMI

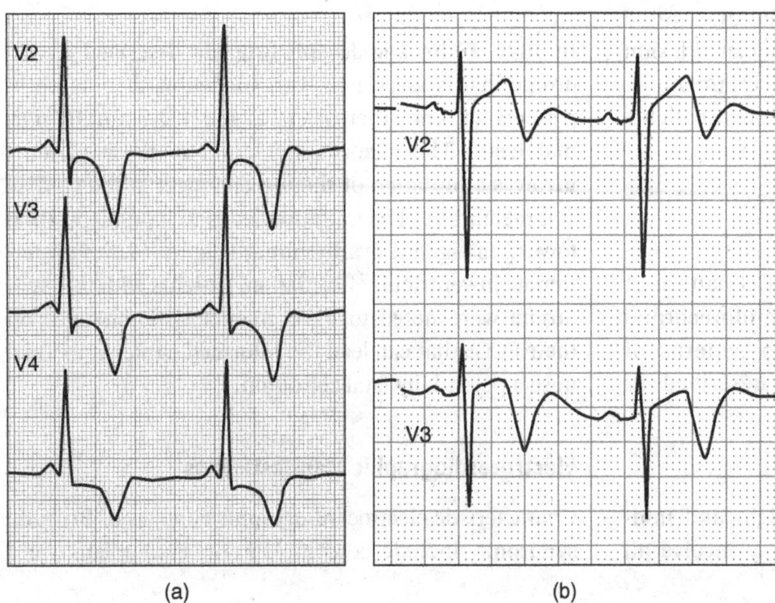

Figure 17.1 T wave morphologies in Wellens' syndrome. (a) Deeply inverted T waves in leads V2–V4. (b) Biphasic T wave (upright and inverted T waves) in the right to midprecordial leads.

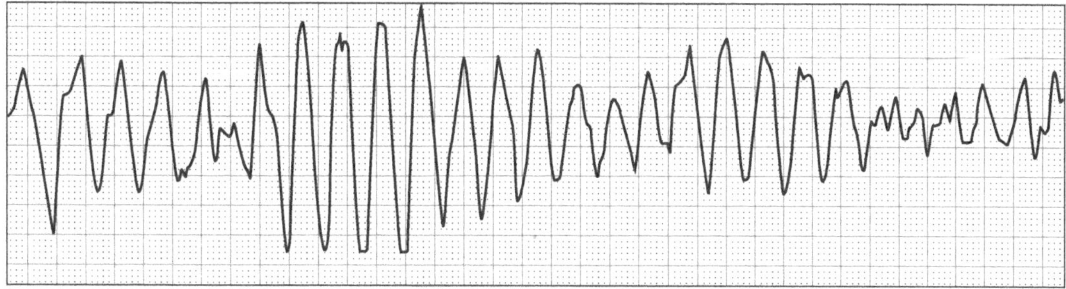

Figure 17.2 Polymorphic ventricular tachycardia, seen in patients with the Brugada syndrome, hypertrophic cardiomyopathy (HCM), and long QT syndrome (LQTS), among many other entities.

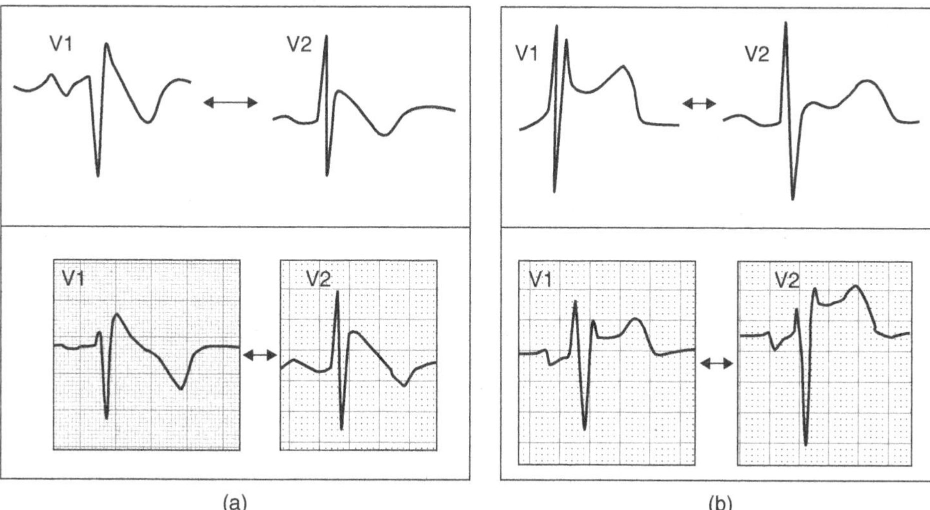

Figure 17.3 Brugada syndrome. (a) The convex/upward "coved" type precordial ST segment elevation with incomplete RBBB pattern. (b) The concave/upward "saddle type" precordial ST segment elevation with incomplete RBBB pattern.

bundle branch block and ST segment elevation in the right precordial leads (leads V1–V3; Figure 17.3). There are two types of ST segment morphologies that have been described:

Convex upward "coved" elevation

- It has a positive terminal R wave and characteristic slurring of the S wave that may be either straight or convex (Figure 17.3a). It has an appropriately discordant (negative) T wave.

Concave upward "saddle-type" elevation

- It is more easily identified by the "horse's saddle" appearance of the ST segment elevation (Figure 17.3b). The terminal R wave is positive but the S wave forms a concave appearance with a positive T wave.

Clinicians should be aware that the characteristic patterns are not fixed but may change with influences such as fever, medications, and age.

Hypertrophic Cardiomyopathy

Hypertrophic cardiomyopathy (HCM) is primarily a disorder of the myocardium (Box 17.2). At rest, most patients with HCM are asymptomatic. Symptoms usually manifest as patients are subjected to conditions producing

Box 17.2 Clinical Consideration – Diagnostic Keys to Hypertrophic Cardiomyopathy

- Young athlete with syncope during exertion or other young person with "adrenergic-mediated" syncope (i.e. fear or anger related).
- Family history of sudden death in family members.
- Systolic murmur worsened with decreased preload (Valsalva) – at times, difficult to detect in the often chaotic emergency situation.
- 12-lead ECG "suggestive" of LVH.

decreased preload, afterload, or contractility – physical exertion, significant emotional distress, and so on. The most feared complication of HCM involves the development of malignant ventricular dysrhythmias, such as polymorphic ventricular tachycardia (Figure 17.2) or ventricular fibrillation. Such events occur most frequently in the setting of exertion – thus, exertional syncope is a typical presentation.

Electrocardiographic manifestations: The two ECG findings consistent with HCM are as follows:

QRS complex morphology

- Large amplitude QRS complexes that are consistent with left ventricular hypertrophy (LVH) with associated ST segment and T wave abnormalities (Figure 17.4). The Sokolow–Lyon index can be used to determine LVH from the ECG. LVH is diagnosed when the S wave in V1 + R wave in V_5 or V_6 (whichever is larger) ≥35 mm or solely by the R wave in aVL ≥ 11 mm.

Q waves morphology

- Deep and very narrow Q waves are the most characteristic and most specific finding of HCM (Figure 17.4). This Q wave morphology is seen in the lateral leads more commonly than in the inferior leads. They may appear in all of the lateral leads – I, aVL, V5, and V6 or in one section of the lateral leads (leads I and aVL or leads V5 and V6); the Q waves of HCM are rarely wide, usually less than 0.04 seconds in width.

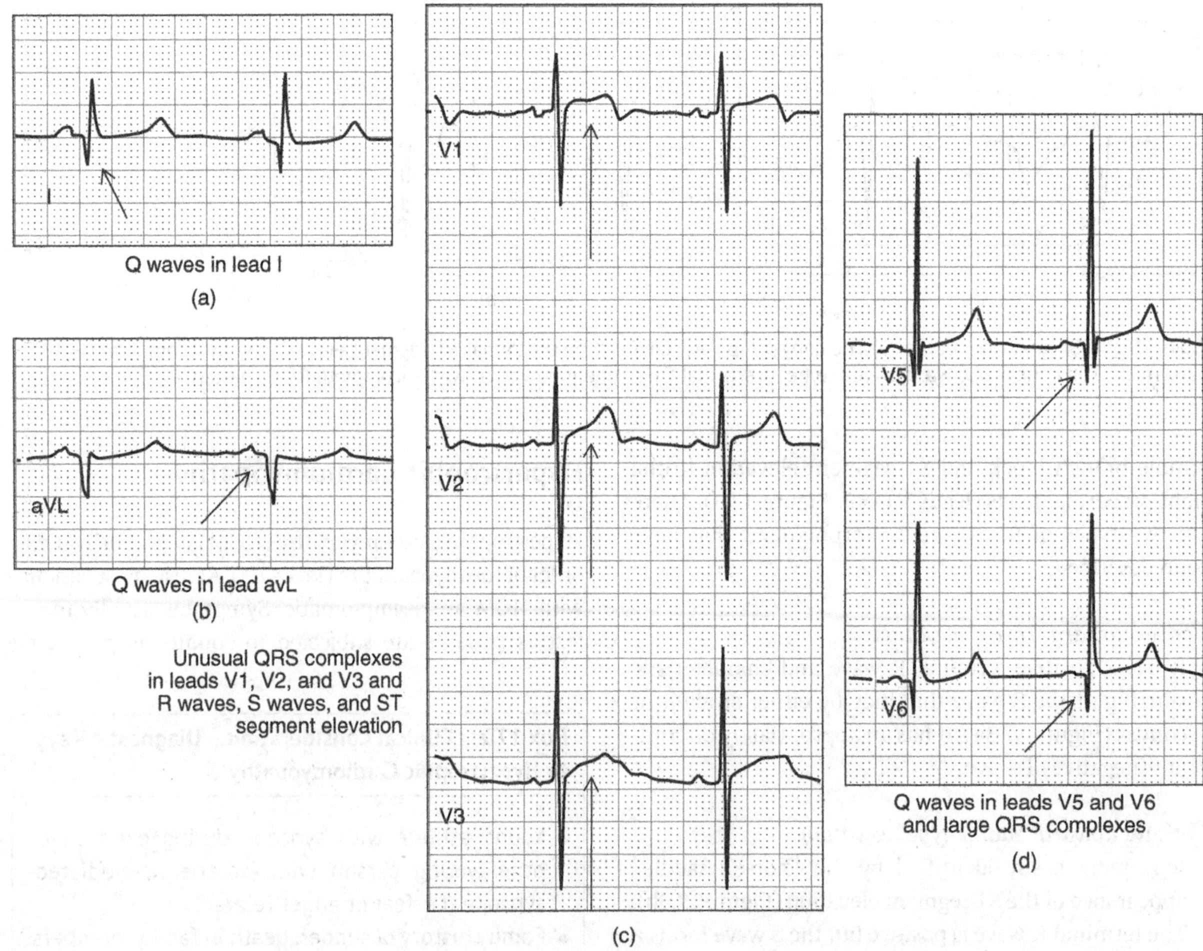

Figure 17.4 The 12-lead with findings suggestive of hypertrophic cardiomyopathy (HCM), including Q waves in the lateral leads (I, aVl, V5, and V6) in (a, b, d). Also note the prominent R waves in leads V1–V3 in (c) as well as ST segment elevation. Finally, note the prominent QRS complexes in the precordial leads consistent with LVH, including large, negative QRS complexes in leads V1–V3 (c) and large, positive QRS complexes in leads V5 and V6 (d). The small arrows denote the Q waves, while the large arrows denote the ST segment elevation.

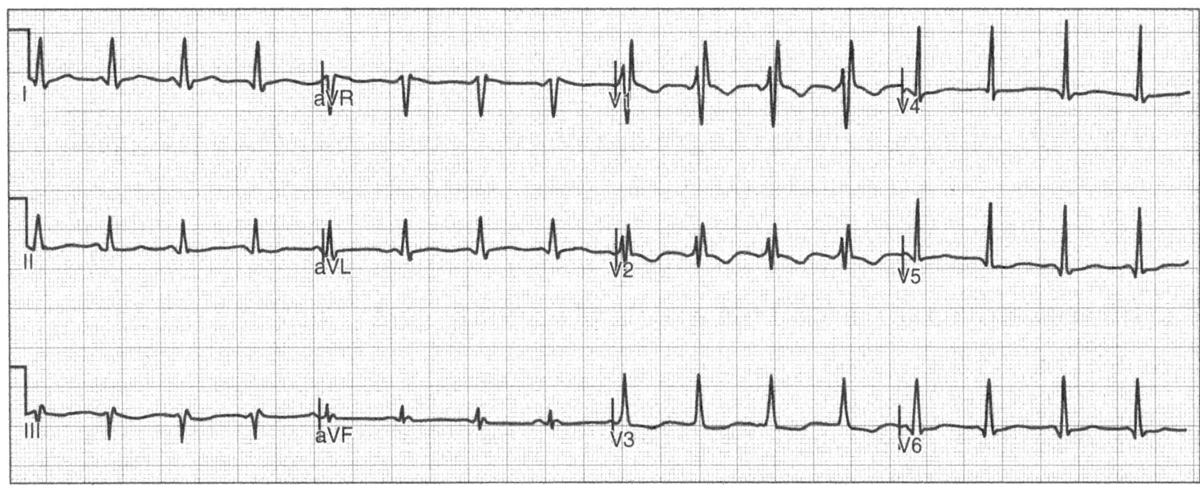

Figure 17.5 Normal sinus rhythm with prolonged QT syndrome with QTc interval of 505 ms; also note the incomplete RBBB pattern. This ECG is an example of prolonged QT interval, illustrating the rather subtle appearance of such an ECG abnormality.

Long QT Syndrome

Long QT syndrome (LQTS) is an electrophysiologic disorder of the heart caused by an abnormality of the repolarization phase of the ventricular action potential. It manifests as a prolongation of the QT interval (Figure 17.5) and can lead to the development of polymorphic ventricular tachycardia (torsades de pointes), ventricular fibrillation, and death (Figure 17.2).

Electrocardiographic Manifestations

QT interval prolongation is considered to occur when the corrected QT (QTc) interval is greater than 440 ms in men and 460 ms in women; in general, a QTc interval greater than 450 ms should be considered abnormal for all patients. Most clinicians, however, do not become concerned until the QTc interval is greater than 500 ms; at this level of prolongation, the chance for dysrhythmias becomes significant. In many instances, the QT interval, even when quite abnormal, is not obvious on the 12-lead ECG. Thus, for clinical presentations that can involve ventricular dysrhythmia (near syncope, syncope, palpitations, etc.), the clinician should review the QT interval.

The QT interval is influenced by the patient's heart rate. Thus, a QT interval cannot simply be measured on the ECG; rather, it should be measured and considered relative to the patient's heart rate. The QT interval is measured from the beginning of the QRS complex to the end of the T wave. The QTc interval is determined using the RR interval (RR). Bazett's formula ($QTc = QT/RR^{1/2}$) is the most commonly utilized formula for determination of the QTc interval.

An easy, bedside determination of the QT interval involves a consideration of the RR interval. When evaluating a rhythm strip, a QT interval that is greater than one-half the accompanying R wave to R wave period, or RR interval, can indicate QT interval prolongation. Similarly, a QT interval that is less than one-half the accompanying RR interval is normal for that particular heart rate. This determination is most appropriately made for supraventricular rhythms with rates from 60 to 100 bpm.

18

The Electrocardiogram in Patients with Implanted Devices

Amita Sudhir[1] *and William J. Brady*[2]

[1] *Department of Emergency Medicine, University of Virginia School of Medicine, Charlottesville, VA, USA*
[2] *Departments of Emergency Medicine and Medicine, University of Virginia School of Medicine, Charlottesville, VA, USA*

Permanent cardiac pacemakers are increasingly encountered in clinical medicine. A basic familiarity with the devices and their electrocardiographic (ECG) findings is essential for clinicians treating both hospitalized patients and patients in the clinic or outpatient setting. The "modern" pacemaker infrequently malfunctions yet a review of the types of pacemaker dysfunction is still appropriate. There are several types of pacemakers, and they are identified according to a universally accepted 3, 4, or 5 designation alphabetical position code. The pacemaker's abilities are described with this coding sequence using various letter designations as described in Table 18.1 and Boxes 18.1 and 18.2.

The Paced Electrocardiogram

A pacer spike is a narrow-appearing electrical discharge on the ECG (Figure 18.1). It can be very large with high amplitude or very small with minimal amplitude. In certain leads, a pacer spike may not be evident. With atrial pacing, a pacer spike can be seen just before the P wave, and both the P wave and the QRS complex appear normal. The ECG appears to be in normal sinus rhythm with the exception of a pacing spike preceding the P wave. With ventricular pacing, a pacer spike can be seen just before the QRS complex, and the QRS complex appears wide. The overall ECG looks similar to a left bundle branch block (LBBB) with the presence of pacer spikes before the QRS complexes. Figure 18.1 demonstrates atrial, ventricular, and atrioventricular pacing.

Pacer spikes may not be visible on a rhythm strip, nor may they be seen on all leads on an ECG. To differentiate between a ventricular paced rhythm (VPR) and LBBB (or other ventricular rhythm), one should consider lead V6. The QRS complex in lead V6 is usually upright with an LBBB, but negative with a VPR.

Pacemaker Malfunction

Pacemaker malfunction can be classified in a number of categories. The issues most often producing ECG abnormality include the following: pacemaker unit malfunction (i.e. battery depletion or component failure), transvenous lead problems, and pacemaker lead–myocardial interface problems. The following pacemaker malfunctions can be seen via the ECG in the clinical setting.

Failure to Pace

The pacemaker does not fire when it should; thus the pacemaker fails to pace (Figure 18.2). On the ECG, pacer spikes are absent. The cardiac rhythm is dependent on the patient's native, or underlying, cardiac rhythm.

Failure to Capture

The pacemaker is firing (i.e. a pacer spike is seen), but no myocardial depolarization occurs (Figure 18.3). Pacer spikes can be seen on the ECG, but without an associated P wave or QRS complex. Again, the cardiac rhythm is dependent on the patient's underlying cardiac rhythm.

The Electrocardiogram in Emergency and Acute Care, First Edition.
Edited by Korin B. Hudson, Amita Sudhir, George Glass, and William J. Brady.

Table 18.1 Pacemaker coding sequence and letter designations.

I – Chamber paced	II – Chamber sensed	III – Sensing response	IV – Programmability	V – Antidysrhythmic functions
A = atrium	A = atrium	T = triggered	P = simple	P = pacing
V = ventricle	V = ventricle	I = inhibited	M = multiprogrammable	S = shock
D = dual	D = dual	D = dual (A and V inhibited)	R = rate adaptive	D = dual (shock and pace)
O = none	O = none	O = none	C = communicating O = none	

Box 18.1 Clinical Consideration – Common Pacemaker Settings

AAIR

- Atria are paced/atria are sensed.
- Pacing is inhibited/rate is adaptive.
- If atrial activity is sensed, pacemaker inhibits itself from pacing.
- Rate depends on the patient's physiologic state.

VVIR

- Ventricles are paced/ventricles are sensed.
- Pacing is inhibited.
- If ventricular activity is sensed, pacemaker inhibits itself from pacing.
- Rate depends on patient's physiologic state.

DDD

- Atria and ventricles are paced/atria and ventricles are sensed.
- Pacing is inhibited in both atria and ventricles.
- If no atrial activity is sensed, the pacemaker generates an atrial beat.
- Subsequently, if no ventricular activity is sensed, the pacemaker generates a ventricular paced beat.

Box 18.2 Clinical Consideration – Automated Internal Cardiac Defibrillators

- Implanted under the skin similar to pacemaker.
- Primary role is defibrillation of VT and/or VF.
  - May also function as pacemaker if so programmed.
- Management of a patient in whom the automated internal cardiac defibrillators (AICD) has fired.
  - Monitor cardiac rhythm via ECG.
  - If normal sinus rhythm or paced rhythm, no further intervention needed.
  - Transport as appropriate.
  - Maintain monitoring.
  - If continued dysrhythmia, initiate appropriate advanced life support therapy.
  - Avoid delivering external shocks directly over AICD unit.
  - AICD generated shocks will display as a large pacer spike on cardiac monitor or ECG.
- AICD function (i.e. continued electrical defibrillation) can be terminated by placing a magnet over the unit.
  - Such a maneuver will not affect the bradycardia pacing function of the AICD.
  - Such a maneuver should only be performed by knowledgeable personnel in situations involving recurrent, inappropriate electrical defibrillations.

Undersensing

The pacemaker does not detect normal cardiac activity and fires when it does not need to (Figure 18.4). On the ECG, pacer spikes can be seen after a normal P or QRS complex, and can result in a paced complex in addition to the native one.

Dysrhythmias

Malfunctioning pacemaker may itself cause abnormal cardiac rhythm. Pacemaker mediated tachycardia occurs when retrograde P waves are sensed by the pacemaker as native, normal P waves, and result in ventricular pacing, causing a reentrant loop and a rapid, wide-QRS complex rhythm.

The Paced Rhythm and Acute Myocardial Infarction

It can be difficult to detect the presence of acute coronary syndrome (ACS) (ischemia or infarction) when a patient has a VPR. In fact, the VPR is said to "confound"

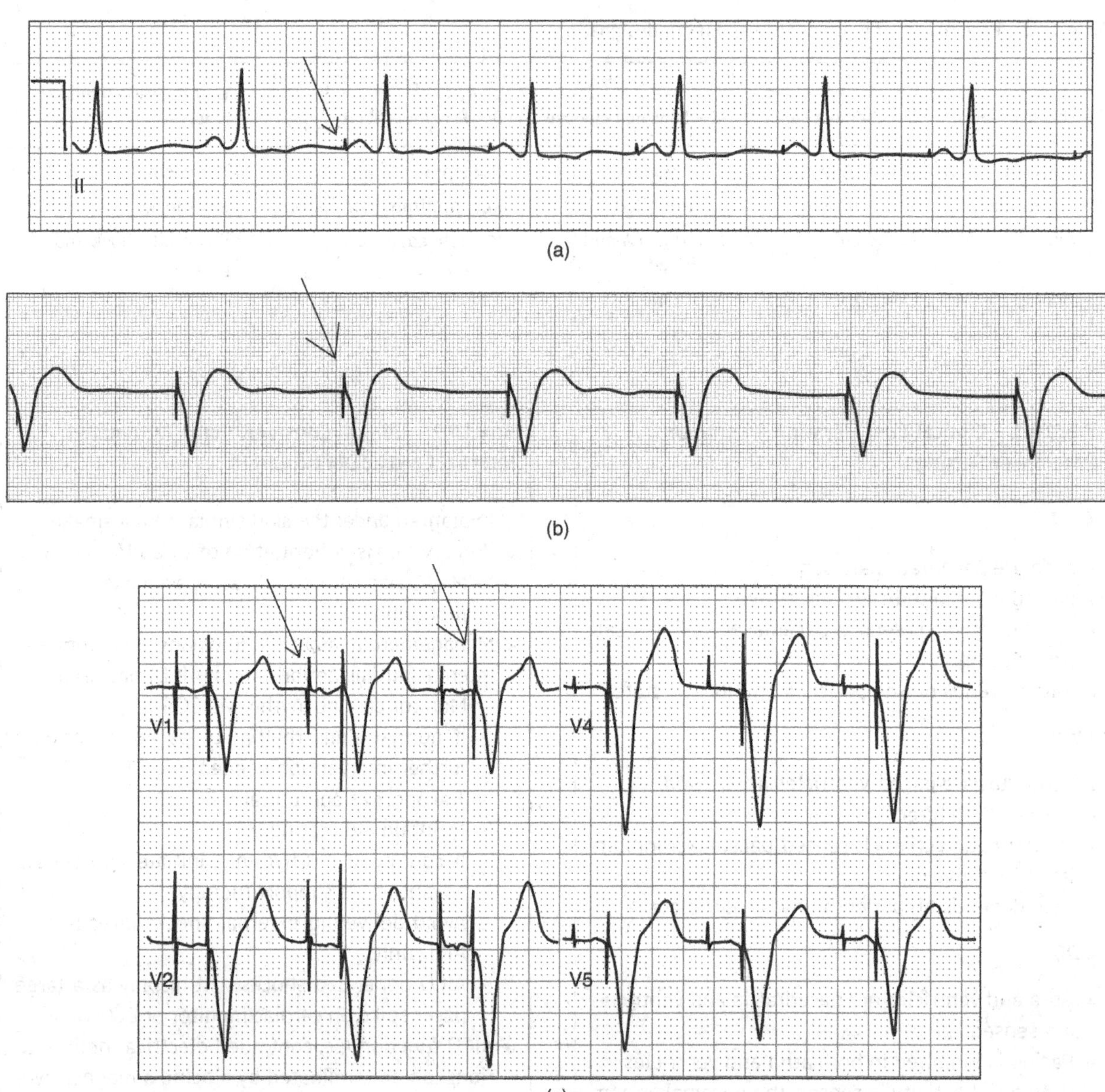

Figure 18.1 (a) Atrial paced rhythm. Note the pacer spike (small arrow) immediately preceding the P wave. (b) Ventricular paced rhythm. Note the pacer spike (large arrow) immediately preceding the widened QRS complex. (c) Atrioventricular paced rhythm. Note the pacer spikes immediately preceding the P wave (small arrow) and QRS complex (large arrow).

the ability of the ECG to detect ACS events. While this statement is largely true, certain patients can demonstrate abnormalities on the ECG that can suggest acute myocardial infarction (AMI).

The concept of appropriate discordance (Figure 18.5) can be used to review the ECG, looking for evidence of AMI. This concept states, in the normal setting, that the major, terminal portion of the QRS complex is located on the opposite side of the baseline from the ST segment; when this situation occurs, the relationship is termed discordance and considered normal. An exception to this statement is found when the degree of discordant elevation is greater than 5 mV; in this setting, the discordant ST segment elevation is considered potentially abnormal. If the ST segment and the major, terminal portion of the QRS complex are found on the same side of the baseline, the relationship is considered concordant and most often abnormal.

As with the LBBB pattern, Sgarbossa and colleagues have developed criteria for the ECG diagnosis of AMI in the presence of VPR pattern; this criteria is very similar to that seen in the LBBB Sgarbossa criteria, including the following findings, referred to as the original VPR Sgarbossa criteria: (i) ST segment elevation of at least 5 mm discordant with the QRS complex; (ii) ST segment elevation of at least 1 mm concordant with the QRS

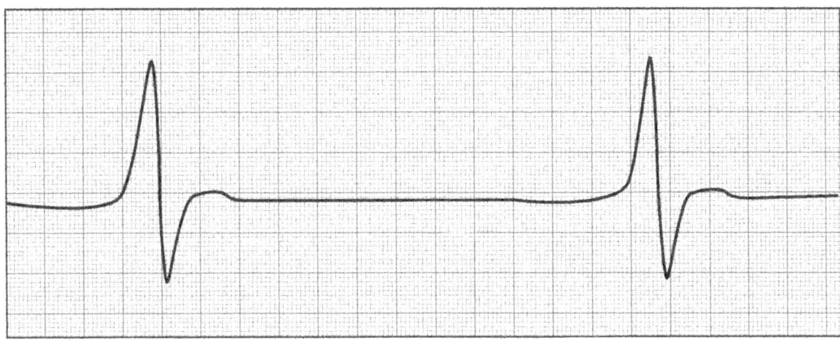

Figure 18.2 Failure to pace. The pacemaker is not functioning properly – in this case, a pacer stimulus (i.e. pacer spike) is not delivered; thus no evidence of pacing occurs. The patient's native rhythm, in this case, an accelerated idioventricular rhythm, is seen.

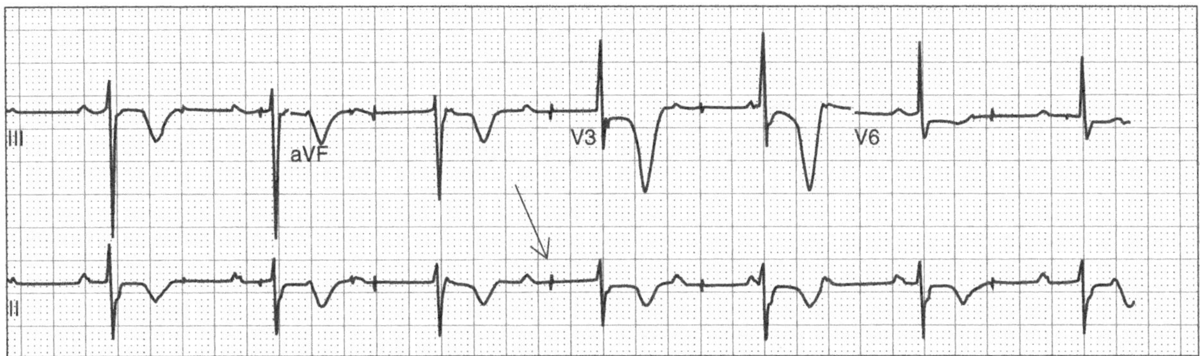

Figure 18.3 Failure to capture. The pacemaker is firing (i.e. a pacer spike is seen [arrow]), but no myocardial depolarization occurs. Pacer spikes can be seen on the ECG, but without an associated P wave or QRS complex. Again, the cardiac rhythm is dependent on the patient's underlying cardiac rhythm.

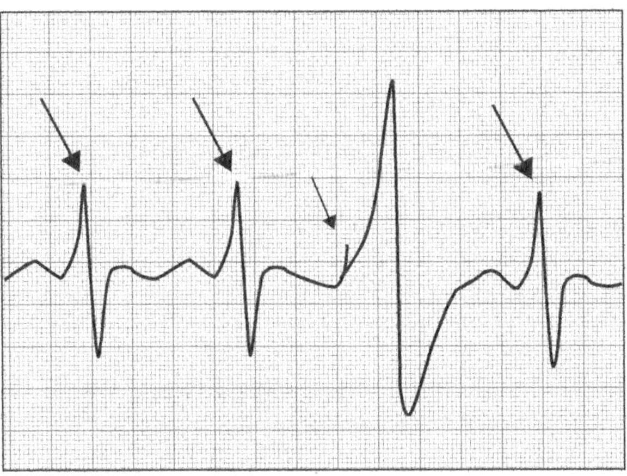

Figure 18.4 Undersensing. The pacemaker does not detect normal cardiac activity and fires when it does not need to. On the ECG, pacer spikes (small arrow) can be seen in the setting of a normal, or native, rhythm (large arrows); the pacer spike results in a paced beat.

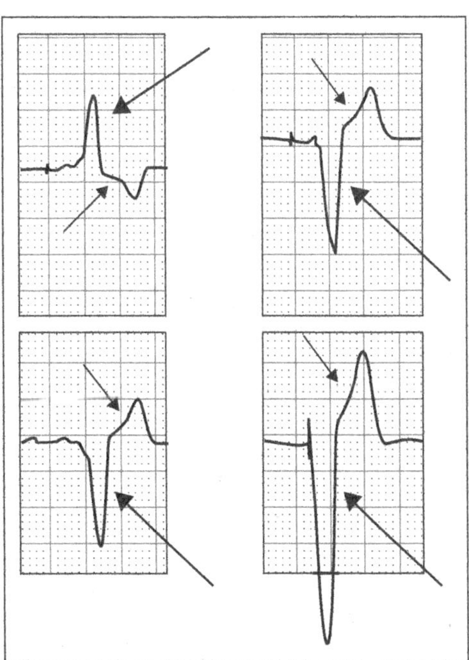

Figure 18.5 The concept of appropriate discordance in ventricular paced rhythms. The large arrows denote the major, terminal portion of the QRS complex, while the small arrows denote the ST segment. These two structures of the P-QRS-T cycle, the QRS complex and the ST segment, are located on the opposite sides of the isoelectric baseline.

complex; and (iii) ST segment depression of at least 1 mm in lead V1, V2, or V3 (Sgarbossa et al. 1996). Recently, the modified Sgarbossa criteria (Dodd et al. 2021) has been validated in the VPR presentation and includes the following three findings, all suggestive of AMI: (i) ST segment elevation of at least 1 mm concordant with the QRS complex; (ii) ST segment depression of at least 1 mm in leads V1–V6; (iii) ST segment elevation of at least 5 mm discordant with the QRS complex. The modified Sgarbossa criteria were more sensitive than the original Sgarbossa criteria of AMI diagnosis; the specificity for AMI diagnosis, however, was very high for both sets of criteria, the original and modified decisions rules. As with the Sgarbossa criteria in the LBBB patient, only one ECG lead need demonstrate such abnormality to support the ECG diagnosis of AMI (Figure 18.6).

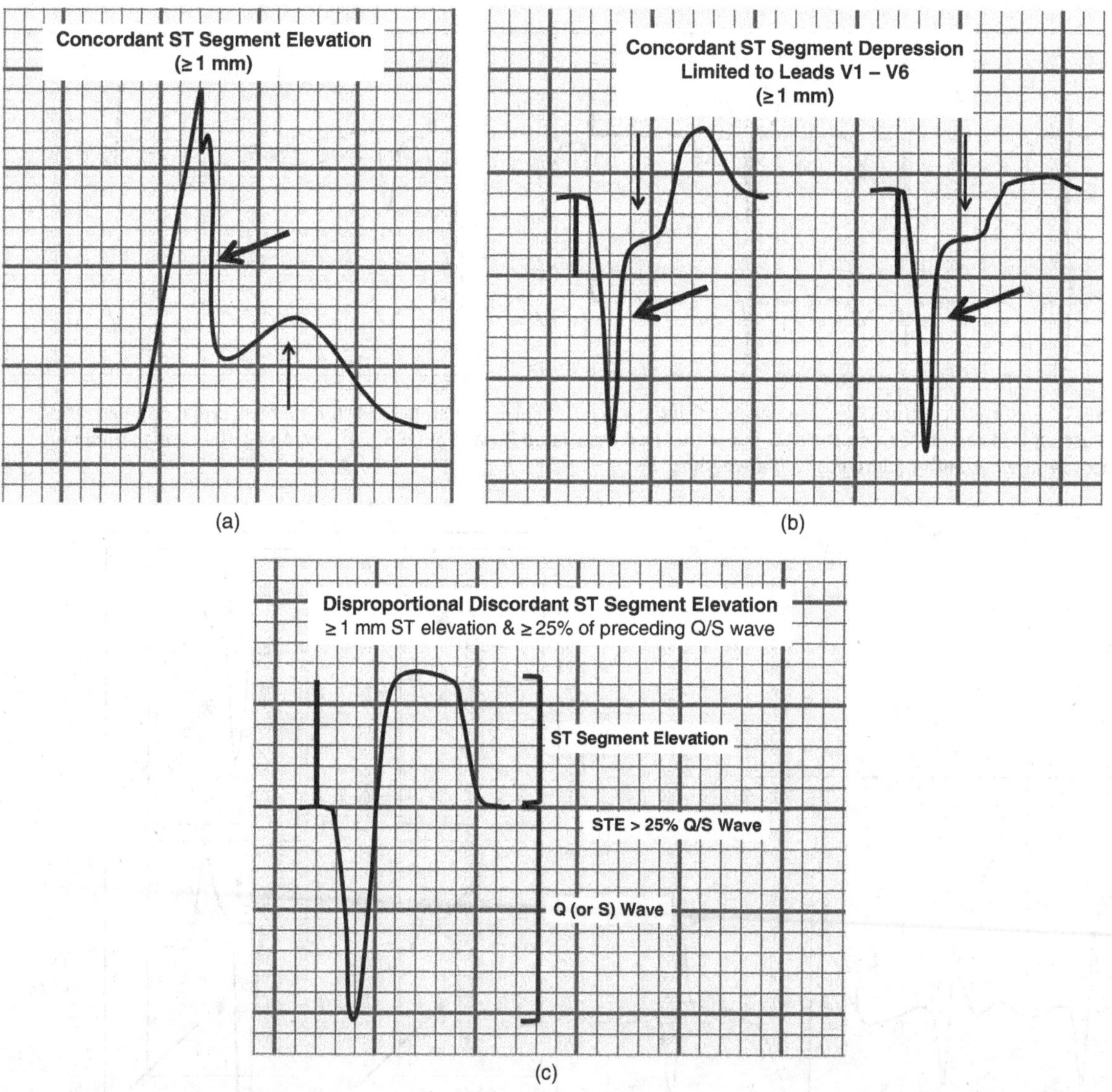

Figure 18.6 The modified Sgarbossa criteria in the right ventricular paced pattern (from an implanted pacemaker). These three findings, if noted in a patient with a clinical presentation consistent with AMI, are suggestive of acute myocardial infarction and provide ECG evidence of acute infarction. Importantly only one lead need demonstrate any of these findings to support the ECG diagnosis of AMI. (a) Concordant ST segment elevation is noted when the ST segment is elevated ≥1 mm and located on the same side of the isoelectric baseline as the major terminal portion of the QRS complex. (b) Concordant ST segment depression is noted when the ST segment is depressed ≥1 mm and located on the same side of the isoelectric baseline as the major terminal portion of the QRS complex. This finding is validated only in leads V1–V6. (c) Disproportional, or excessive, discordant ST segment elevation is noted when the ST segment is elevated ≥1 mm and, when compared to the magnitude of the negative portion of the QRS complex, is ≥25% the accompanying negative QRS complex.

References

Sgarbossa, E.B., Piniski, S.L., Gates, K.B. et al. (1996). Early electrocardiographic diagnosis of acute myocardial infarction in the presence of ventricular paced rhythm. *Am. J. Cardiol.* 77: 423–424.

Dodd, K.W., Zvosec, D.L., Hart, M.A. et al. (2021). Electrocardiographic diagnosis of acute coronary occlusion myocardial infarction in ventricular paced rhythm using the modified Sgarbossa criteria. *Ann. Emerg. Med.* 78: 517–529.

19

Electrocardiographic Tools in Clinical Care

Robin Naples[1], Alvin Wang[2], and William J. Brady[3]

[1] *Thomas Jefferson University, Philadelphia, PA, USA*
[2] *Division of EMS, Jefferson Health System, Philadelphia, PA, USA*
[3] *Departments of Emergency Medicine and Medicine, University of Virginia School of Medicine, Charlottesville, VA, USA*

Cardiac rhythm monitoring and interpretation has evolved from single-lead rhythm strips to advanced multilead ECGs, which can now be rapidly performed, interpreted, and digitally transmitted to specialists and transfer centers. Accurate interpretation of the ECG enables medical providers to rapidly diagnose and treat cardiac arrhythmias, myocardial ischemia, and infarction and an array of metabolic emergencies. Adjuncts to the standard 12-lead ECG may further aid the clinician during the care of the patient, including additional ECG leads and serial electrocardiography.

Additional Electrocardiographic Leads

Two anatomic regions of the heart, the posterior wall of the left ventricle and the entire right ventricle, are less well imaged by the standard 12-lead ECG (Table 19.1). Both of these anatomic regions of the heart are susceptible to infarction. The clinician should consider evaluating these regions in selected situations, including high clinical suspicion for acute myocardial infarction (AMI) with a non-diagnostic 12-lead ECG and certain ST segment depression patterns (Box 19.1).

Posterior Electrocardiographic Leads – Posterior Wall (of the Left Ventricle) Electrocardiographic Imaging

Posterior leads are particularly useful in the diagnosis of posterior wall myocardial infarction; the posterior ECG leads consist of leads V7–V9. Lead V8 is placed on the patient's back at the lower pole of the left scapula and lead V9 is placed half-way between lead V8 and the left paraspinal muscles. Lead V7 is placed on the posterior axillary line (Figure 19.1). In most instances, leads V8 and V9 are used and are adequate; lead V7 is less commonly employed.

ECG lead findings suggestive of acute posterior infarction include ST segment elevation in leads V7, V8, and/or V9 (Figure 19.2). The degree of elevation can be minimal because of the relative distance from the surface electrode to the infracting myocardium. ECG findings other than ST segment elevation in these additional leads have not been defined.

Indirect signs of posterior wall infarction can be present on the standard 12-lead ECG (Figure 19.3). Leads V1–V4 indirectly image the posterior LV from an anterior perspective; thus, the clinician must consider the ECG findings in a "reciprocal manner." In other words, when leads V1–V4 show ST segment depression that is flat or horizontal in configuration and accompanied by a positive QRS complex (i.e. R wave) and upright T wave on a standard 12-lead ECG, the reciprocal perspective from the posterior wall is ST segment elevation with a Q wave and T wave inversion. If one considers all patients suspected of acute coronary syndrome (ACS) who have ST segment depression in leads V1–V4 distribution, approximately 50% of these individuals will be diagnosed with posterior wall ST segment elevation myocardial infarction (STEMI) and the rest with anterior wall ischemia.

The most appropriate indication for obtaining posterior leads is ST segment depression in leads V1, V2, and/or V3 in a patient who is suspected of experiencing an ACS event. Patients with ST segment depression in

The Electrocardiogram in Emergency and Acute Care, First Edition.
Edited by Korin B. Hudson, Amita Sudhir, George Glass, and William J. Brady.

Table 19.1 ECG leads, anatomic segment, and coronary anatomy.

Primary chamber	Cardiac segment	ECG leads	Coronary artery
Left ventricle	Posterior wall	V1–V4 indirectly V8 and V9 directly	Posterior descending branch (RCA) or left circumflex artery
Right ventricle	Right ventricle	RV4 (RV1–RV4)	Right ventricular branch (RCA)

Box 19.1 Clinical Consideration – Diagnosing Acute Myocardial Infarction by Additional Leads

Posterior wall infarction

- In isolation
  - Potential indication for fibrinolytic therapy or emergent revascularization
- In combination with lateral or inferior wall STEMI
  - Higher acute complication rate than lateral or inferior wall STEMI alone
    - Acute heart failure
    - Dysrhythmias

RV infarction

- In isolation
  - Rare
- In combination with inferior wall AMI
  - Poorer prognosis than inferior wall AMI alone
  - Hypotension is common; management issues based upon awareness of RV infarction include:
    - Judicious used of vasodilatory agents (i.e. nitroglycerin and morphine)
    - Aggressive use of normal saline to increase preload

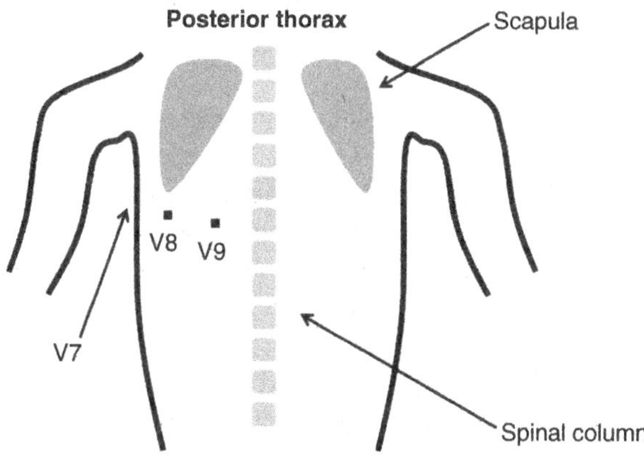

Figure 19.1 Placement of the ECG posterior leads V7–V9.

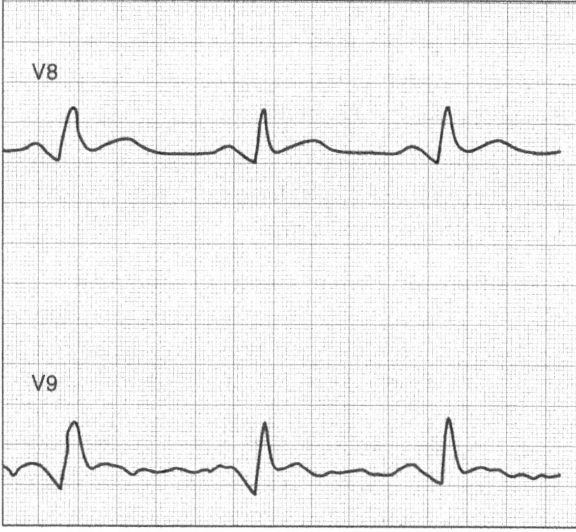

Figure 19.2 The posterior wall of the left ventricle is imaged with leads V7–V9. In this case, only leads V8 and V9 are employed, which demonstrate ST segment elevation. In most instances, leads V8 and V9 are adequate.

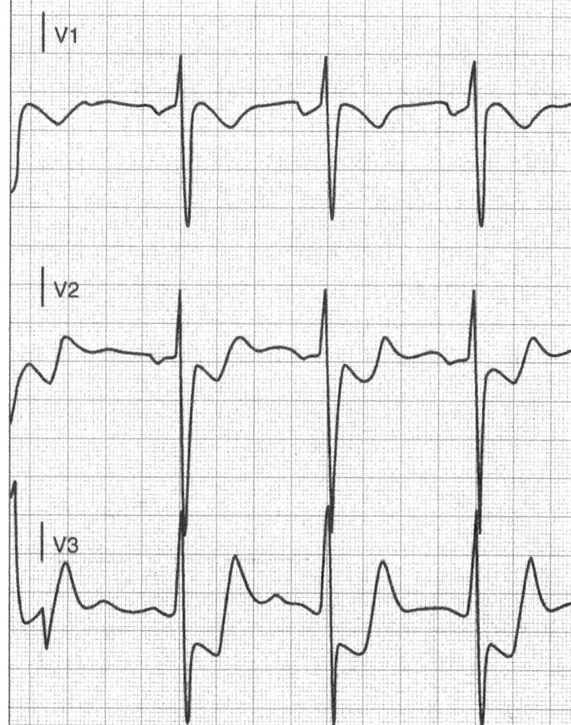

Figure 19.3 ECG leads V1–V3 in a patient with posterior wall acute myocardial infarction. Note the prominent R wave in all three leads and ST segment depression in leads V2 and V3 with upright T waves, all findings consistent with acute posterior wall AMI.

leads V1–V3 resulting from bundle branch block or other instances of abnormal intraventricular conduction are not included in this indication. Posterior wall infarction is not infrequently associated with inferior and/or lateral wall STEMI, which will present with typical ST segment elevation in these regions. Posterior leads may be helpful in this instance to define the full extent of myocardial involvement.

Right-Sided Leads – Right Ventricular Electrocardiographic Imaging

The right-sided ECG leads consist of leads V1R, V2R, V3R, V4R, V5R, and V6R. These leads are also referred to as lead RV1–RV6. They are placed in a mirror image of the traditional left-sided precordial leads and are useful in detecting ST segment elevation associated with right ventricular (RV) myocardial infarction. The most sensitive lead for detecting an RV infarction is lead V4R, which is placed at the fifth intercostal space on the midclavicular line (Figure 19.4). Certain authorities advocate for collection of this lead alone to detect acute RV infarction in the appropriate clinical setting (inferior STEMI with hypotension).

If one adds two posterior ECG leads (V8 and V9) and one right-sided lead (lead V4R) to the standard 12-lead ECG, the 15-lead ECG is produced. The 15-lead ECG is the most commonly used additional lead ECG used in clinical medicine today.

The finding suggestive of RV infarction in the right-sided leads is ST segment elevation (Figure 19.5), irrespective of whether the single lead RV4 (Figure 19.5a) or the entire right-sided array (leads RV1–RV6, Figure 19.5b) of leads is used. Similar to the posterior wall STEMI, the magnitude of the elevation in these leads is usually less pronounced. In the case of RV infarction, the decreased magnitude is due to the relatively small amount of muscle comprising the right ventricle – less myocardium generates a lower current (voltage) of injury, which is manifested by lesser degrees of ST segment elevation – not the distance to the leads.

From the 12-lead ECG perspective, a number of findings are suggestive of RV infarction, including inferior STEMI, excessive ST segment elevation in lead III compared to leads II and/or aVf, and ST segment elevation in lead V1. Right-sided lead placement can be considered in the setting of an inferior wall infarction; in fact, approximately 33% of all inferior wall myocardial infarctions will involve the right ventricle. Indirect signs of RV infarction may be seen on the standard 12-lead ECG. When the RV is involved, the magnitude of ST segment elevation is usually greatest in lead III compared to leads II or aVF (Figure 19.6a,b) – this finding results from the fact that lead III most directly images the right ventricle of the inferior leads; thus ST segment elevation is usually most pronounced in this lead when an RV infarction is present. Furthermore, lead V1 can also demonstrate ST segment elevation.

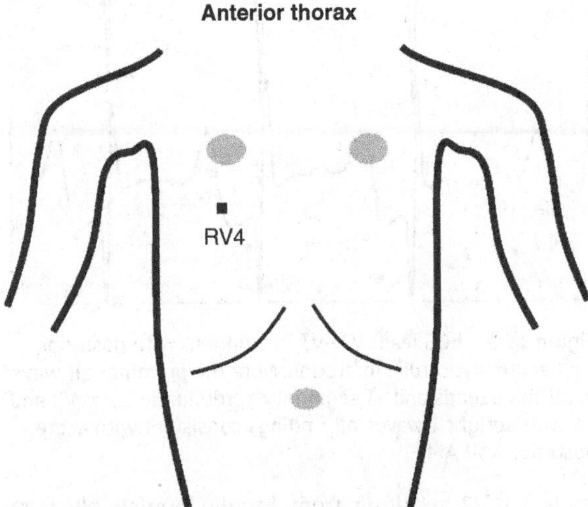

Figure 19.4 Placement of lead RV4, the lead that will directly image the right ventricle. This lead is also referred to as lead V4R.

Serial Electrocardiography

Acute coronary ischemia is a dynamic process involving intracoronary plaque rupture, thrombus formation, and vasospasm. While the myocardium is constantly remodeling in response to the injury, the ECG is a single snapshot in time, recording only several seconds of activity. It can image the heart at a moment in which no acute ischemic changes are taking place while, seconds later, the process can intensify and produce ECG abnormality. The interval at which to perform these repeat ECGs is best determined by the on-scene provider. If the time and the clinical situation permit, repeating the 12-lead ECG in high suspicion patients may increase the rate of ACS diagnosis via the serial ECG (Box 19.2); of course the need for serial ECGs is best determined by the clinician caring for the patient.

A transient, large-amplitude, hyperacute T wave that is asymmetric and broad-based is the earliest manifestation of STEMI (Figure 19.7a). It appears within 30 minutes of coronary occlusion and may also be associated with an R wave of increased amplitude. The T wave broadens as infarction continues and leads to ST segment elevation (Figure 19.7b).

The initial ST segment changes begin as a flattening of the initial upsloping portion as well as a loss of the usual ST segment–T wave angle (Figure 19.8a). Gradually, the ST segment loses its normal concavity and develops a

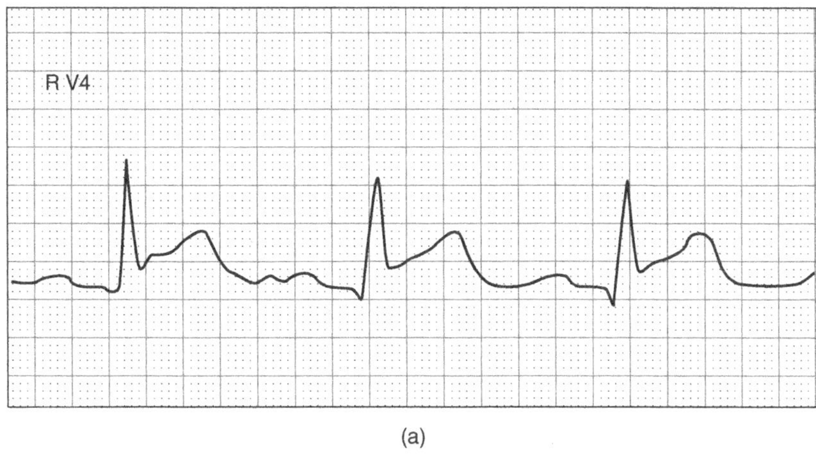

(a)

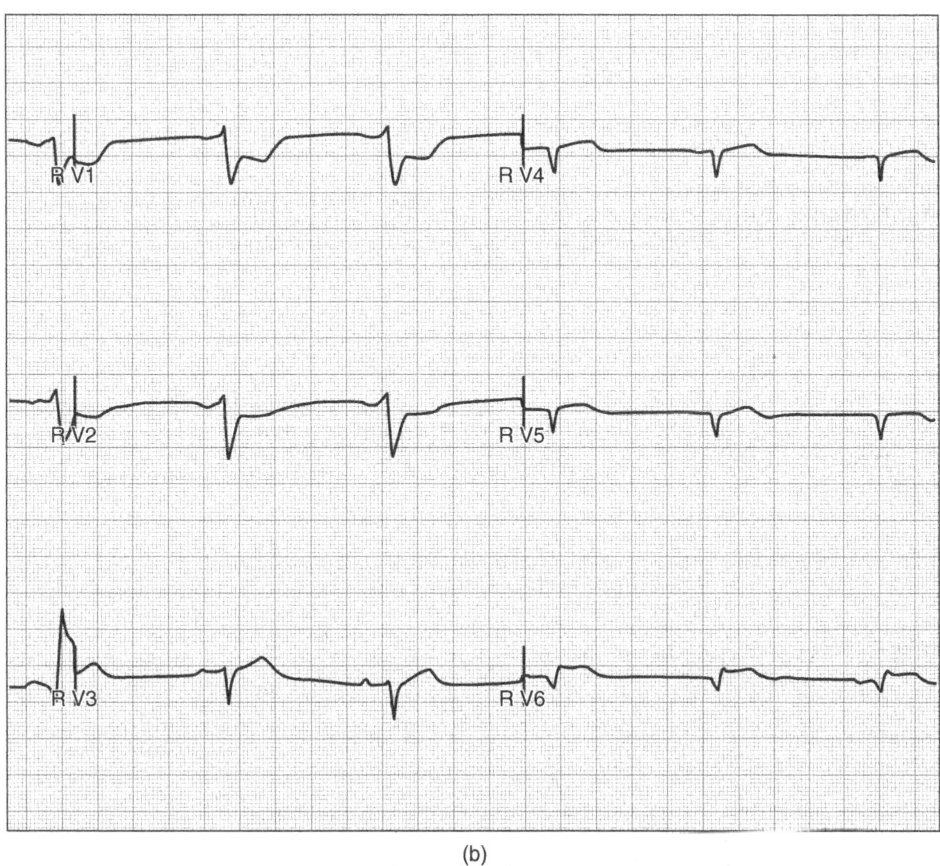

(b)

Figure 19.5 Right-sided ECG leads. (a) Lead RV4 with ST segment elevation consistent with right ventricular acute myocardial infarction. (b) Leads RV1–RV6 in a patient with acute right ventricular infarction. In this case, subtle ST segment elevation is noted in leads RV3–RV6.

convex or obliquely straight orientation as it begins to elevate in relation to the J-point (Figure 19.8b). This may be a subtle elevation or the classic "tombstone" morphology where the ST segment and T wave have become indistinguishable. Reciprocal ST segment depression may become more prominent in anatomically opposing leads as ST segment elevation evolves.

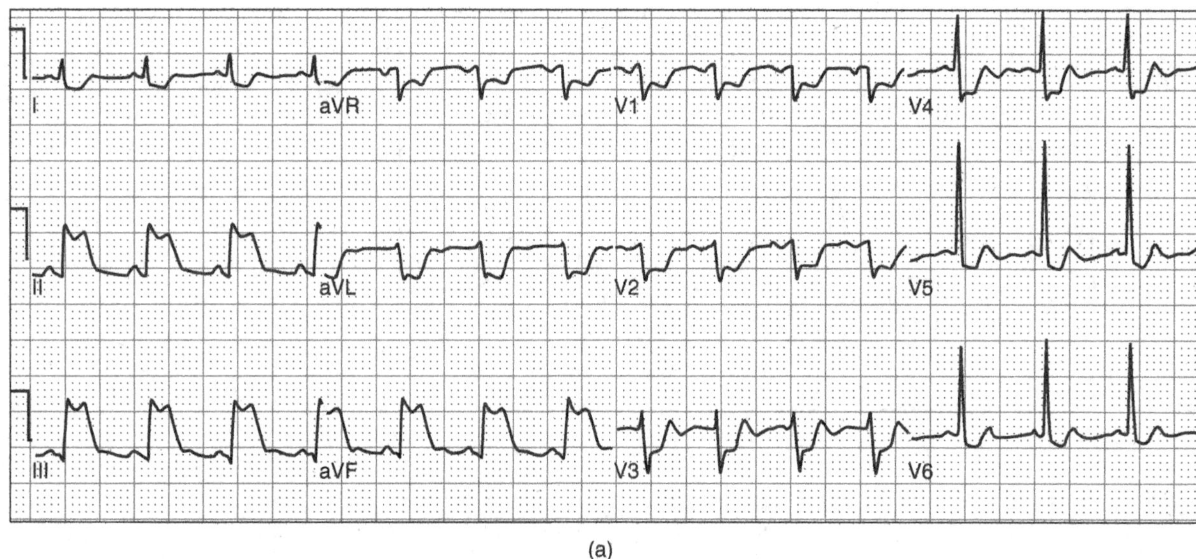

(a)

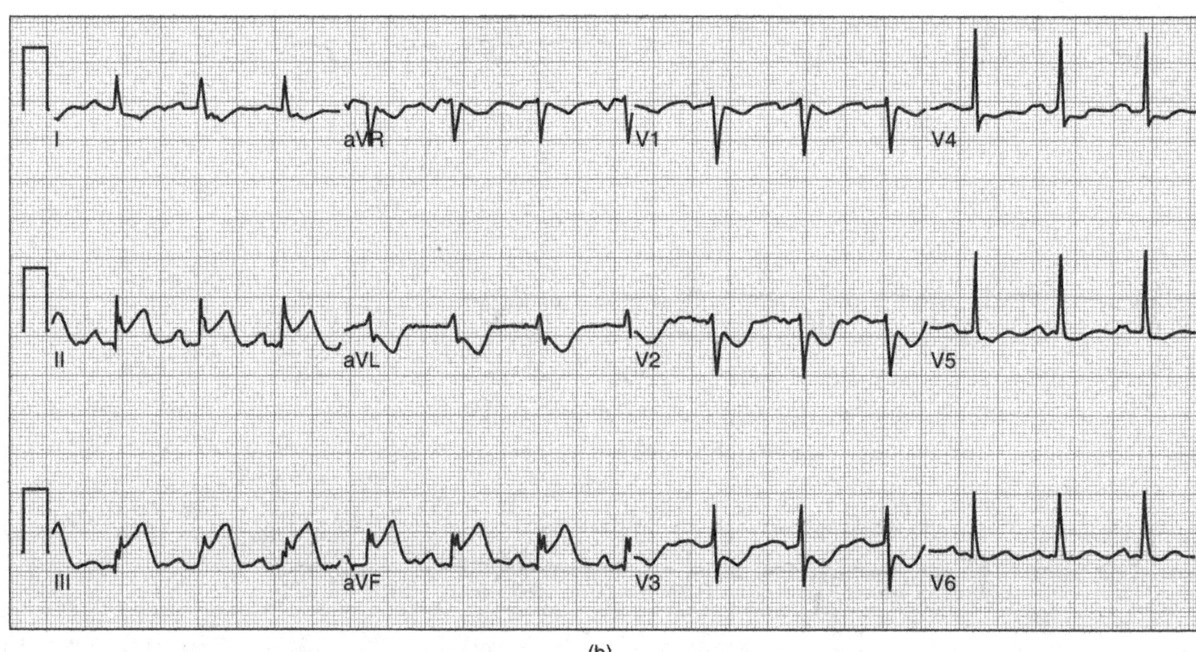

(b)

Figure 19.6 (a) Inferior STEMI with RV and posterior wall infraction. This patient presented with hypotension, which is very common with RV infarction. In addition, the degree of ST segment is greatest in lead III compared to the other inferior leads; RV infraction is likely present based upon the hypotension and disproportionate amount of ST segment elevation in lead II – all of which is occurring within the setting of an inferior STEMI. ST segment depression is seen in leads V1–V3, which is likely consistent with posterior wall myocardial infarction. (b) ECG findings similar to those in (a) in a patient with inferoposterior infarction with RV involvement.

Box 19.2 Clinical Consideration – Potential Indications for Serial Electrocardiogram

- High suspicion for ACS
  - Non-diagnostic ECG
  - Ongoing discomfort
  - Change in clinical status
- Resolution of pain in STEMI patient

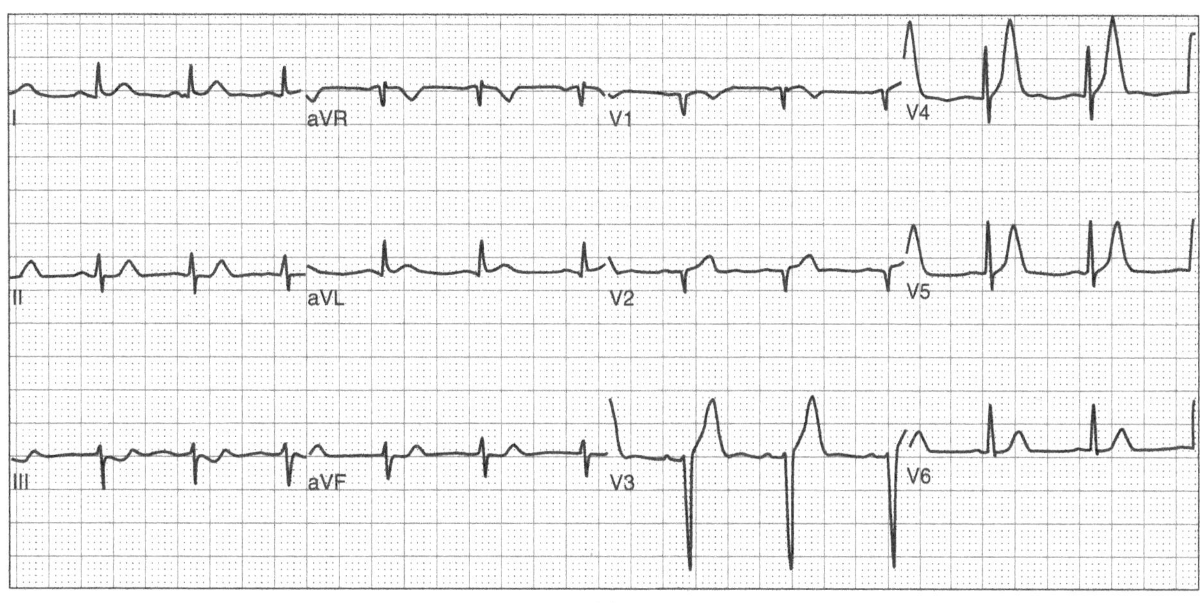

(a)

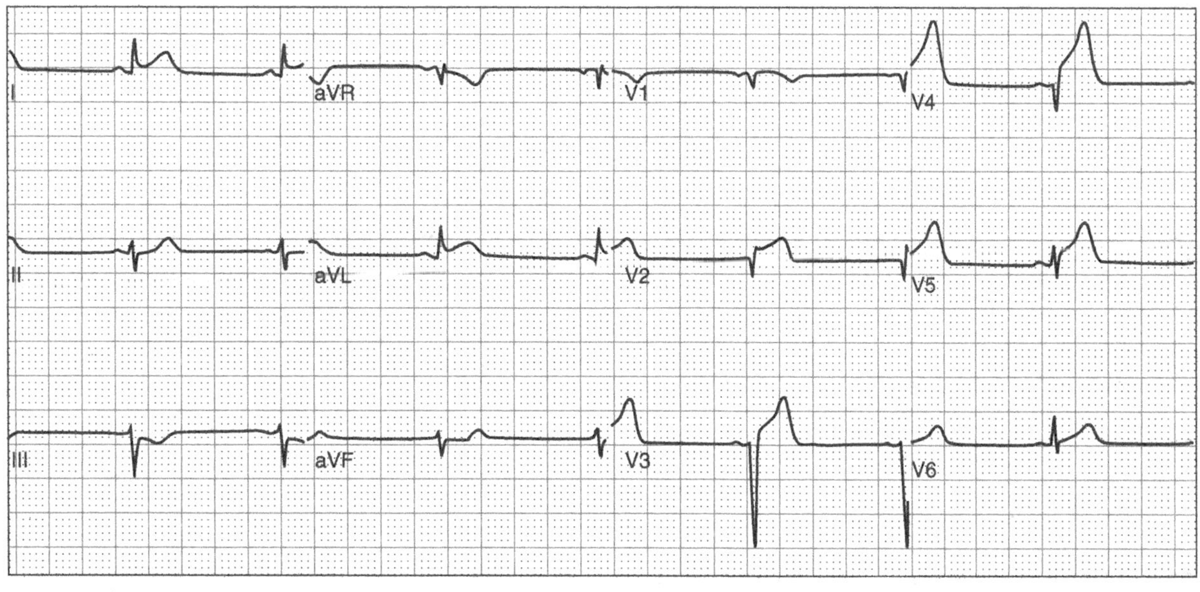

(b)

Figure 19.7 Serial ECGs. (a) 12-lead ECG with concerning findings for early ACS, including borderline ST segment elevation in leads I, aVl, V1, and V2 as well as prominent, hyperacute T waves in leads V3–V5. (b) Repeat ECG over approximately seven minutes from (a) demonstrating an anterolateral STEMI with ST segment elevation in leads V2–V6 as well as in leads I and aVL. Reciprocal ST segment depression is also seen here in leads III and aVf.

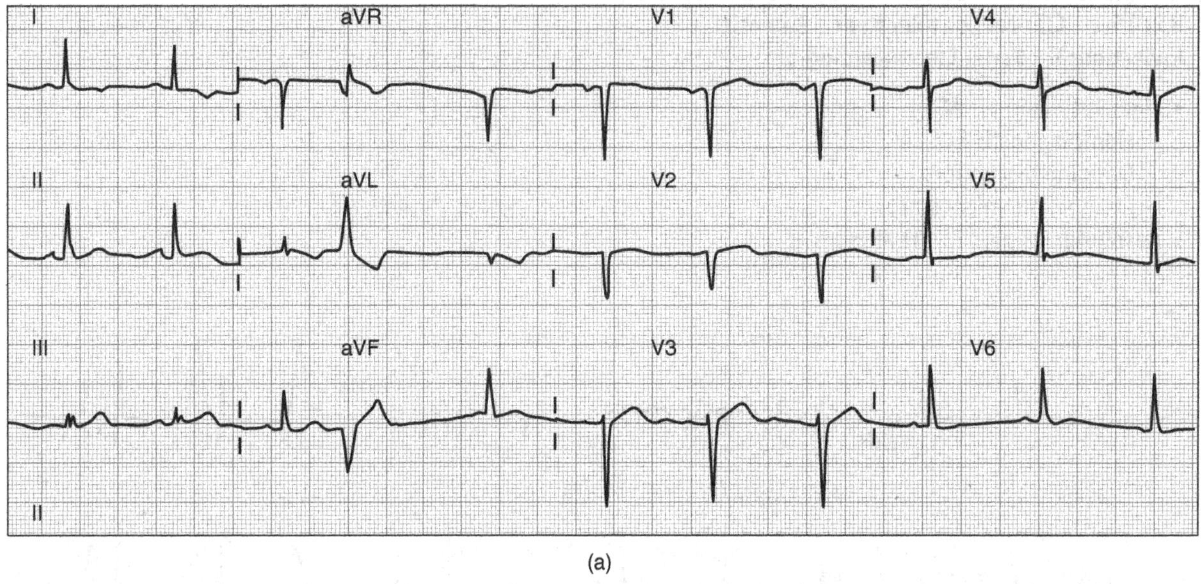

(a)

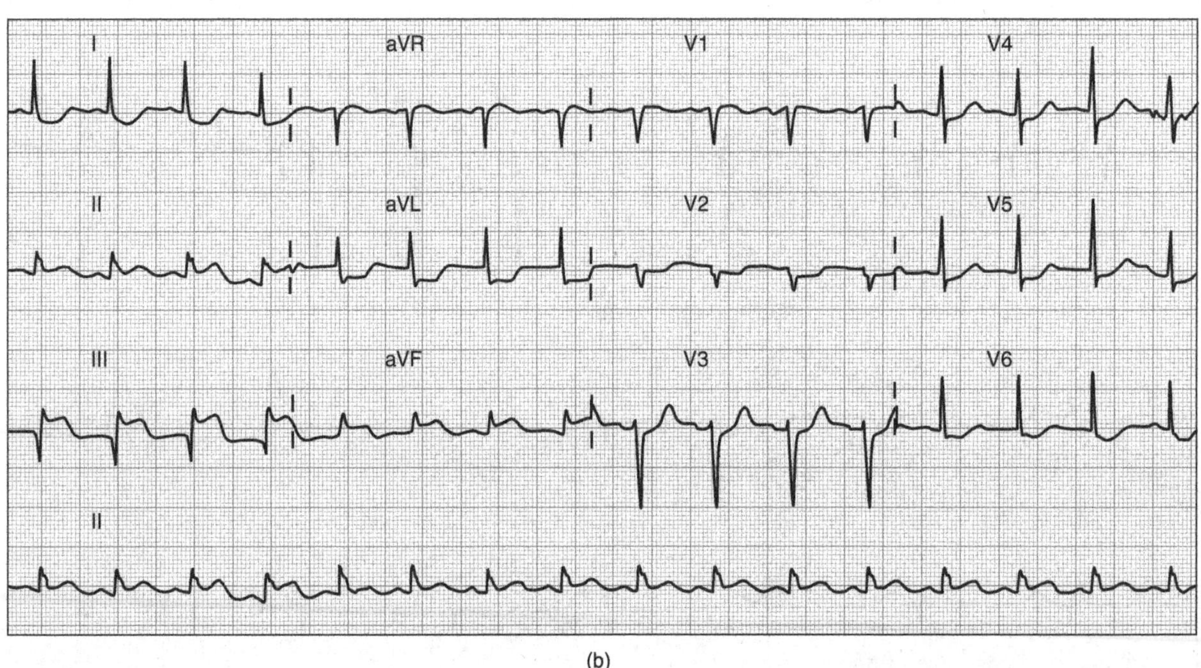

(b)

Figure 19.8 Serial ECGs. (a) Borderline, or subtle, ST segment elevation in leads III and aVf, concerning for an early inferior STEMI. (b) Repeat ECG for (a) approximately 12 minutes later with obvious inferior STEMI.

20

Wolff–Parkinson–White Syndrome

William J. Brady

Departments of Emergency Medicine and Medicine, University of Virginia School of Medicine, Charlottesville, VA, USA

The Wolff–Parkinson–White syndrome (WPW) is a ventricular preexcitation syndrome involving the electrocardiographic combination of bundle branch block and shortened PR interval; a number of these patients, who are healthy with otherwise normal hearts, experience recurrent episodes of supraventricular tachycardias (Box 20.1). The basic issue responsible for these clinical findings is the accessory pathway, an abnormal electrical connection that bypasses the atrioventricular (AV) node and creates a direct electrical connection between the atria and ventricles. Electrical impulses within the atria bypass the AV node and His-Purkinje system using this accessory pathway, activating the ventricular myocardium both directly and earlier than expected. The resultant ventricular depolarization is due to a combination of impulses traveling through both the AV node and the accessory pathway. Aside from establishing the abnormal electrical connection between the atria and the ventricles, the accessory pathway also provides uncontrolled conduction; this "uncontrolled conduction" means that any and all electrical impulses that arrive at the accessory pathway will be transmitted to the ventricle without delay. This "uncontrolled conduction" produces the risk of extremely rapid ventricular rates and the loss of protection by the AV node (which limits the number of impulses that travel to the ventricle via the AV node).

When in sinus rhythm, the classic electrocardiographic triad of WPW includes the following features (Figure 20.1):

1) PR interval less than 0.12 seconds;
2) Initial slurring of the QRS complex, known as a delta wave; and
3) Widened QRS complex with a duration greater than 0.12 seconds.

The PR interval is shortened because the impulse progressing down the accessory pathway is not subjected to the physiological slowing that occurs in the AV node (Figure 20.1). Thus, the ventricular myocardium is activated by two separate pathways, resulting in a fused, or widened, QRS complex. The initial part of the QRS complex, the delta wave, represents aberrant activation through the accessory pathway; the terminal portion of the QRS complex represents activation of the remaining ventricular myocardium, via both the accessory pathway and the His-Purkinje system (Figure 20.1).

To be diagnosed with the WPW syndrome, the patient must demonstrate the electrocardiographic findings in sinus rhythm noted above as well as symptomatic tachydysrhythmias, including paroxysmal supraventricular tachycardia (PSVT, including both the NCT and wide complex tachycardia [WCT] varieties) (70%), atrial fibrillation (25%), atrial flutter (5%), and ventricular fibrillation (rare). The most common tachycardia in WPW is PSVT; from an electrophysiologic perspective, this form of tachycardia is termed an *atrioventricular reentrant tachycardia*. WPW PSVT can present in one of two types as separated by and identified via the width of the QRS complex: narrow and wide QRS complex tachycardias. Narrow complex tachycardia (NCT), the most common dysrhythmia of symptomatic WPW, is characterized by the following conduction features: forward electrical conduction from the atria to the ventricle through the AV node and retrograde movement of the impulse via the accessory pathway from the ventricle to the atria (Figure 20.2a). The QRS complex is narrow because of the depolarization wave's use of the ventricular conduction pathway, producing rapid, efficient movement of the impulse throughout the ventricles.

The Electrocardiogram in Emergency and Acute Care, First Edition.
Edited by Korin B. Hudson, Amita Sudhir, George Glass, and William J. Brady.

Box 20.1 Clinical Considerations – The Patient with Wolff–Parkinson–White Syndrome

- *Patient age at presentation ranges from neonatal to geriatric.*
- *Patients have structurally normal hearts.*
- *ECG triad in normal sinus rhythm.*
  - Shortened PR interval
  - Delta wave
  - Minimally widened QRS complex
- *Dysrhythmias*
  - Narrow QRS complex tachycardia (rapid and regular)
  - Wide QRS complex tachycardia (rapid and regular)
  - Atrial fibrillation (rapid, irregular, and bizarre QRS complex morphologies)

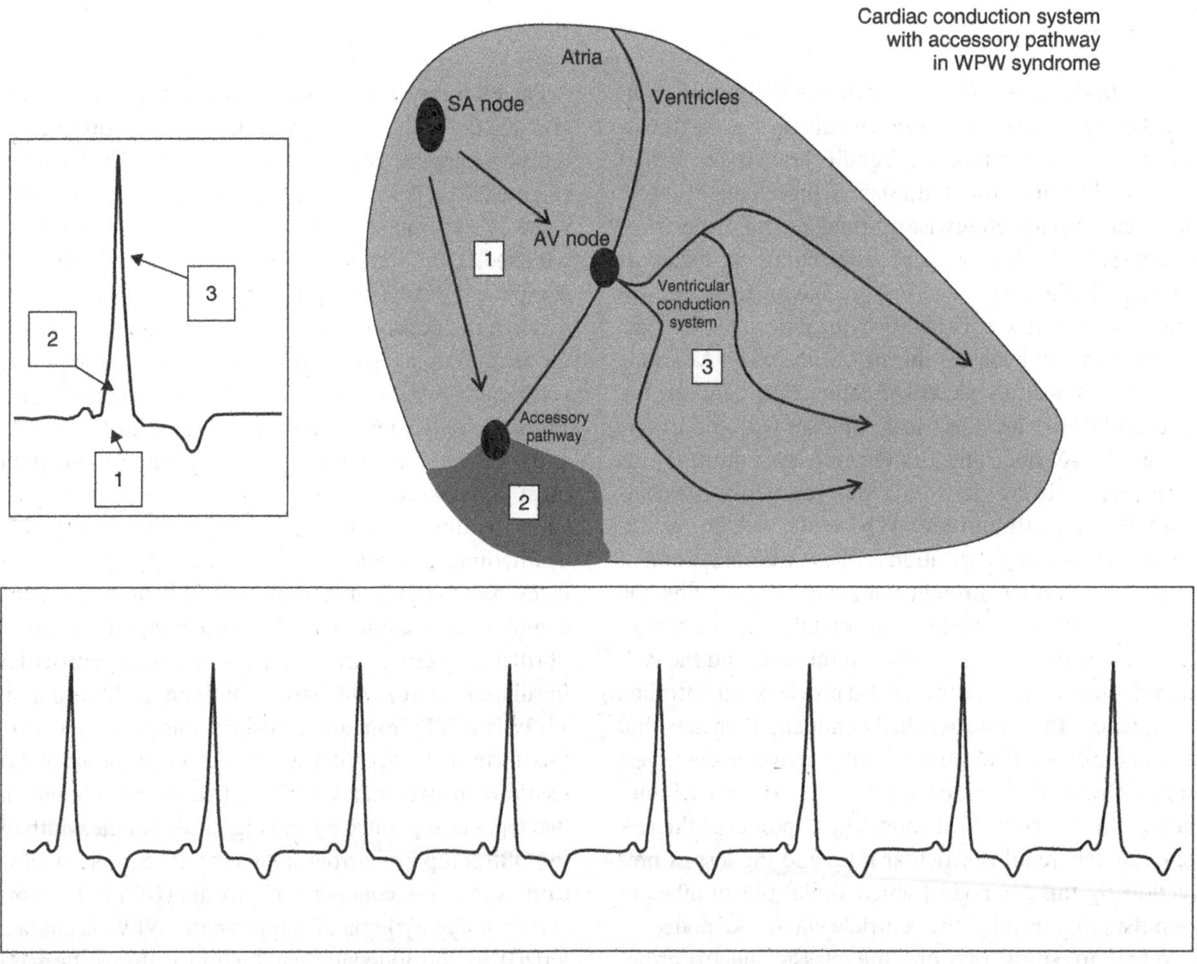

Figure 20.1 The ECG in the patient with WPW syndrome while in normal sinus rhythm (NSR). Note the classic triad of ECG findings, including the shortened PR interval (denoted by "1"), the delta wave (the initial slurring of the QRS complex, "2"), and the minimally widened QRS complex ("3"). While in NSR, the impulse travels through the atrial tissues and is transmitted to the ventricle via both the AV node and accessory pathway. The impulse arrives earlier than anticipated to the ventricular myocardium thus the PR interval is shorter ("1") than the normal lower range of 0.12 seconds. The impulse travels into the ventricle via both the AV node and accessory pathway. The portion of the ventricular myocardium that depolarizes as a result of the impulse traveling through the accessory pathway is manifested on the ECG by the delta wave ("2"). Then, as the impulse moves into the ventricle via the accessory pathway and intraventricular conduction system, the QRS complex is minimally widened ("3"). This widening results from the inefficient conduction of the accessory pathway-transmitted impulse throughout the ventricular myocardium (i.e. the intraventricular conduction system is not used).

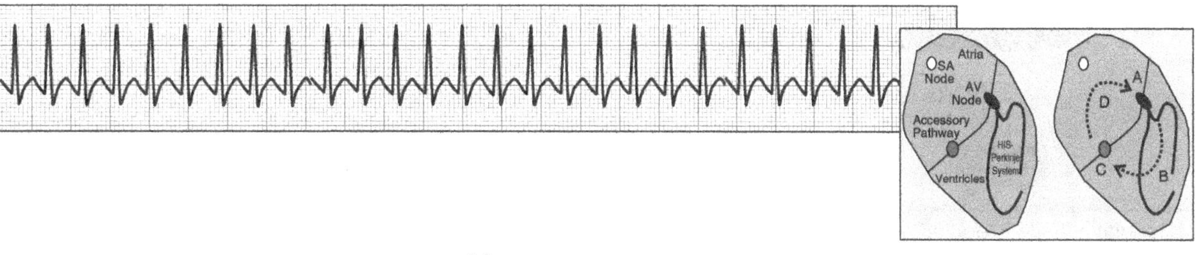

(a)

(b)

(c)

Figure 20.2 (a) Narrow QRS complex tachycardia (rapid and regular). The impulse moves forward from the atria into the ventricle via the AV node (depicted by "A") and returns to the atria from the ventricles via the accessory pathway (depicted by "C"). The QRS complex is narrow in that the impulse travels throughout the ventricular myocardium via the ventricular conduction system (depicted by "B"). The impulse then moves through atrial myocardium (depicted by "D") and reenters the AV node, repeating the reentry loop and sustaining the dysrhythmia. This rhythm is difficult, if not impossible, to distinguish from typical paroxysmal supraventricular tachycardia. (b) Wide QRS complex tachycardia (rapid and regular). The impulse moves forward from the atria into the ventricle via the accessory pathway (depicted by "A") and returns to the atria from the ventricles via the AV node (depicted by "C"). The QRS complex is wide in that the impulse does not use the ventricular conduction system thus the impulse is inefficiently transmitted throughout the ventricular myocardium (depicted by "B"). The impulse travels through the atrial myocardium from the AV node to the accessory pathway (depicted by "D"), reentering the ventricle and completing the reentry loop. This rhythm is difficult to distinguish from ventricular tachycardia. (c) Atrial fibrillation. The impulse moves forward from the atria into the ventricle via both the accessory pathway (depicted by "B") and the AV node (depicted by "A"). The impulse that arrives at the ventricular myocardium via the accessory pathway (depicted by "C") produces an earlier than anticipated depolarization of a portion of the ventricular myocardium; this area of early ventricular depolarization is manifested on the ECG as the delta wave. The rate is extremely rapid because of the loss of impulse conduction control provided by the AV node. The QRS complex varies in shape from beat to beat; this variation in QRS complex morphology results from a combination of the impulse arriving via the AV node and the accessory pathway (depicted by "D") – each beat results from a fusion of these two impulses.

This conduction loop, if sustained, will produce a rapid, regular, narrow QRS complex tachycardia (Figure 20.2a).

The other form of the WPW PSVT, an uncommon dysrhythmia, presents with a wide QRS complex, producing a WCT. Its conduction pattern is the reverse of the NCT variety described above: forward electrical conduction from the atria to the ventricle through the accessory pathway and retrograde movement of the impulse via the AV node from the ventricle to the atria (Figure 20.2b). The QRS complex is wide in that the ventricular conduction system is not used to spread the impulse throughout the ventricular myocardium.

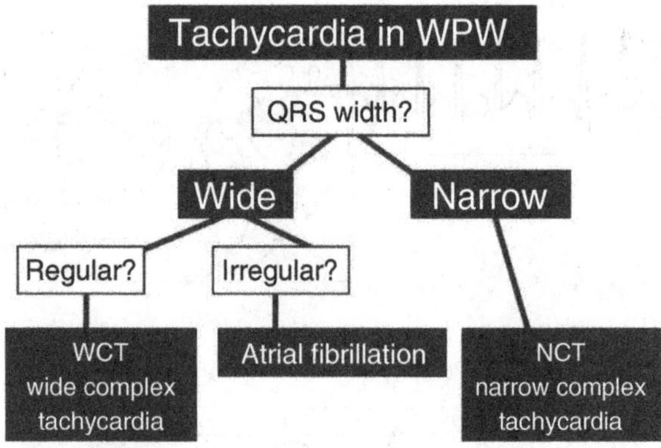

Figure 20.3 Algorithm for the differentiation of the three dysrhythmias seen in the WPW patient using simple observations, including rate, QRS complex width, and regularity.

The electrocardiogram (ECG) will demonstrate a rapid, regular, wide QRS complex tachycardia (Figure 20.2b).

Atrial fibrillation is also seen in the WPW patient; it is the second most frequent rhythm disturbance encountered in these patients. In this setting, the supraventricular impulses are transmitted simultaneously from the atria to the ventricles via both the accessory pathway and the AV node. As noted, the loss of rate limiting protection by the AV node subjects the ventricle to the extremely rapid rates in this form of atrial fibrillation. Also, the electrical impulse arrives at the ventricle by both conduction pathways (AV node and accessory pathway). The end result of these two physiologic properties is an extremely rapid, irregular, wide QRS complex tachycardia; further, the various QRS complexes vary in appearance with different morphologies from beat-to-beat (Figure 20.2c).

Box 20.2 Clinical Considerations – Urgent Treatment of Wolff–Parkinson–White-Related Dysrhythmias

- *Narrow QRS complex tachycardia*
  - *Unstable*
    - Electrical cardioversion
    - Adenosine
  - *Stable*
    - Adenosine
    - Procainamide
    - β-Blocker/calcium channel blocker
- *Wide QRS complex tachycardia*
  - *Avoid all AV node blocking medications*
  - *Unstable*
    - Electrical cardioversion
  - *Stable*
    - Procainamide
- *Atrial fibrillation*
  - *Avoid all AV node blocking medications*
  - *Unstable*
    - Electrical cardioversion
  - *Stable*
    - Procainamide

Figure 20.3 provides a simplified approach to rhythm differentiation in the WPW syndrome. Obviously, ventricular fibrillation is life threatening – whether it is related to WPW or not. If one considers the other three forms of tachycardia, all three have the possibility of cardiovascular decompensation, yet atrial fibrillation and the WCT forms of the PSVT are the most dangerous. Refer to Box 20.2 for a review of the major treatment issues in WPW dysrhythmias.

21

Cardiac Arrest Rhythms

Amita Sudhir[1] *and William J. Brady*[2]

[1] *Department of Emergency Medicine, University of Virginia School of Medicine, Charlottesville, VA, USA*
[2] *Departments of Emergency Medicine and Medicine, University of Virginia School of Medicine, Charlottesville, VA, USA*

In a cardiac arrest, there are several possible rhythms that may result in loss of spontaneous perfusion, including asystole, pulseless electrical activity (PEA) rhythm presentations, pulseless ventricular tachycardia (VT), and ventricular fibrillation (VF).

Asystole

Asystole is a complete lack of electrical activity in the heart, resulting in pulselessness. Primary asystole occurs when there is a problem with the electrical system of the heart and no electrical impulses can be generated. It can be caused by a structural defect affecting the sinoatrial (SA) node, atrioventricular (AV) node, or other part of the conduction system; acute myocardial infarction or non-ischemic disease such as a tumor or cardiac trauma may be the cause. Primary asystole usually begins as a bradycardia caused by heart block, then proceeds to asystole. Alternatively, a patient who is dependent on his or her pacemaker may develop primary asystole if the pacemaker malfunctions and stops working.

Secondary asystole is caused by factors outside the heart's electrical system that affect its ability to generate depolarization. Electrolyte abnormalities and acidosis resulting from systemic illnesses can cause this type of asystole; toxicologic issues also can ultimately produce asystole. Untreated VF or pulseless VT can also result in this type of asystole.

Electrocardiographic Manifestations

In either type of asystole, the electrocardiogram (ECG) demonstrates the complete absence of cardiac electrical activity (Figure 21.1) – in essence, the ECG is a "flat line." The clinician should determine that the equipment, including ECG cables, is functioning appropriately. Furthermore, asystole should be determined in three separate leads since fine VF can mimic asystole in certain ECG leads.

Pulseless Electrical Activity

PEA features the unique combination of no discernible cardiac mechanical activity (i.e. a "pulseless" state) with a persistent, identifiable cardiac electrical activity (i.e. the cardiac rhythm). *Electromechanical dissociation*, an older term used for PEA, is another descriptive phrase for this malignant cardiac presentation – the complete dissociation of electrical and mechanical activity of the cardiovascular system.

PEA is usually caused by two major mechanisms (Table 21.1):

Decreased Preload

1) There is an inadequate blood return to the heart. Cardiac cells cannot contract optimally, nor is there enough blood to generate an adequate blood pressure. This decreased "effective" preload can occur in the setting of pericardial tamponade, tension pneumothorax, large pulmonary embolus (PE), or significant volume loss from trauma or severe dehydration.

Metabolic Dysfunction

2) A metabolic problem interferes with the ability of the cardiac muscle cells to contract: hypoxia, metabolic acidosis, hyper- or hypokalemia, hypoglycemia, hypothermia, myocardial infarction, or toxin effects.

The Electrocardiogram in Emergency and Acute Care, First Edition.
Edited by Korin B. Hudson, Amita Sudhir, George Glass, and William J. Brady.

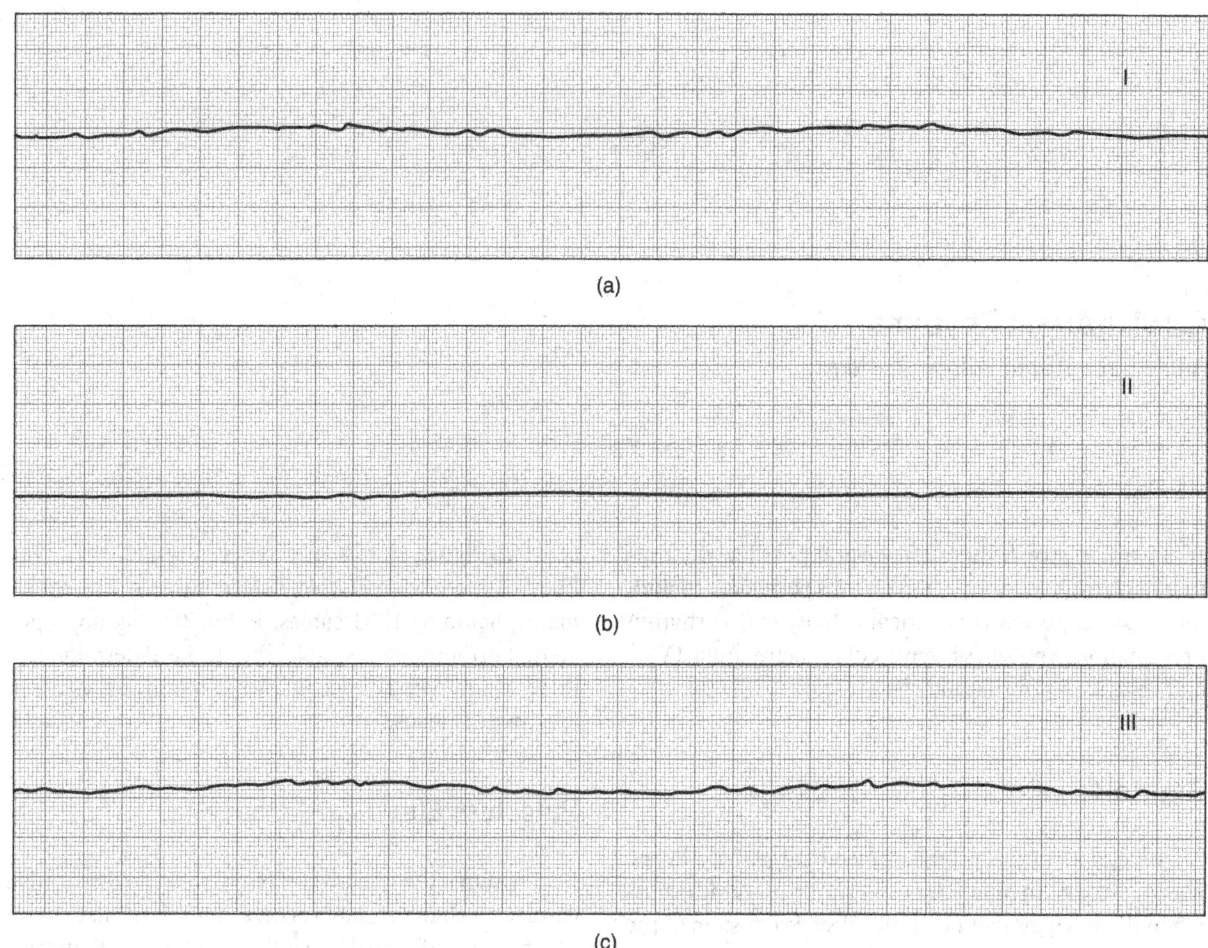

Figure 21.1 Asystole noted in the three limb leads, as seen in (a–c).

Table 21.1 Pulseless electrical activity cardiac arrest: causes and primary treatment considerations.

Causes	Primary treatment
Hypovolemia	IV fluid and/or blood product administration
Hypoxia	Airway support and oxygen therapy
Hypothermia	External and active rewarming
Hypoglycemia	IV dextrose
Hyper- or hypokalemia	Directed therapy
Hydrogen ion (i.e. acidosis)	IV sodium bicarbonate, respiratory support
Tamponade	Pericardiocentesis, IV fluid
Tension pneumothorax	Needle thoracostomy (decompression)
Thrombosis (pulmonary or coronary)	IV fluid, IV thrombolytics
Toxins	Supportive care, specific antidote as indicated
Trauma	IV fluid, advanced trauma life support (ATLS) management as indicated

Basic management considerations are listed.

Electrocardiographic Manifestations

Any cardiac rhythm other than VT or VF can be encountered in a PEA arrest presentation. In a general sense, the rate and QRS complex width can predict outcome in a PEA cardiac arrest. PEA tachydysrhythmias are associated with a less dismal prognosis, while bradydysrhythmias are associated with a very poor prognosis. Common rhythms encountered are as follows:

Sinus Tachycardia

The rate is greater than 100 beats per minute (bpm) (Figure 21.2a). The impulse is generated at the SA node.

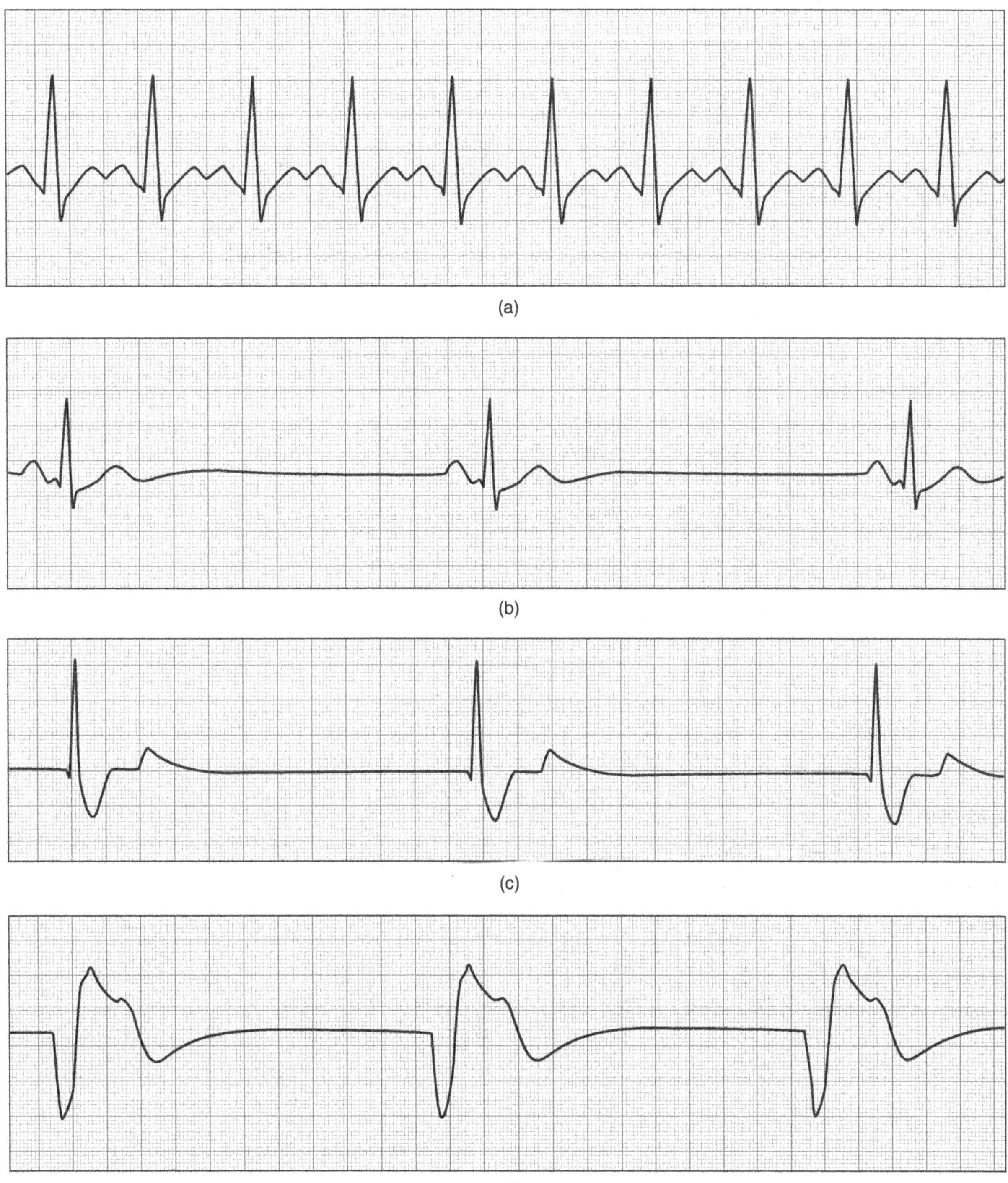

Figure 21.2 Pulseless electrical activity potential rhythm presentations. (a) Sinus tachycardia. (b) Sinus bradycardia. (c) Junctional bradycardia. (d) Idioventricular rhythm.

A P wave is present for every QRS and a QRS is present for every P wave. The R–R interval is regular and the QRS complex is less than 120 ms.

Sinus Bradycardia

The rate is less than 60 bpm with all other criteria as noted above for sinus tachycardia (Figure 21.2b).

Atrial Fibrillation with Rapid Ventricular Response

The rate is greater than 100 bpm. The impulse is generated in the atria. P waves are not discernable. The R–R interval is irregular and the QRS complex is less than 120 ms.

Junctional Bradycardia

The rate is usually 40–60 bpm (Figure 21.2c). The impulse is generated within the AV node or proximal Bundle of His. Retrograde (non-conducting) P waves may or may not be present. The R–R interval is regular. The QRS complex is less than 120 ms.

Idioventricular Rhythm

The rate is usually less than 40 bpm (Figure 21.2d). The impulse is generated within the ventricles. Retrograde P waves may be present. R-R interval is irregular. The QRS complex is wide with a duration usually greater than 120 ms.

Pulseless Ventricular Tachycardia

VT may or may not be a perfusing rhythm. Pulseless VT is most often seen in patients with coronary artery disease or cardiomyopathies, early in cardiac arrest. Pulseless VT, however, can be encountered in any range of clinical settings, particularly early in a cardiac arrest event.

Electrocardiographic Manifestations

The ventricular rate is usually between 100 and 200 bpm, frequently 170–180 bpm. On occasion, P waves are identified but they are completely dissociated from the QRS complex. A discernable QRS complex is seen that is wide (>120 ms and usually 140 ms). On the basis of the morphology of the QRS complexes (Figure 21.3), VT can be described as either monomorphic (Figure 21.3a,b) or polymorphic (Figure 21.3c,d) being the two choices. Monomorphic VT (Figure 21.3a,b) is a regular rhythm with one consistent QRS complex morphology. Polymorphic VT (Figure 21.3c,d) has more than one QRS complex morphology and can be regular or irregular. If the polymorphic VT demonstrates a consistent pattern of "twisting about a point," then the rhythm is likely a subset of polymorphic VT known as *torsades de pointes* (TdP; Figure 21.3d). Additional evidence of TdP includes the demonstration of a prolonged QT interval on the ECG while the patient is in a supraventricular, perfusing rhythm (e.g. sinus rhythm) either before arrest or after successful resuscitation.

Ventricular Fibrillation

VF is an irregular, disorganized rhythm originating in the ventricles. Because of the irregular electrical activity, the ventricles cannot contract effectively so patients with VF lack any form of spontaneous perfusion, that is, they are pulseless. Patients with a primary cardiac cause of cardiac disease frequently will present initially with VF; other non-cardiac cardiac arrest events can present with VF but have a higher rate of either asystole or PEA as the presenting rhythm.

Electrocardiographic Manifestations

In VF (Figure 21.4), the ECG does not demonstrate discernible P waves, QRS complexes, or any other structure. The electrocardiographic baseline is irregular with no obvious pattern to any structure – it is completely chaotic. The baseline pattern can be fine or coarse – these descriptors speak to the amplitude of the ventricular activity. The "coarse" pattern (Figure 21.4a) is seen when large amplitude ventricular activity occurs; "fine" (Figure 21.4b) denotes markedly lower amplitude ventricular activity and, in extreme cases, can be confused with asystole. Early in a VF cardiac arrest, coarse VF is seen with high amplitude (high voltage) undulations of the ECG; as cardiac arrest progresses without either intervention or response to therapy, the rhythm will progress to fine VF with a markedly lower voltage.

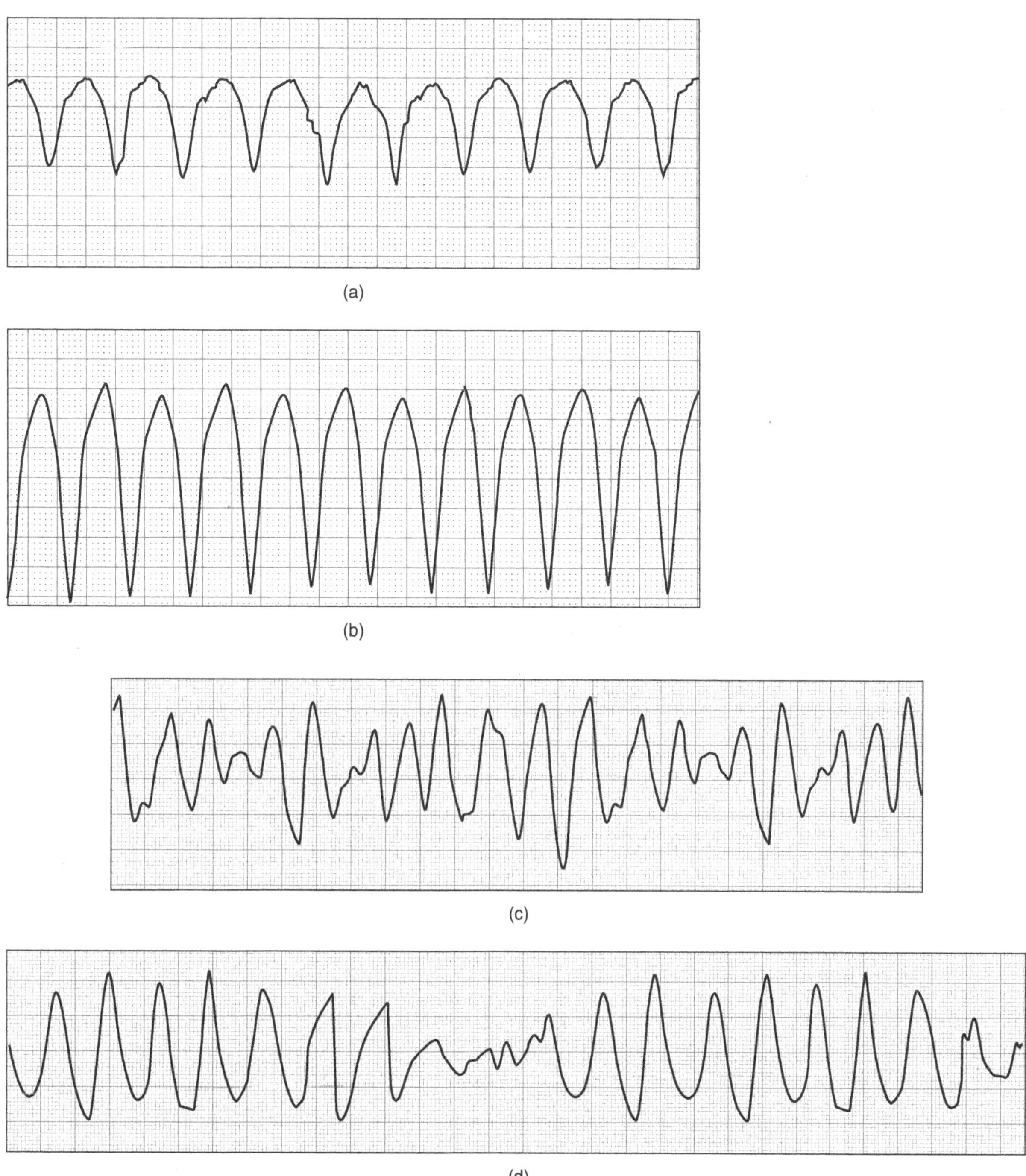

Figure 21.3 Ventricular tachycardia. (a) Monomorphic VT. (b) Monomorphic VT. (c) Polymorphic VT. (d) Torsades de pointes form of polymorphic VT.

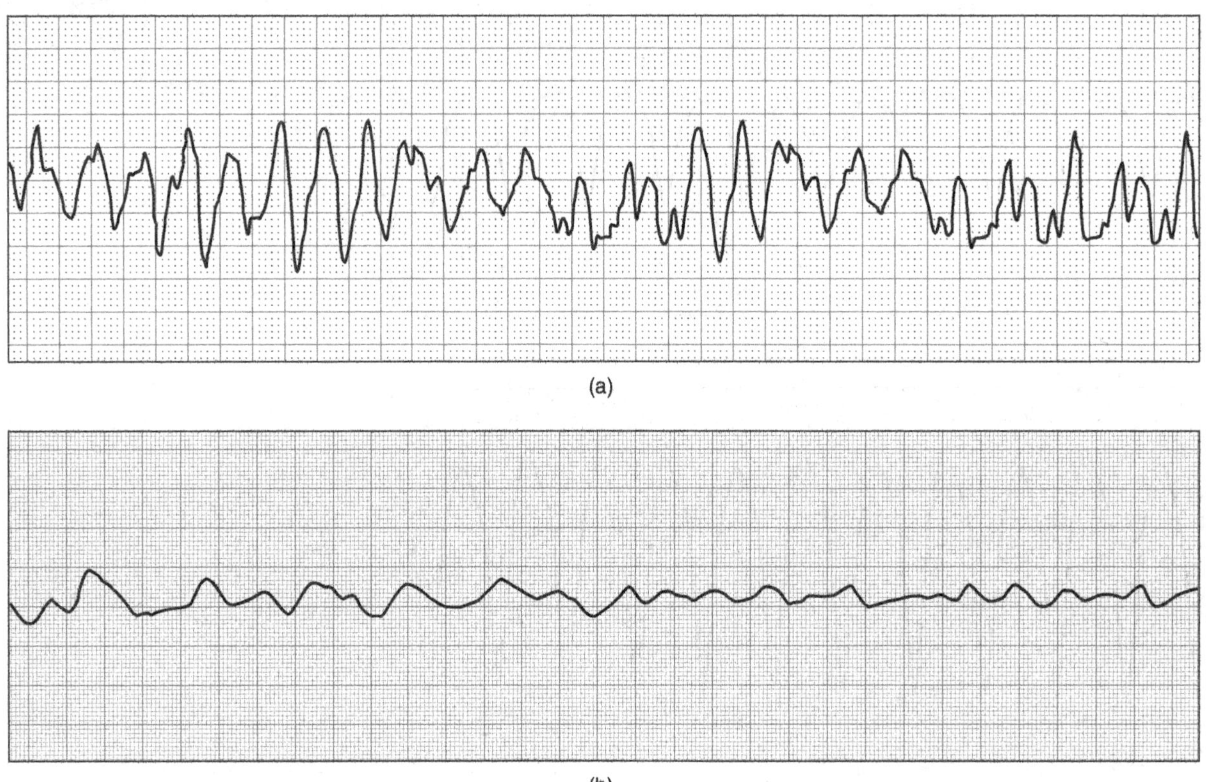

(a)

(b)

Figure 21.4 Ventricular fibrillation (VF). (a) Coarse VF. "Coarse" indicates large amplitude waveforms. (b) Fine VF. "Fine" indicates lower amplitude waveforms.

Section V

Electrocardiographic Differential Diagnosis of Common ECG Presentations

22

Electrocardiographic Differential Diagnosis of Narrow Complex Tachycardia

Megan Starling[1,2] *and William J. Brady*[3]

[1] *Department of Emergency Medicine, University of Virginia School of Medicine, Charlottesville, VA, USA*
[2] *Department of Emergency Medicine, Culpeper Memorial Hospital, Culpeper, VA, USA*
[3] *Departments of Emergency Medicine and Medicine, University of Virginia School of Medicine, Charlottesville, VA, USA*

Multiple types of narrow complex tachycardia (NCT) are encountered in the acute care setting, the vast majority of which originate above the ventricles and have a rate over 100 bpm with a QRS complex duration less than 120 ms; the single exception to this statement is the ventricular-based NCT called *fascicular tachycardia* or *fascicular ventricular tachycardia* – this rhythm is quite rare and is usually encountered in medication toxicity presentations. Any tachycardic rhythm originating above the ventricles is technically a supraventricular tachycardia (SVT); thus the term *SVT* is a general category of tachydysrhythmias. A distinction must be made between SVT and paroxysmal supraventricular tachycardia (PSVT); PSVT is a commonly used term to describe a specific type of NCT with an abrupt onset and resolution. Most of the NCTs described below tend to be regular, with the exception of atrial fibrillation and multifocal atrial tachycardia (MAT).

The differential diagnosis of the NCT (Table 22.1) includes sinus tachycardia, atrial fibrillation, atrial flutter, PSVT, MAT, and paroxysmal atrial tachycardia (PAT). In addition, the Wolff–Parkinson–White syndrome can present with a NCT similar in appearance to PSVT. Lastly, the rare fascicular ventricular tachycardia should also be considered in the differential diagnosis of the NCT.

Sinus tachycardia is a common finding in response to physiologic stress and is identified on the electrocardiogram (ECG) (Figure 22.1) by a regular NCT with identical, upright P wave for each QRS complex; importantly, the P waves are upright in leads I, II, and III. Sinus tachycardia has both a gradual onset and a gradual "termination." Rates range from 100 to approximately 160 bpm in the adult; age-related rates are seen in children, with maximum rates approaching 200 bpm in the infant and young child. Sinus tachycardia should be considered a "reactive rhythm" in that it is usually secondary to a primary physiologic event such as hypovolemia, hypoperfusion, hypoxia, fever, pain, anxiety, and medication effect (Clinical Presentation Box 22.1). Treatment is rarely required for the tachycardia itself; rather, attention and potential therapy should be paid to the cause of the sinus tachycardia (Management Box 22.1).

Atrial fibrillation is a result of multiple ectopic foci in the atrium firing simultaneously at atrial rates of up to nearly 600 bpm. When an occasional impulse reaches the atrioventricular (AV) node, conduction of a ventricular impulse occurs. The resulting ventricular rate is very irregular and can range from severely bradycardic to extremely tachycardic with rates up to 150–250 or even higher in the presence of accessory AV tracts (i.e. the Wolff–Parkinson–White syndrome). The usual rate of atrial fibrillation without medication effect or other active disease impact is approximately 170 bpm. ECG (Figure 22.2) tracings reveal absent P waves and a chaotic (wavy, bumpy) baseline caused by the multiple small atrial firings. The QRS complex is narrow except at extreme high rates or in patients with coexistent intraventricular conduction delays or accessory pathways (APs). Importantly, the rhythm pattern is irregular in an irregular fashion, thus the irregularly irregular pattern of atrial fibrillation (Management Box 22.2).

Atrial flutter is caused by rapid firing of a single, ectopic atrial focus that is continuously restimulated by an aberrant reentry loop within the atrium. The atrial rate is generally 250–350 bpm with only a portion of these atrial impulses proceeding through the AV node to cause ventricular depolarization. The ventricular rate

The Electrocardiogram in Emergency and Acute Care, First Edition.
Edited by Korin B. Hudson, Amita Sudhir, George Glass, and William J. Brady.

Table 22.1 Differential diagnosis of narrow complex tachycardia (NCT).

Sinus tachycardia
Atrial fibrillation
Atrial flutter
Paroxysmal supraventricular tachycardia (PSVT)
Multifocal atrial tachycardia (MAT)
Paroxysmal atrial tachycardia (PAT)
Wolff–Parkinson–White syndrome NCT
Fascicular ventricular tachycardia

depends on the ratio of atrial impulses generated to ventricular impulses sensed. Commonly, atrial flutter is seen with 2:1 atrioventricular (A:V) conduction causing a regular NCT with a rate of approximately 150 bpm (Clinical Presentation Box 22.2). The ECG (Figure 22.3) demonstrates regular, identical "flutter" waves (the P waves) which appear as pointed, asymmetric structures. With 2:1 block, there will be two flutter waves for every one generated QRS. If uncertain whether flutter waves are present, performing vagal maneuvers may momentarily slow the A:V conduction to 3:1 (ventricular rate of 100 bpm) or 4:1 (ventricular rate of 75 bpm), thus making the flutter waves more apparent. The clinician should consider atrial flutter (Figure 22.3) in patients with NCT and fixed (i.e., non-varying) ventricular rates of approximately 150 bpm.

Clinical Presentation Box 22.1 Sinus Tachycardia

Sinus tachycardia should be considered a "reactive rhythm."

Consider the underlying causes of sinus tachycardia:
- hypovolemia (dehydration, hemorrhage)
- hypoperfusion (sepsis, anaphylaxis)
- hypoxia
- fever
- pain
- anxiety
- medication effect (both medicinal and illicit substances)

Management Box 22.1 Sinus Tachycardia

Primary treatment of sinus tachycardia itself is rarely required.

Rather, treatment interventions should be potentially applied to the underlying cause of the sinus tachycardia.

If the patient has no signs of heart failure such as rales or peripheral edema, administration of an IV fluid bolus is a reasonable starting point.

Rate controlling medications should be avoided since the tachycardia is often a compensatory mechanism for relative hypovolemia or increased oxygen demand.

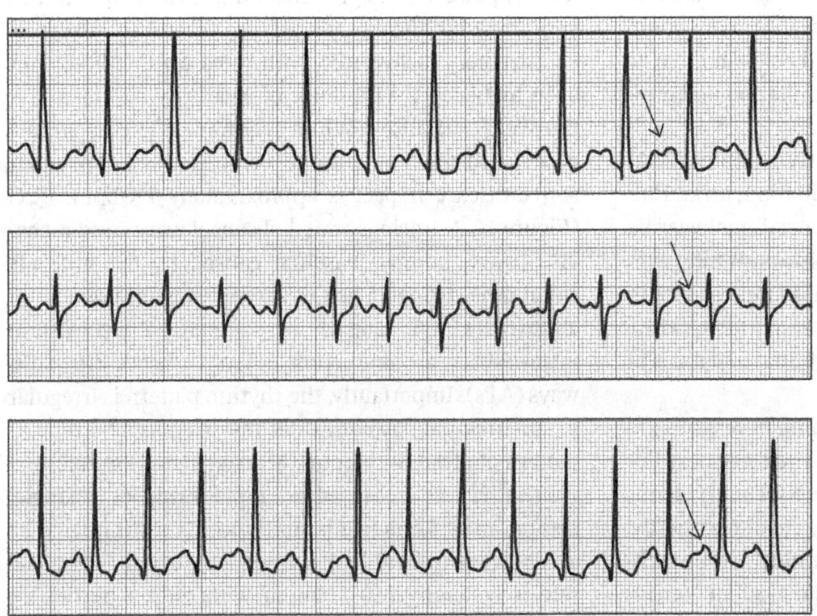

Figure 22.1 Sinus tachycardia, three examples in lead II. Note the P wave preceding each QRS complex (arrow), suggesting a sinus origin to the tachycardia. Importantly, the P wave is upright in these examples of sinus tachycardia. P waves are upright in leads I, II, and III.

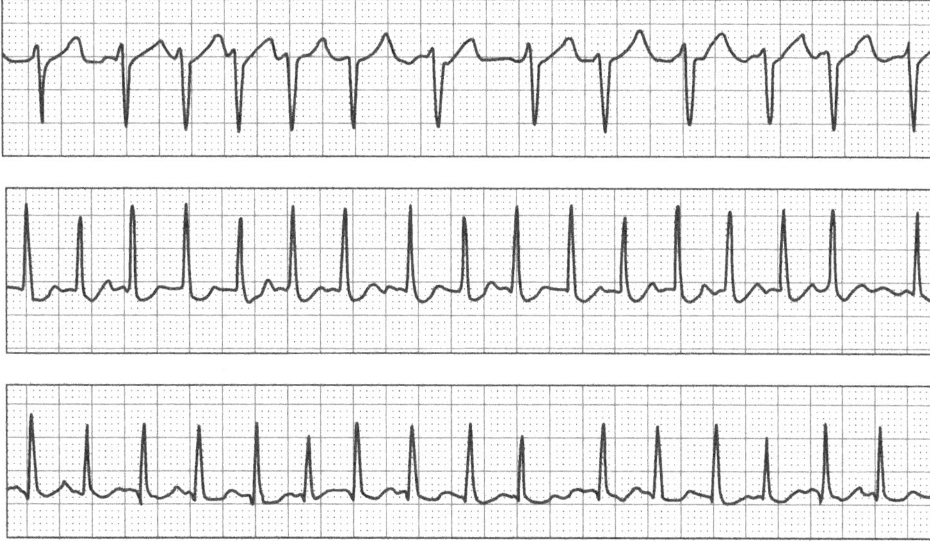

Figure 22.2 Atrial fibrillation with rapid ventricular response.

> **Clinical Presentation Box 22.2 Atrial Flutter**
>
> A NCT with a consistent ventricular rate of approximately 150 bpm should suggest atrial flutter.
>
> Of course, many forms of SVT can demonstrate ventricular rates of 150 bpm yet the natural history rate of atrial flutter is 150 bpm.

> **Management Box 22.2 Atrial Fibrillation**
>
> Atrial fibrillation can be a difficult NCT to manage.
>
> The primary goal of treatment is to control the ventricular response (i.e. the ventricular rate).
>
> Emergent electrical cardioversion is not always the initial therapy in patients with hemodynamic compromise.
>
> Rather, the cause of the instability must be considered with appropriate therapy aimed at the underlying issue.
>
> Most often, atrial fibrillation with rapid ventricular response and accompanying hypotension results from another clinical issue, such as dehydration, sepsis, or other primary non-cardiac event.

PSVT is a common form of NCT encountered in many clinical settings. The focus can be in the atrial tissues or AV node itself – thus, PSVT is a group of similar appearing SVTs; in most cases, the focus is found in the AV node. The various forms as defined by the focus are largely indistinguishable in the early phases of patient care, such as in the prehospital and emergency department (ED) settings. In both adult and pediatric patients, the atrial rate is generally 150–250 bpm, most often with 1 : 1 A : V conduction. The ECG tracings (Figure 22.4) reveal a sudden onset, regular NCT with either no P waves or abnormally positioned P waves (Figure 22.4c); the abnormally positioned P wave includes inverted P waves preceding the QRS complex and varying polarity P waves following the QRS complex – these P waves are termed "retrograde" P waves.

A NCT resembling *PSVT is seen in the Wolff–Parkinson–White (WPW) syndrome.* The WPW syndrome is a form of ventricular preexcitation involving an accessory conduction pathway between the atria and ventricles. In the WPW patient, the accessory pathway bypasses the AV node, creating a direct electrical connection between the atria and ventricles – and therefore removing the ventricles' protection against excessively rapid rates, which is provided by the AV node in patients without WPW. WPW patients are prone to develop a variety of supraventricular tachyarrhythmias, including the most common NCT, seen in approximately 70% of cases. This *NCT* is termed an orthodromic (anterograde) reciprocating tachycardia; the impulse pathway allows for anterograde, or forward, conduction through the AV node followed by retrograde conduction via the AP. With this pathway, the QRS complexes appear normal (i.e. narrow) and the ECG displays a very rapid, narrow-complex tachycardia that is nearly indistinguishable from that of PSVT (Figure 22.4d) (Management Box 22.3).

MAT is the result of three or more ectopic atrial foci initiating impulses that are conducted through the AV

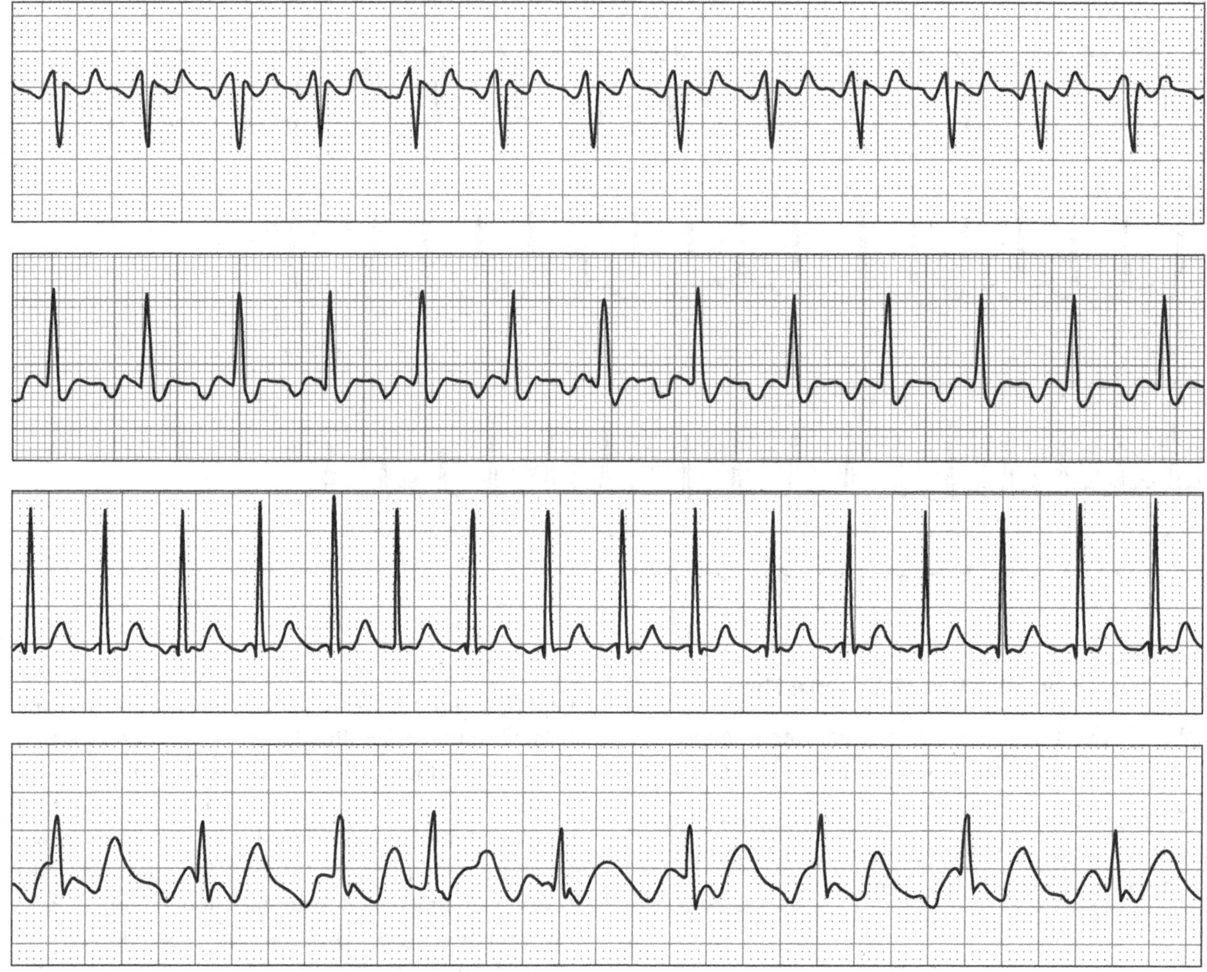

Figure 22.3 Atrial flutter with rapid ventricular rates.

node, causing subsequent ventricular depolarization. ECG tracings (Figure 22.5) reveal an irregular NCT with a rate greater than 100 bpm and a P wave before each QRS. There must be at least three morphologically distinct P waves present in a single ECG lead. MAT is usually caused by an underlying respiratory pathology such as chronic obstructive pulmonary disease (COPD). Management is aimed at correcting the underlying cause (Management Box 22.4).

PAT is caused by rapid firing of an irritable ectopic focus in the atrium similar to atrial flutter but often without an identifiable reentry circuit. The atrial rate generally ranges from 150 to 250 bpm and most often there is 1:1 A:V conduction, thus producing a ventricular rate of 150–250 as well. In some circumstances, such as digitalis poisoning, there may be an AV block leading to 2:1 AV conduction. In PAT without conduction block, ECG tracings reveal a sudden onset of regular, identical P waves with an accompanying QRS complex (i.e., one P wave for each QRS complex) at a rate of 150–250 bpm. The P waves present during the tachyarrhythmia are distinct from the P waves seen, while in a sinus rhythm, though this distinction may not always be possible unless the clinician has the "luxury" of a rhythm strip in sinus rhythm.

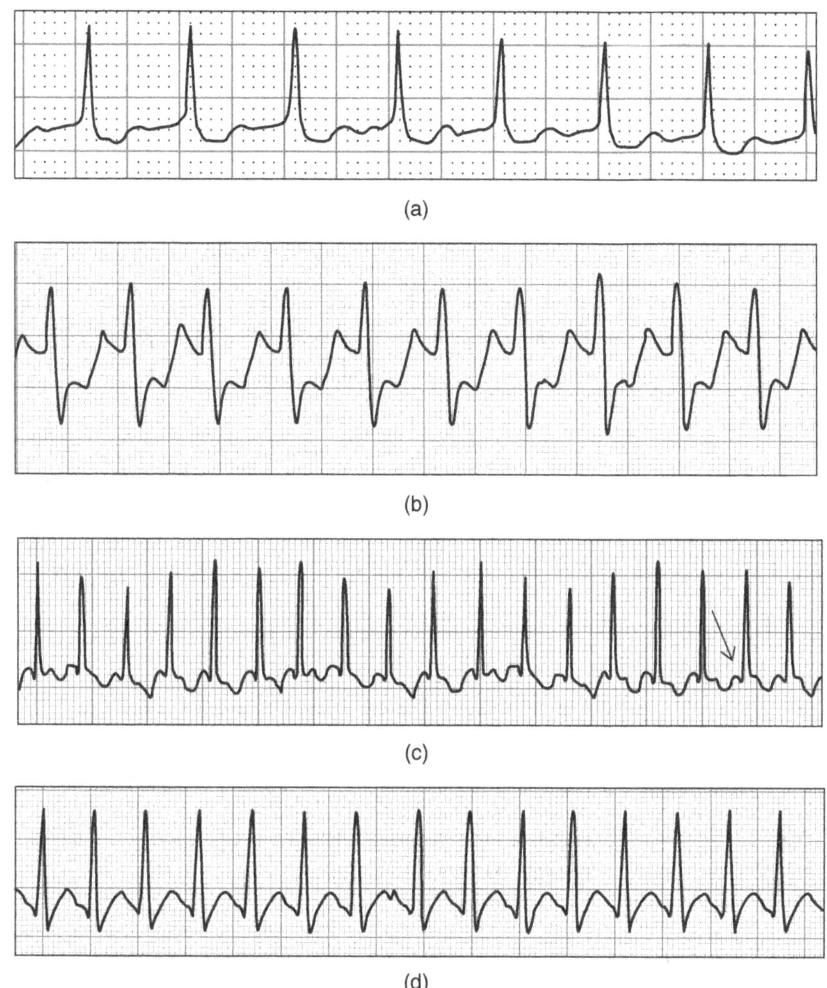

Figure 22.4 Paroxysmal supraventricular tachycardia (PSVT). (a) PSVT with a relatively slower rate of approximately 150 bpm. (b) PSVT at approximately 170 bpm; the ST segment depression is likely a rate-related phenomenon and not indicative of coronary ischemia. (c) PSVT in a neonate with an approximate rate of 260 bpm; note the retrograde P wave (arrow) preceding the QRS complex. (d) PSVT in the Wolff–Parkinson–White syndrome. Other than a more rapid rate, this form of PSVT is indistinguishable from non-WPW-related PSVT.

Management Box 22.3 Narrow Complex Tachycardia in the Wolff–Parkinson–White Syndrome

The NCT seen in the WPW syndrome patient is difficult to distinguish from PSVT.

Management of this form of WPW-related dysrhythmia is similar to that of typical PSVT, that is, the use of AV nodal blocking agents is correct and appropriate.

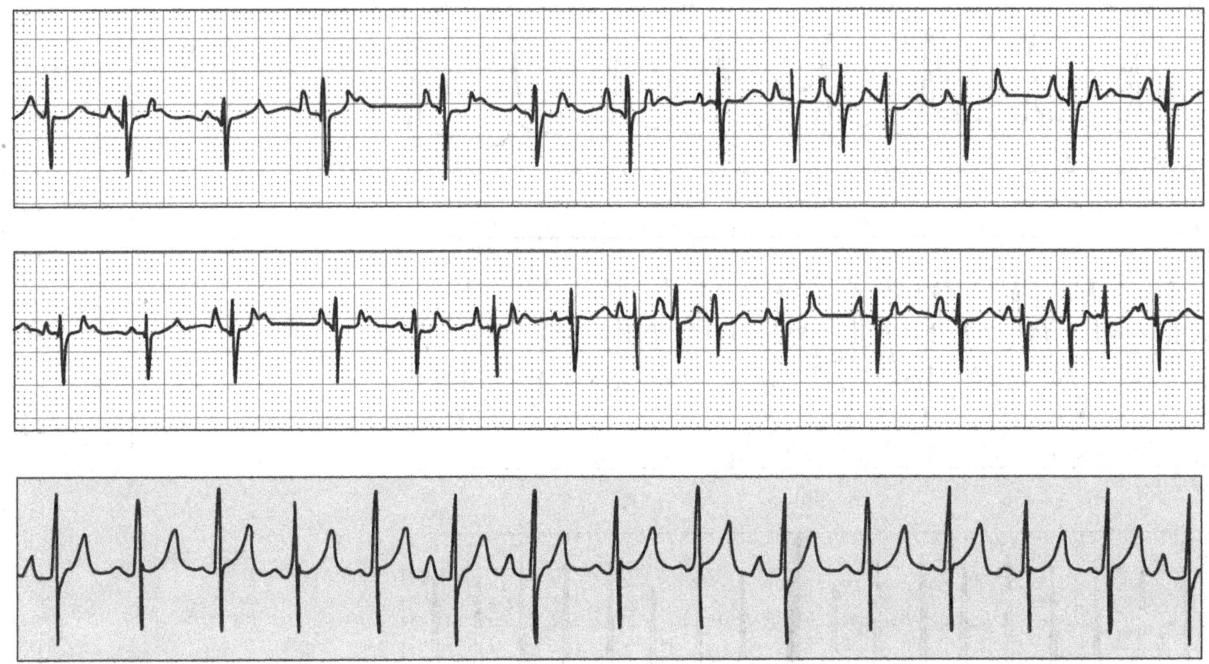

Figure 22.5 Multifocal atrial tachycardia (MAT). Note the presence of at least three different P waves in any single lead.

Management Box 22.4 Multifocal Atrial Tachycardia
Primary treatment of MAT itself is rarely required. Rather, treatment should be aimed at the underlying cause which is most often an acute exacerbation of chronic heart or lung disease.

23

Electrocardiographic Differential Diagnosis of Wide Complex Tachycardia

Amita Sudhir[1] *and William J. Brady*[2]

[1] *Department of Emergency Medicine, University of Virginia School of Medicine, Charlottesville, VA, USA*
[2] *Departments of Emergency Medicine and Medicine, University of Virginia School of Medicine, Charlottesville, VA, USA*

Wide complex tachycardia (WCT) is an abnormally fast heart rate, demonstrating a widened QRS complex. In the adult patient, the ventricular rate is usually over 120 bpm and the QRS complex is prolonged to greater than 0.12 second in duration or width. In the infant and young child, the clinician should use age-specific norms for rates when interpreting the electrocardiogram (ECG). The wide QRS complex is caused by abnormal depolarization of the ventricles because of one of three mechanisms – ectopic ventricular foci (i.e. premature ventricular contraction [PVCs] and/or ventricular tachycardia [VT]), aberrant conduction (i.e. supraventricular tachycardia [SVT] with aberrant conduction), or ventricular preexcitation (i.e. Wolff–Parkinson–White [WPW] syndrome). Thus, the differential diagnosis for WCT (Table 23.1) includes VT, SVT with aberrant conduction, and ventricular preexcitation syndrome-related tachycardia. WCTs may be either regular or irregular. See Clinical Presentation Box 23.1.

See Management Box 23.1.

Ventricular Tachycardia

VT almost always presents with a widened QRS complex. In the adult, the QRS complex is most often greater than 0.12 second in width; in infants and very young children, the QRS complex may not appear "wide" by adult standards when, in fact, it is. In VT, the QRS complex can be described as monomorphic (i.e. one predominant shape for the QRS complexes; Figure 23.1) or polymorphic (more than one shape for the QRS complexes; Figure 23.2). The focus of VT is found most often in the ventricular myocardium. The very rare form of fascicular tachycardia is a form of VT with a narrow QRS complex; the QRS complex is narrow in this instance because of the rhythm focus being in the intraventricular conduction system. Monomorphic VT demonstrates QRS complexes that are uniform in appearance (i.e. all appear the same or very similar). This rhythm is often seen in patients with ischemic heart disease or in the setting of an active myocardial infarction. The wide complex is caused by depolarization occurring at an ectopic ventricular focus, outside the normal conducting system. Monomorphic VT is always regular (Figure 23.1).

Polymorphic VT is a form of VT in which the morphology of the QRS complexes varies from beat to beat (Figure 23.2). The variation in the QRS complexes can be minimal or maximal. One subtype of polymorphic VT is Torsades de Pointes (TdP) in which the QRS complexes appear to be twisting around an electrical baseline (Figure 23.2b and c). If the patient's cardiac rhythm can be viewed in a supraventricular setting either before or after the TdP occurs, the QTc interval is usually prolonged. Polymorphic VT, including TdP, is generally irregular. This rhythm is seen in a range of settings, including acute coronary syndrome, toxicologic presentations, and early in cardiac arrest.

Supraventricular Tachycardia with Aberrancy

If there is a dysfunction (i.e. a block or delay in activation) in the intraventricular conduction system, then the electrical impulse is delayed or slowed as it passes through the ventricular myocardium, thus widening the QRS complex. For instance, a left bundle branch block (LBBB) can be present in a patient with an SVT. Owing

The Electrocardiogram in Emergency and Acute Care, First Edition.
Edited by Korin B. Hudson, Amita Sudhir, George Glass, and William J. Brady.

Table 23.1 Differential diagnosis of wide complex tachycardia (WCT).

Ventricular tachycardia
- Monomorphic ventricular tachycardia
- Polymorphic ventricular tachycardia

Supraventricular tachycardia (SVT) with aberrant conduction
- Sinus tachycardia
- Atrial fibrillation
- Atrial flutter
- Paroxysmal supraventricular tachycardia (PSVT)
- Multifocal atrial tachycardia (MAT)
- Paroxysmal atrial tachycardia

Ventricular preexcitation-related tachycardia
- Atrial fibrillation
- Wide complex tachycardia (antidromic tachycardia)

Other wide complex tachycardias
- Pacemaker-mediated tachycardia
- Artifact mimicking WCT

Clinical Presentation Box 23.1 Clinical Features Associated with Ventricular Tachycardia as the Rhythm Diagnosis in Wide Complex Tachycardia Presentations

Clinical features associated with VT:

- Age over 50 years
- History of myocardial infarction
- History of significant CHF
- Absence of these findings does not rule out VT

Clinical instability (i.e. hypotension and pulmonary edema) is encountered in both VT and SVT with aberrant conduction.

to the presence of the LBBB, the SVT, even though it arises above the ventricles, will demonstrate a widened QRS complex. The SVT can include any supraventricular rhythm that is tachycardic, including sinus tachycardia, atrial fibrillation, paroxysmal supraventricular tachycardia (PSVT), and so on (Figures 23.3–23.5). The malfunction in the intraventricular conduction system can be permanent, as with a bundle branch block, or temporary because the abnormal conduction may only occur at higher heart rates. SVT with aberrancy may be regular or irregular, depending on the origin of the rhythm; sinus tachycardia and PSVT will be regular, while atrial fibrillation and multifocal atrial tachycardia (MAT) will be irregular.

Management Box 23.1 Management of Wide Complex Tachycardia Presentations

Rhythm diagnosis often is not possible with WCT presentation.

Management should focus on ECG and clinical findings.

In unstable patients, synchronized electrical cardioversion is frequently appropriate.

Specific management considerations:

- Avoid AV nodal-blocking agents in extremely rapid atrial fibrillation with widened QRS complex with varying morphologies.
- Avoid AV nodal-blocking agents in most regular WCT presentations.
- Consider sodium bicarbonate therapy in WCT with overdose.
- Consider therapy for hyperkalemia in patients with significant renal failure and WCT.

Ventricular Tachycardia versus Supraventricular Tachycardia with Aberrant Conduction

For treatment purposes, it is important to attempt to differentiate between VT and SVT with aberrancy. In some cases, this distinction is not possible; thus, management decisions must be made based on the patient's clinical situation and the ECG rhythm. The following are some signs that favor VT as the rhythm diagnosis in the setting of a WCT and can quickly be identified on an ECG or a rhythm strip:

- QRS complex width is extremely wide (>0.14–0.16 seconds in duration).
- Atrioventricular (AV) dissociation (Figure 23.6) in which P waves do not correlate with the QRS complexes.
- Capture beats (Figure 23.7), where some impulses are conducted normally from the atria, are seen as the occasional narrow QRS complex.
- Fusion beats (Figure 23.8), which occur when an impulse conducted from the atria fuses with a ventricular-generated impulse, creating a QRS complex with a new morphology and intermediate width.
- The QRS complexes in leads V1–V6 will be concordant in orientation, i.e. all QRS complexes are either positive or negative in polarity (Figure 23.9).

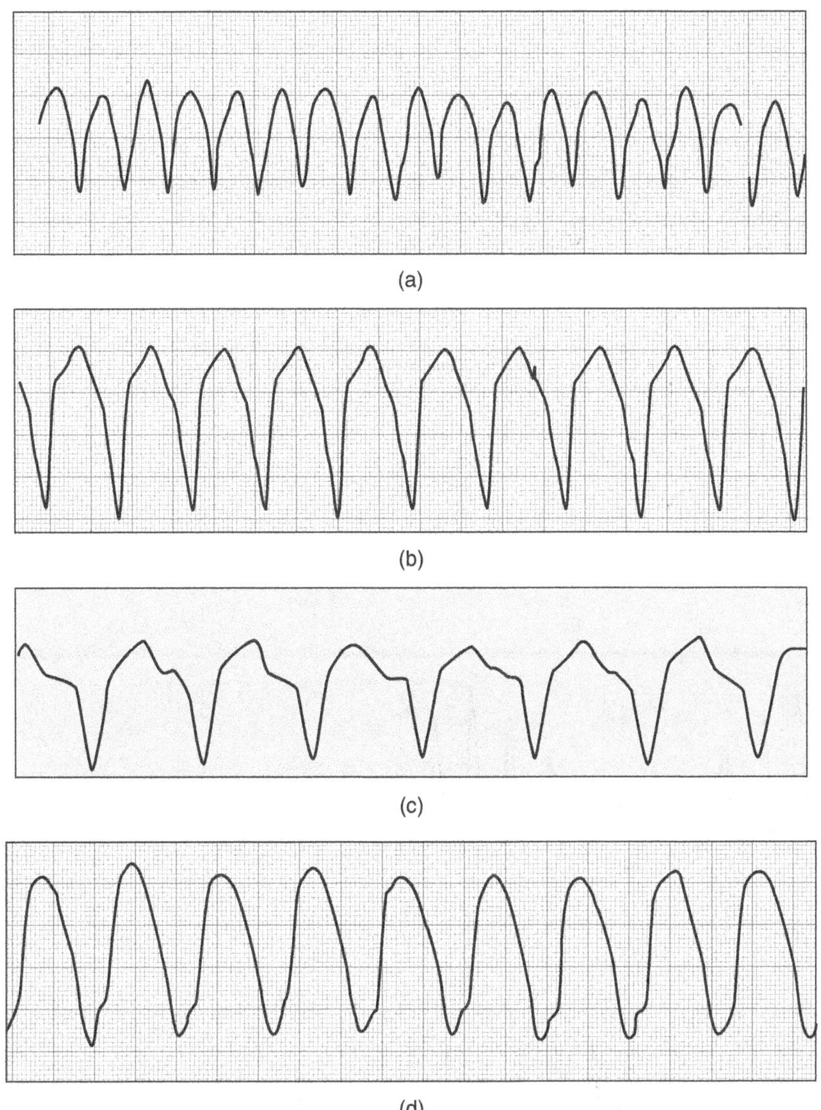

Figure 23.1 Ventricular tachycardia – monomorphic. (a) Monomorphic VT with a rate of approximately 180 bpm. (b) Monomorphic VT with a rate of approximately 170 bpm. (c) Monomorphic VT with a markedly slower rate of approximately 130 bpm; this patient is using amiodarone, which can markedly slow the rate of VT. (d) Monomorphic VT with a rapid rate of approximately 220 bpm.

Significant irregularity of the rhythm can suggest atrial fibrillation with preexisting or rate-related bundle branch block. The degree of irregularity is usually very obvious.

In addition, several clinical features, such as patient age and medical history, can suggest the diagnosis. For instance, age over 50 years and a past history of myocardial infarction and/or significant congestive heart failure (CHF) strongly suggest VT as an etiology, while SVT with aberrancy is more likely in a young, healthy patient.

Ventricular Preexcitation (Wolff–Parkinson–White Syndrome)

The WPW syndrome is a form of ventricular preexcitation involving an accessory conduction pathway between the atria and the ventricles. WPW patients are prone to develop a variety of supraventricular tachyarrhythmias, including two WCT subtypes: WPW-related atrial fibrillation (Figure 23.10) and a WCT (Figure 23.11).

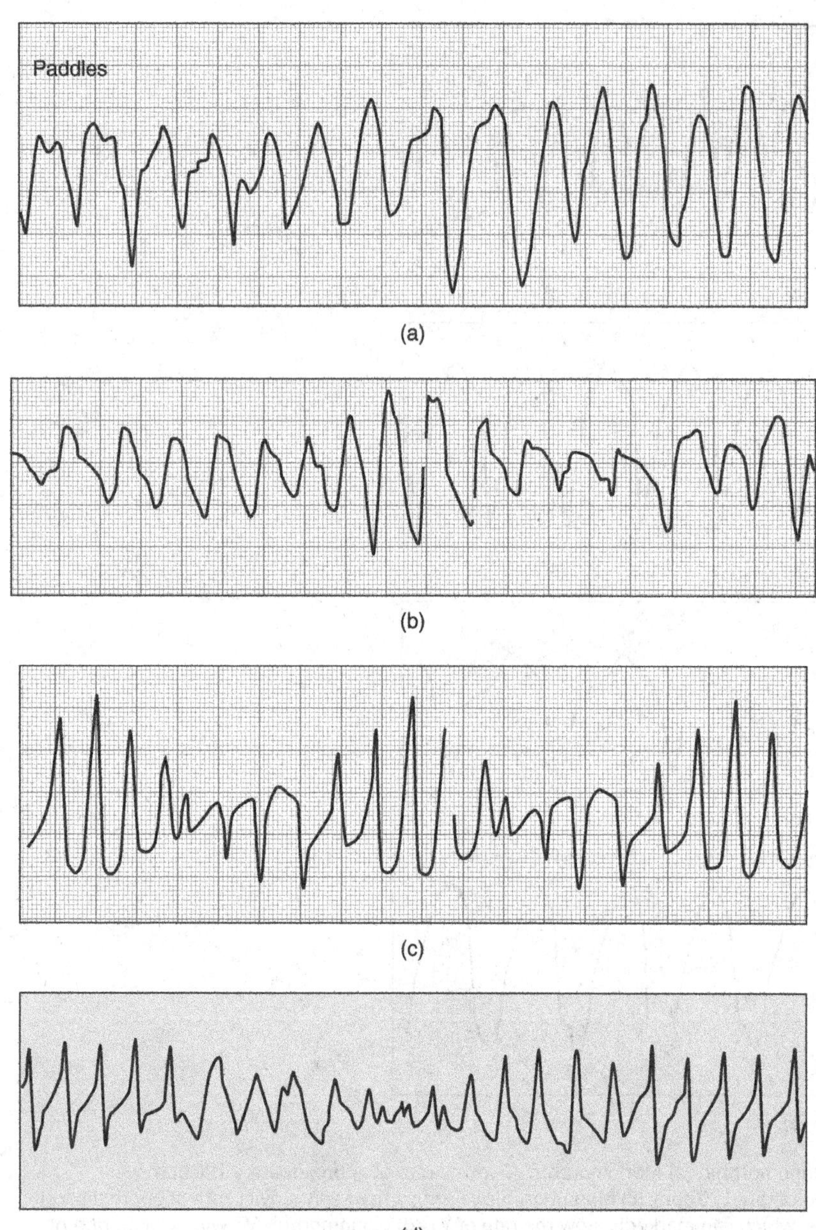

Figure 23.2 Polymorphic VT. (a) polymorphic VT, (b) polymorphic VT, (c) polymorphic VT – Torsade de pointes variety of VT, and (d) polymorphic VT – Torsade de pointes variety of VT.

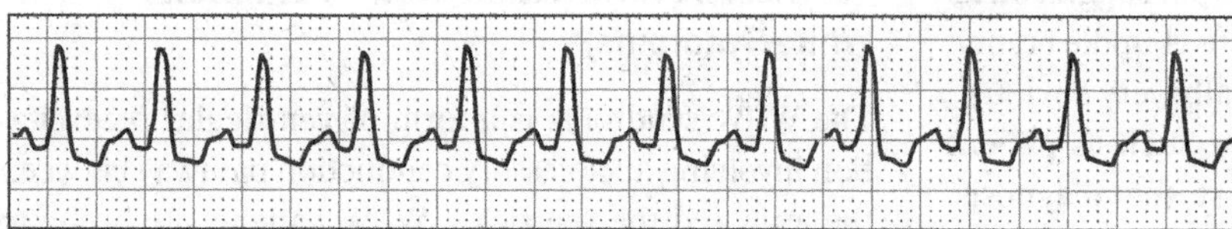

Figure 23.3 Supraventricular tachycardia (SVT) with aberrant ventricular conduction – sinus tachycardia with bundle branch block morphology.

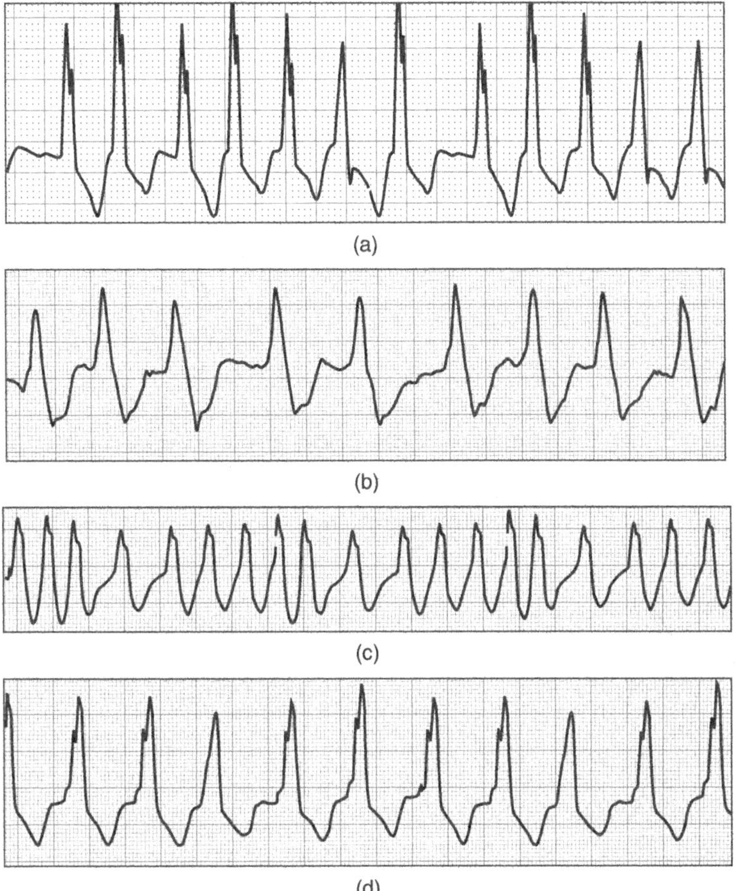

Figure 23.4 Supraventricular tachycardia (SVT) with aberrant ventricular conduction – atrial fibrillation with widened QRS complex. (a) Atrial fibrillation with bundle branch block; (b) atrial fibrillation with bundle branch block; (c) atrial fibrillation with bundle branch block. The rate was extremely rapid, producing bundle branch fatigue and resulting in the widened QRS complex. (d) Atrial flutter with bundle branch block.

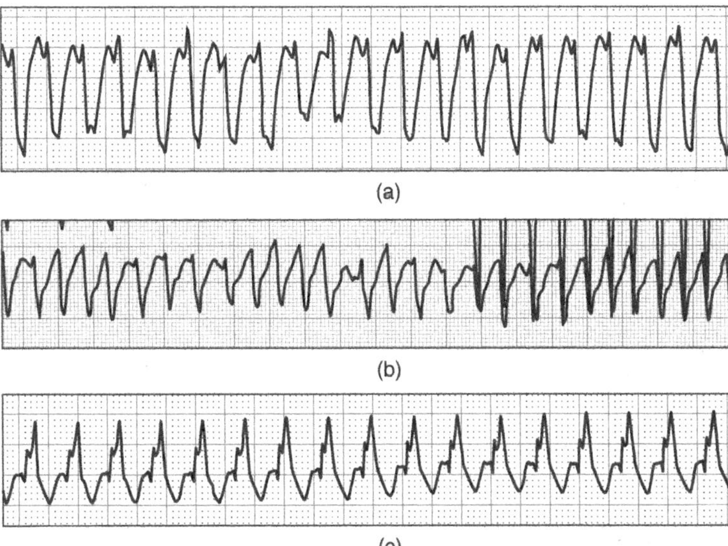

Figure 23.5 Supraventricular tachycardia (SVT) with aberrant ventricular conduction – PSVT with aberrant conduction. (a) PSVT with widened QRS complex due to preexisting bundle branch block. (b) PSVT with two forms of QRS complex width – wide (left side of rhythm strip) and narrow (right side of rhythm strip). The rate was extremely rapid, producing bundle branch fatigue and resulting in the widened QRS complex because of preexisting bundle branch block. (c) PSVT with widened QRS complex because of preexisting bundle branch block.

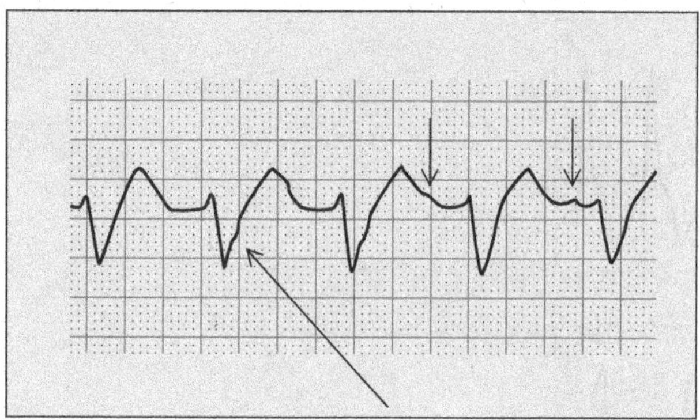

Figure 23.6 Atrioventricular (AV) dissociation. The presence of AV dissociation in the setting of a WCT strongly suggests the presence of ventricular tachycardia. The long arrow indicates the likely presence of a P wave that is "lost" in the larger QRS complex; the small arrows denote P waves. In all instances, these P waves are dissociated from the QRS complex.

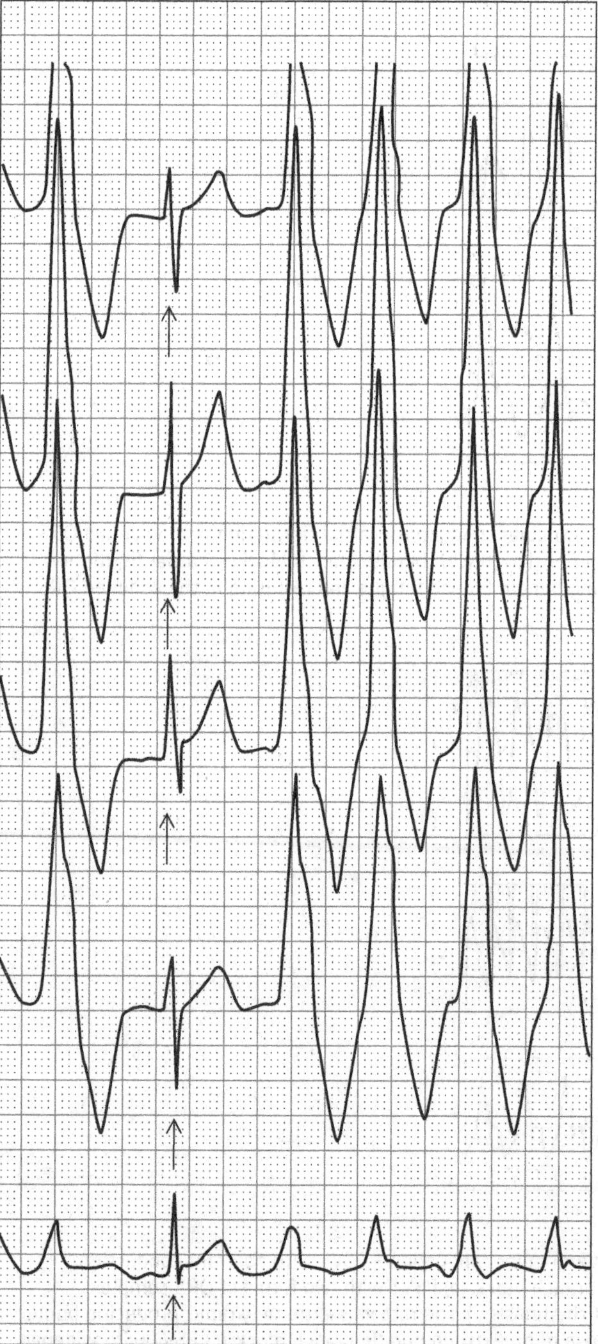

Figure 23.7 Capture beat – the arrows indicate a narrow QRS complex, which results from a supraventricular impulse conducted through the AV node. The presence of a capture beat in the setting of a WCT strongly suggests the presence of ventricular tachycardia.

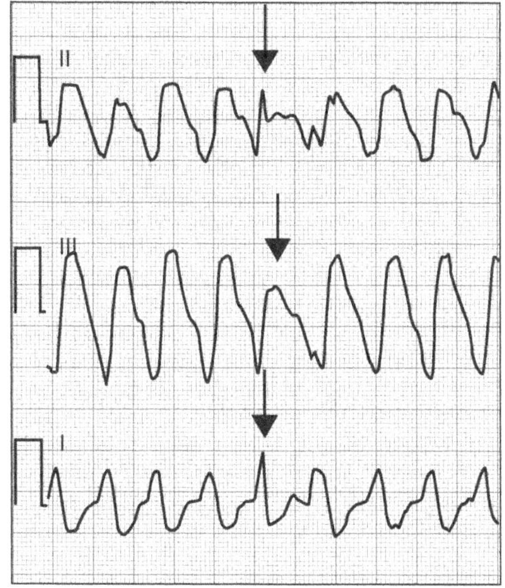

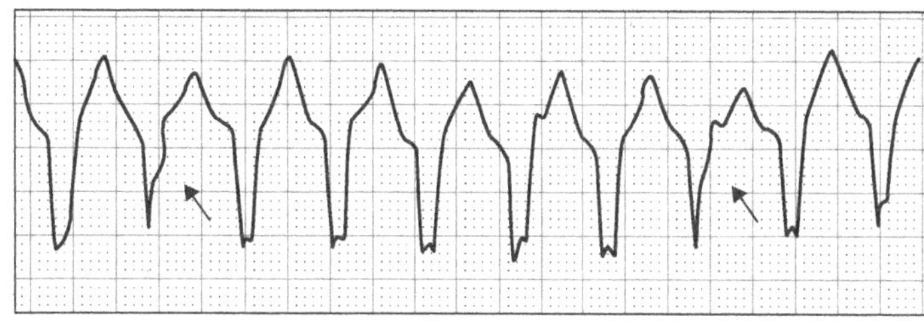

Figure 23.8 Fusion beats – the arrows indicate QRS complexes, which are intermediate in width – between the widened QRS complex of the WCT and a normal QRS complex. A fusion beat results from the fusion of supraventricular impulse and ventricular impulse, producing a unique QRS complex that is intermediate in width. The presence of a fusion beat in the setting of a WCT strongly suggests the presence of ventricular tachycardia.

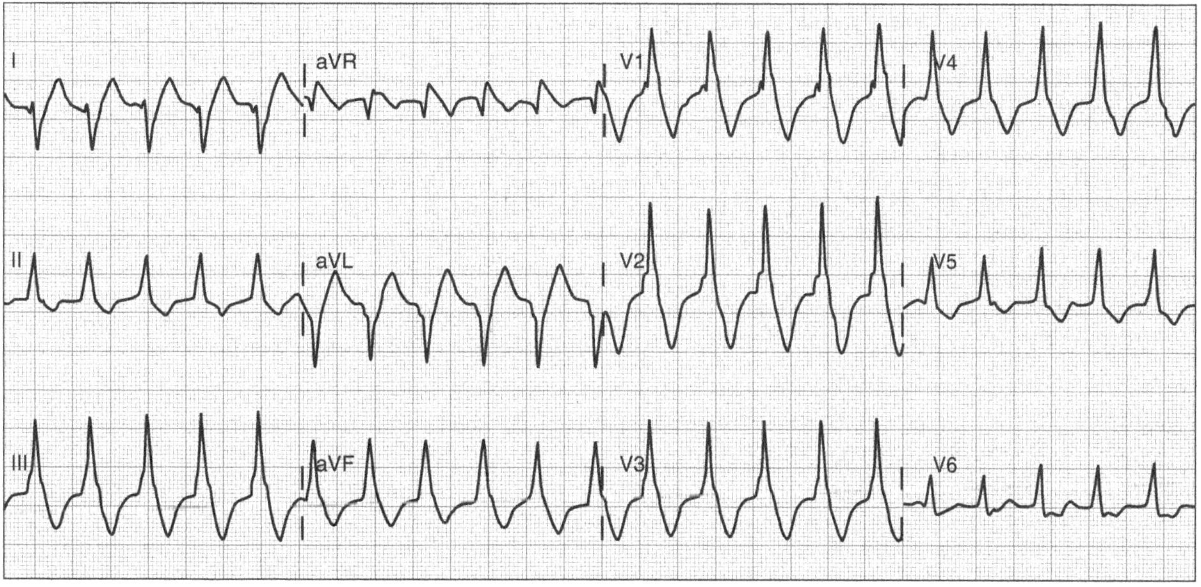

Figure 23.9 Positive concordance. The QRS complexes in leads V1–V6 are all positively oriented – positive concordance. If all QRS complexes are negatively oriented, the ECG is said to demonstrate negative concordance. In either case, concordance is suggestive of ventricular tachycardia as the cause of the WCT.

Other Causes of Wide Complex Tachycardia

Severe hyperkalemia can also cause a rapid, wide complex rhythm that can mimic VT if the rate is rapid (Figure 23.12a). Sodium channel blocking agents, such as tricyclic antidepressants, can cause both tachycardia and widened QRS complexes, resulting in a WCT in overdose situations (Figure 23.12b). Sinus tachycardia with anterior wall ST segment elevation myocardial infarction (STEMI) and the giant R wave (prominent T wave with ST segment elevation of early STEMI) mimic a WCT (Figure 23.12c). Finally, electrocardiographic artifact can be easily mistaken for WCT (Figure 23.13). Patient movement, poor electrode application, equipment malfunction, or electromagnetic interference may all result in a wide complex artifact.

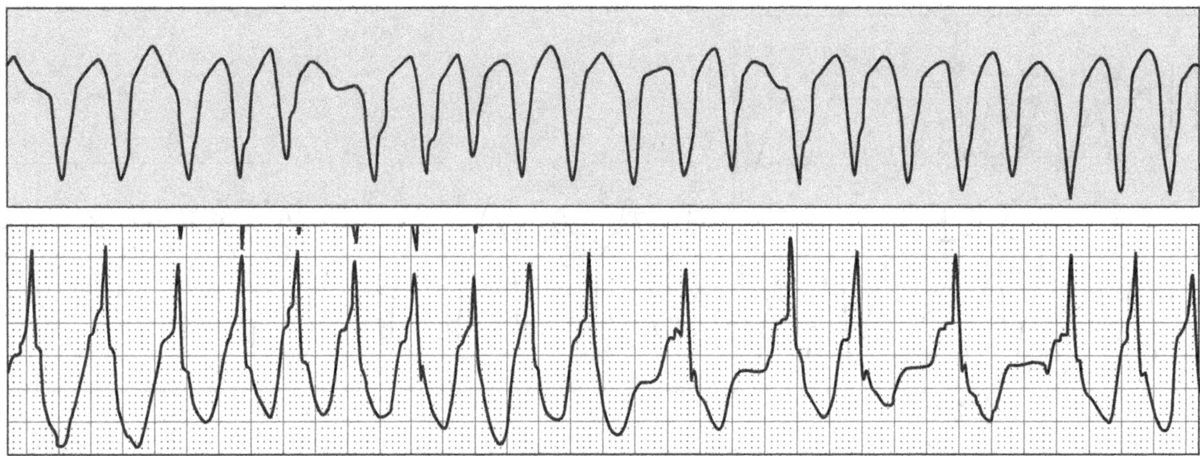

Figure 23.10 Supraventricular tachycardia (SVT) with aberrant ventricular conduction – WPW-related atrial fibrillation. Note the rapid rate, irregular pattern, and varying QRS complex morphology.

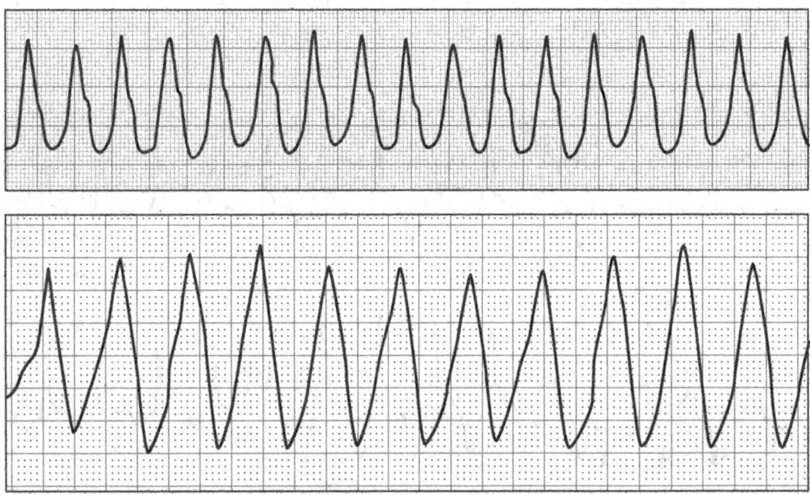

Figure 23.11 Supraventricular tachycardia (SVT) with aberrant ventricular conduction – WPW-related wide complex tachycardia (WCT). Note the extremely rapid rates.

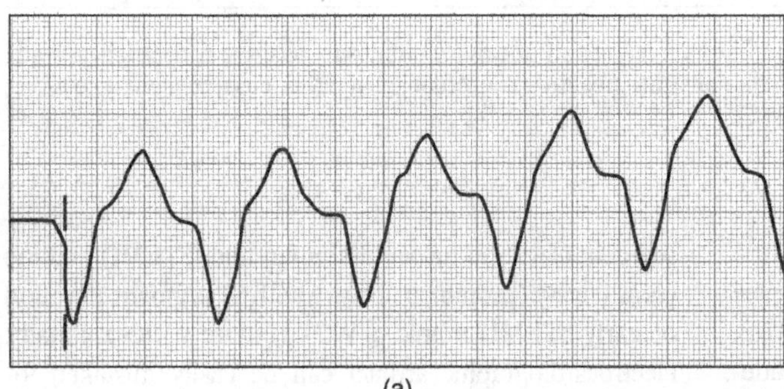

(a)

Figure 23.12 Miscellaneous causes of supraventricular tachycardia (SVT) with aberrant ventricular conduction. (a) Sinoventricular rhythm due to hyperkalemia. (b) Sodium channel blockade due to overdose of an antidepressant medication. (c) Sinus tachycardia with anterior wall STEMI and the giant R wave (prominent T wave with ST segment elevation of early STEMI) mimicking a wide complex tachycardia (WCT).

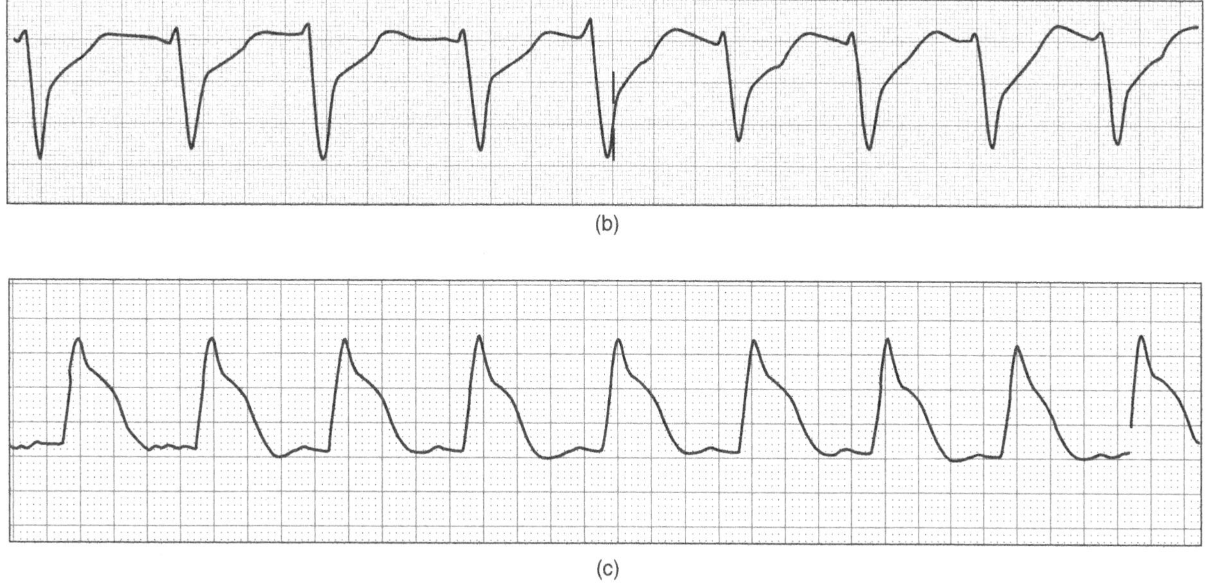

(b)

(c)

Figure 23.12 (Continued)

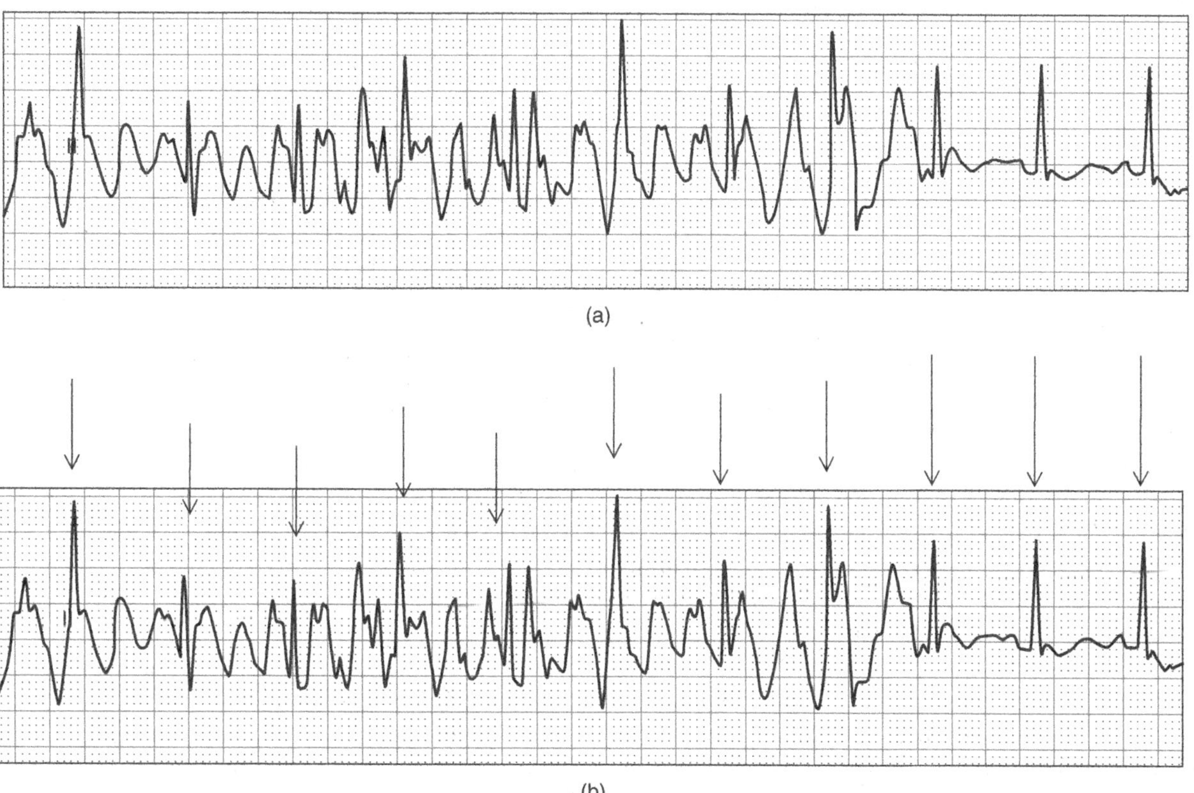

(a)

(b)

Figure 23.13 Artifact mimicking wide complex tachycardia (WCT). (a) Rhythm strip of a patient with motion-related ECG artifact mimicking a WCT. (b) The same rhythm strip from "a." The long arrows on the right of the rhythm strip highlight the actual cardiac rhythm (sinus rhythm), while the small arrows on the remainder of the tracing indicate the normal appearing QRS complexes, which are partially obscured by the artifact. Note that the R–R interval of normal appearing beats (the space between two consecutive QRS complexes) can provide a clue to this diagnosis.

Pacemaker-Mediated Tachycardia

In a patient with an implanted permanent pacemaker that allows for atrial sensing and ventricular pacing, tachycardia may occur because of an SVT-stimulating ventricular pacing or because of retrograde P waves being sensed and resulting in inappropriate ventricular pacing. The ventricular paced QRS complexes produced are wide, and pacer spikes can be seen.

24

Electrocardiographic Differential Diagnosis of Bradyarrhythmia

Megan Starling[1,2] *and William J. Brady*[3]

[1] *Department of Emergency Medicine, University of Virginia School of Medicine, Charlottesville, VA, USA*
[2] *Department of Emergency Medicine, Culpeper Memorial Hospital, Culpeper, VA, USA*
[3] *Departments of Emergency Medicine and Medicine, University of Virginia School of Medicine, Charlottesville, VA, USA*

Bradyarrhythmia is defined as any cardiac rhythm with a slow ventricular response. In the adult patient, a heart rate less than 60 bpm is considered "slow" and thus a bradyarrhythmia; infants and young children, of course, have age-related rate definitions for bradycardia. Bradycardic rhythms include a broad range of diagnoses such as sinus bradycardia, junctional and idioventricular rhythms, advanced atrioventricular (AV) block with varying escape rhythms (i.e. second- and third-degree AV blocks), atrial rhythms with heightened AV block (i.e. atrial fibrillation with slow ventricular response), and rhythms related to metabolic issues (i.e. hyperkalemia). In most instances, a slow heart rate is indicative of pathology; sinus bradycardia, however, can be encountered in high endurance athletes, among other patient types, representing a normal variant finding.

The differential diagnosis of bradycardia is listed in Table 24.1.

Sinus bradycardia is a rhythm with a heart rate less than 60 bpm; the impulse originates from the sinus node, demonstrating the characteristics of sinus rhythm, including upright P waves in leads I–III and a 1:1 P wave-to-QRS complex ratio. It is the most common form of bradycardia seen in clinical medicine and has a multitude of causes including acute coronary syndrome (ACS), chronic conduction system disease, medication effect, electrolyte disturbances, and extreme athletic conditioning (Figure 24.1a).

See Management Box 24.1.

Junctional escape rhythms have a cardiac impulse originating from the AV junction. This rhythm occurs when impulses from the sinoatrial (SA) node or other atrial sources are not present, are not functioning properly, or are not being sensed by the AV node; a junctional rhythm is thus an escape rhythm. The AV nodal tissue assumes the pacemaker function of the heart, creating a junctional rhythm, which is bradycardic. It can be identified as regular narrow complex bradycardia (Figure 24.1b) at a rate of 40–60 bpm with absent, misplaced, and/or inverted P waves. The misplaced and/or inverted P waves will be present if there is retrograde transmission of the impulse from the AV node to the atrium and are termed *retrograde P waves*. In the setting of third-degree heart block, a junctional rhythm can be seen as the escape rhythm; in this case, there may also be normal appearing upright P waves occurring at regular intervals but at a rate and rhythm completely detached from the "junctional" QRS complexes. The upright P waves are caused by the SA node-firing impulses that are not being sensed by the AV node and thus are not being transmitted to the ventricles. The junctional rhythm, when encountered, should be considered an escape rhythm, assuming the role of pacemaker if the SA node is non-functional. The clinical causes are similar to those of sinus bradycardia (Clinical Presentation Box 24.1).

Idioventricular rhythm has a cardiac impulse originating from a focus in the ventricles. This rhythm occurs when dysfunction in the conducting system proximal to the ventricles forces a focus in the ventricular myocardium to assume the function as a cardiac pacemaker. This assumption of pace-making function may occur when SA node and all other foci in the atria and AV node fail to either conduct or generate an impulse or when there is complete AV block. Similar to the junctional rhythm, the idioventricular rhythm should be

The Electrocardiogram in Emergency and Acute Care, First Edition.
Edited by Korin B. Hudson, Amita Sudhir, George Glass, and William J. Brady.

Table 24.1 The differential diagnosis of bradycardia.

Sinus bradycardia
Junctional bradycardia
Idioventricular rhythm
Second-degree AV block, type II
Third-degree AV block
Atrial fibrillation/flutter with slow ventricular response
Sinoventricular rhythm of severe hyperkalemia

Management Box 24.1 Bradycardia

Atropine is an effective agent used in patients with compromising bradyarrhythmia.

Atropine is likely more effective in sinus bradycardia compared to idioventricular rhythm; furthermore, higher initial doses (i.e. 1.0 mg in the adult) of atropine are likely to be more effective than lower doses.

Clinical Presentation Box 24.1 Sinus Bradycardia and Junctional Rhythms

Sinus bradycardia and junctional rhythms can be encountered in asymptomatic patients, thus representing normal variants; these patients are usually younger individuals, highly conditioned athletes, etc.

Extreme caution should be applied in considering the bradyarrhythmia to be a normal variant.

The patient should not have any clinical correlation with a bradyarrhythmia, such as syncope, weakness, overdose, and ACS event.

Patients on β-blockers or the non-selective calcium channel blockers may present with a sinus bradycardia caused by these medications even in situations when sinus tachycardia is anticipated (i.e. shock states).

considered an escape rhythm. An idioventricular rhythm (Figure 24.1c) can be identified as a regular, wide complex bradycardia with a rate of 20–40 bpm with absent P waves. Not unlike the situation with the junctional rhythm and complete heart block, an idioventricular rhythm can be the escape rhythm in patients with third-degree AV block; in this situation, there will be regularly spaced, identical appearing upright P waves with no apparent association to the ventricular QRS complexes.

Atrial fibrillation and atrial flutter with slow ventricular response can both present with bradyarrhythmias (Figure 24.2). In most cases, these rhythms will present as tachycardia. Yet, if certain medications or other disease states alter the AV node's ability to transmit impulse, a slow ventricular response – that is, a bradycardia – will be seen in these two rhythm scenarios.

Sick sinus syndrome occurs when there is a dysfunctional sinus node that produces a regular or irregular sinus bradycardia at a rate that would normally trigger atrial, junctional, or ventricular escape rhythms but because of underlying cardiac dysfunction, these escape rhythms do not appear. ECG tracings reveal a regular or irregular wide or narrow complex sinus bradycardia with identical P waves preceding each QRS complex at a rate lower than would be expected with sinus bradycardia in a heart with functional escape mechanisms. In addition to the underlying severe sinus bradycardia in sick sinus syndrome, there may be occasional runs of tachyarrhythmias, atrial, junctional, or ventricular escape beats, and periods of sinus arrest.

Atrioventricular block can be present with bradyarrhythmias, including both forms of second-degree AV block and third-degree AV block (also known as *complete heart block*; Clinical Presentation Box 24.2 and Management Box 24.2). Etiologies of AV block are similar to those seen in patients with bradycardia. First-degree AV block (Figure 24.3a) is diagnosed when a prolonged PR interval is noted, greater than 0.2 second in length, that is unchanging in length from beat to beat. It is less commonly associated with bradycardia.

Second-degree type I AV block (Wenkebach) is identified when the PR interval progressively prolongs to a point at which the impulse cannot reach the ventricles, resulting in a non-conducted P wave (i.e. no QRS complex). On the ECG (Figure 24.3b), it is an irregular, narrow complex rhythm with progressively longer PR interval followed by a P wave with no QRS complex. The degree of block is expressed as a ratio of the P waves to QRS complexes; thus, a pattern with three P waves, the last of which is not conducted but produces three QRS complexes can be termed a *3:2 block*. Second-degree type II AV block is caused by periodic blockage of impulses through the AV node; at times, this form of AV block can cause a bradycardia if there are frequent non-conducted beats. The ECG (Figure 24.3c) demonstrates a consistent, non-changing PR interval; it may be normal in length or prolonged, but it is fixed. Ultimately, a P wave occurs, which is not associated with a QRS complex, resulting in a non-conducted beat. The term *high grade* is used if there are more than one non-conducted P waves occurring sequentially.

Third-degree AV block is caused by complete blockade at the AV node, leading to no impulse conduction from the atria to ventricles. ECG tracings (Figure 24.3d) reveal a regular ventricular or junctional escape rhythm superimposed on regularly occurring identical, upright

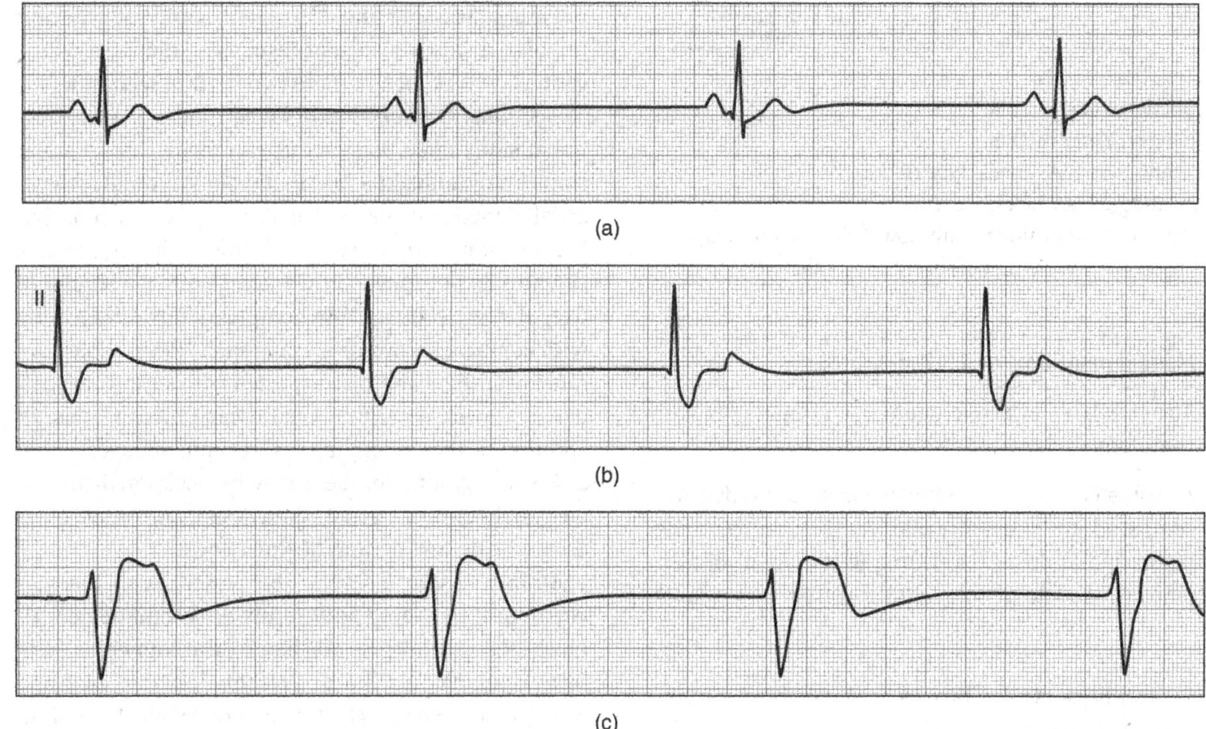

Figure 24.1 Bradycardias. (a) Sinus bradycardia – criteria for sinus rhythm are present with the exception of a rate less than 60 bpm. (b) Junctional bradycardia – a regular, narrow QRS complex rhythm without evidence of obvious P waves. (c) Idioventricular bradycardia – a regular, wide QRS complex rhythm without evidence of P waves.

P waves with no associated QRS complex. The P waves and QRS complexes each have their own, regular rates caused by two separate impulses, sinus node and AV node or ventricular myocardium, respectively.

Hyperkalemia, or elevated serum potassium, can present with bradycardia. Elevated serum potassium slows impulse release and disrupts conduction, resulting in bradycardia, AV block, and intraventricular conduction abnormality. The most concerning hyperkalemia-related bradyarrhythmia is the sinoventricular rhythm (Clinical Presentation Box 24.3) (Figure 24.4). It is diagnosed as follows: absence of P waves, extremely widened QRS complexes (e.g. the sine wave morphology), and slow ventricular rate.

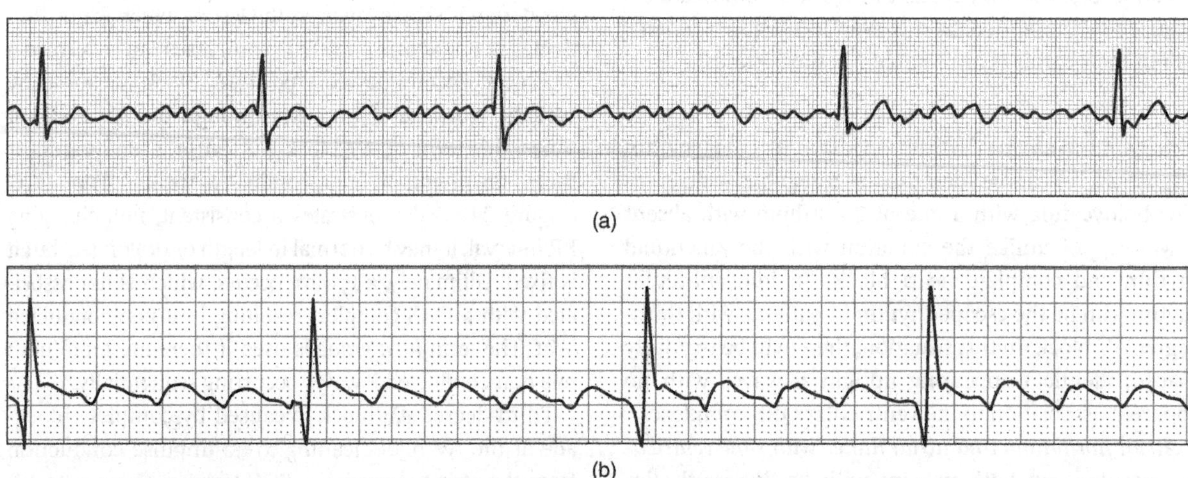

Figure 24.2 (a) Atrial fibrillation with slow ventricular response. (b) Atrial flutter with slow ventricular response; note the appearance of the flutter waves, which are more easily seen with the less frequent appearance of QRS complexes.

Clinical Presentation Box 24.2 Atrioventricular Block

Second-degree type I AV block can be considered a normal variant; extreme caution should be exercised when "normal variant" status is considered – the patient should not have any clinical correlation with a bradyarrhythmia, such as syncope, weakness, overdose, and ACS event.

Second-degree type II and third-degree AV blocks are always pathologic, indicative of significant conduction system dysfunction.

Management Box 24.2 Atrioventricular Block

Atropine is less likely to be effective in more severe forms of AV block, such as second-degree type II and third-degree AV blocks.

Furthermore, certain authorities consider atropine contraindicated in these AV blocks.

Transcutaneous pacing should be considered in these compromised patients.

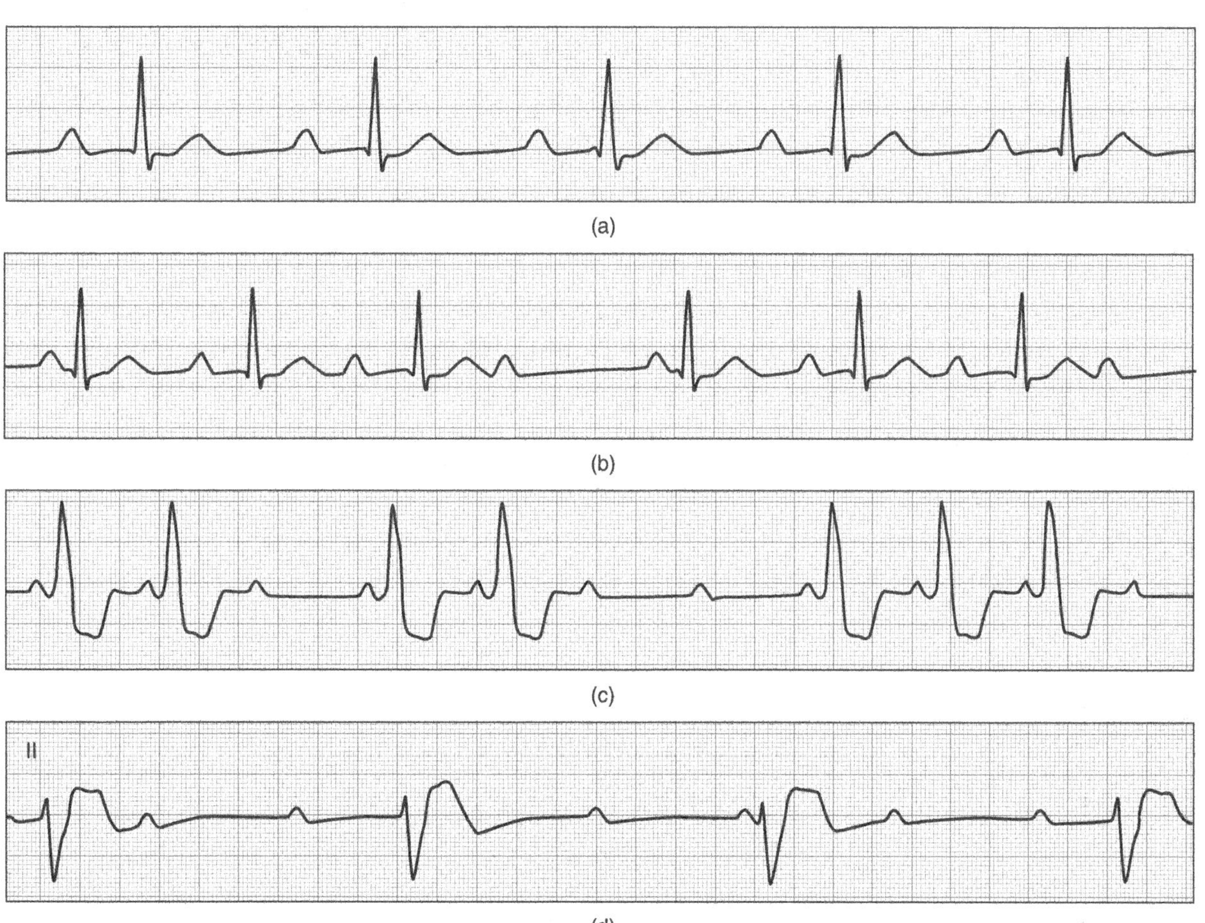

Figure 24.3 Atrioventricular blocks. (a) First-degree AV block. Note the prolonged PR interval, which does not alter from beat to beat. (b) Second-degree type I AV block. Note the progressive lengthening of the PR interval with ultimate dropped beat (i.e. no QRS complex). (c) Second-degree type II AV block. Note the constant length of the PR interval with sudden dropped beat (i.e. no QRS complex). The QRS complex is frequently, but not always, widened in this form of AV block. (d) Third-degree (i.e. complete) AV block. This block is also known as *complete heart block* or *heart block*. There is no association of the P waves to the QRS complexes; the atrial rate is also greater than the ventricular rate.

Clinical Presentation Box 24.3 Sinoventricular Rhythm of Severe Hyperkalemia

In the patient with a wide QRS complex bradycardia, consider the sinoventricular rhythm of hyperkalemia in patients with acute or chronic renal failure, severe liver disease, digitalis poisoning, and salt substitute (e.g. potassium chloride) use.

These patients are at risk for hyperkalemic cardiac arrest.

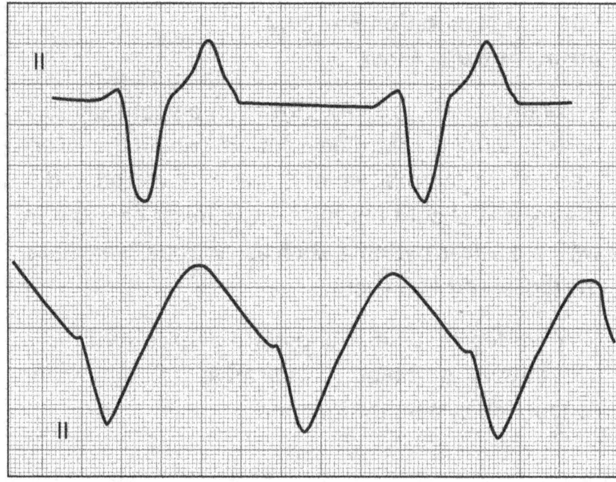

Figure 24.4 The sinoventricular rhythm of severe hyperkalemia. Note the very widened QRS complex, absence of P wave, and overall slow rate.

25

Electrocardiographic Differential Diagnosis of ST Segment Elevation

Megan Starling[1,2] *and William J. Brady*[3]

[1] *Department of Emergency Medicine, University of Virginia School of Medicine, Charlottesville, VA, USA*
[2] *Department of Emergency Medicine, Culpeper Memorial Hospital, Culpeper, VA, USA*
[3] *Departments of Emergency Medicine and Medicine, University of Virginia School of Medicine, Charlottesville, VA, USA*

ST segment elevation is a well-recognized electrocardiographic sign of acute coronary syndrome (ACS), in particular, ST segment elevation myocardial infarction (STEMI). There are, however, many other different clinical situations that are capable of causing ST segment elevation (Figure 25.1 and Table 25.1). The correct management of the patient is dependent on the correct diagnosis.

In certain individuals, ST segment elevation is benign and considered a normal variant; benign early repolarization (BER) is a common cause of non-pathologic ST segment elevation. In other persons, ST segment elevation indicates some form of cardiac illness, whether it be acute or chronic in nature, including STEMI, Prinzmetal's angina, left bundle branch block (LBBB), left ventricular hypertrophy, pericarditis/myopericarditis, left ventricular aneurysm, ventricular paced rhythm, Brugada syndrome, hyperkalemia, and major non-cardiac causes such as intracranial hemorrhage, pulmonary embolism, and aortic dissection.

ST segment elevation myocardial infarction is diagnosed when the patient presents with the appropriate symptoms (e.g. chest pain, dyspnea, etc.) and electrocardiographic ST segment elevation. ST segment elevation seen in STEMI must be at least 1 mm in height above the electrocardiographic baseline and present in at least two anatomically contiguous leads; note that the baseline is defined as the TP segment. The morphology of the ST segment (Figures 25.2 and 25.3) is commonly convex (or "bulging upward"), although it may often be straight (flat) or concave (or "sagging downward"). Other ECG findings associated with STEMI include new T wave inversion, ST segment depression in leads opposite to those with elevations (i.e. reciprocal change or reciprocal ST segment depression), evolving/changing ST segment and T wave morphologies with serial ECGs, and the presence or development of Q waves. Figures 25.4–25.6 present different forms of ST segment elevation associated with STEMI.

Prinzmetal's angina is a cause of ST segment elevation that may appear identical to STEMI. In this case, the ischemia is generally reversible as it is caused by coronary artery vasospasm as opposed to the acute plaque rupture with thrombus formation and blockage of arterial flow seen in STEMI. Resolution is often spontaneous, although treatment with nitroglycerin or calcium channel blockers can hasten resolution. This entity should be considered in patients with typical symptoms and ECG findings of STEMI that resolve before reperfusion treatment (e.g. fibrinolytic agents or percutaneous coronary intervention). The distinction between the ST segment elevations seen in STEMI and Prinzmetal's angina is extremely difficult, if not impossible, based on initial assessment and ongoing evaluation and serial ECGs may be required with a low threshold to default to the more serious condition (STEMI) if there are ongoing symptoms, concerns, or doubts as to the diagnosis.

LBBB and ventricular paced rhythms are both common causes of ST segment elevation, both generally discordant to the QRS complex (Figure 25.7). The ST segment elevation of LBBB is generally concave in shape and discordant to the QRS complex (Figure 25.8). "Discordant to the QRS complex" means that the ST segment elevation is directed in the opposite direction (discordant) from the major terminal portion of the QRS complex; thus, a patient with LBBB-related ST segment elevation will demonstrate a predominantly or entirely negatively oriented QRS

The Electrocardiogram in Emergency and Acute Care, First Edition.
Edited by Korin B. Hudson, Amita Sudhir, George Glass, and William J. Brady.

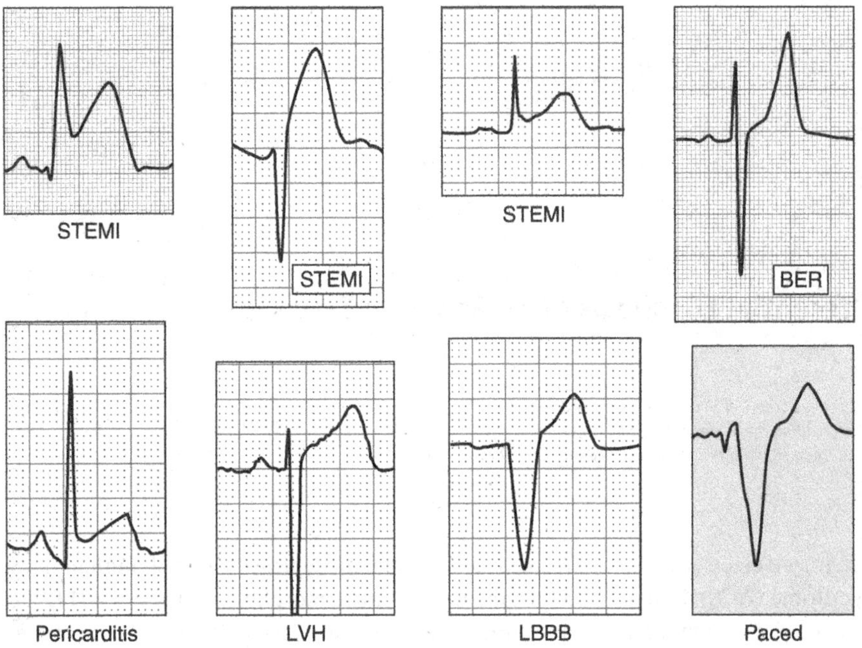

Figure 25.1 Various causes of ST segment elevation in adults with chest pain. LVH, left ventricular hypertrophy.

Table 25.1 Differential diagnosis of ST segment elevation.

More common causes:
- STEMI
- Left bundle branch block (LBBB)
- Left ventricular hypertrophy
- Ventricular paced rhythm
- Acute pericarditis
- Benign early repolarization (BER)
- Left ventricular aneurysm

Less common causes:
- Myocarditis
- Brugada syndrome
- Cardiomyopathy
- Hyperkalemia
- Intracranial hemorrhage
- Pulmonary embolism
- Aortic dissection

complex – such is the case in leads V1–V3. Although some ST segment elevation is normal in LBBB, excessive ST segment elevation (>5 mm) in patients with a convincing clinical presentation for ACS should prompt consideration of acute myocardial infarction (MI). Similar findings are noted in the patient with a ventricular paced rhythm (Figure 25.9; Clinical Presentation Box 25.1).

Left ventricular hypertrophy may also cause concave ST segment elevation, especially in leads V1–V3 (Figure 25.10). Like LBBB, these ST segment elevations are discordant with the major portion of the QRS complex – that is, directed opposite to a negatively oriented QRS complex. These elevations are typically less than 5 mm and do not evolve, or change, with serial ECG evaluation.

Acute pericarditis (or acute myopericarditis) can be present with diffuse concave ST segment elevation (Figure 25.11). In acute pericarditis, ST segment elevation is usually less than 5 mm in height and widely distributed across the ECG, seen in all leads except leads aVR and V1. Other ECG clues to acute pericarditis include the absence of ST segment depression, the presence of PR segment changes (depression in the inferior leads and lead V6) and elevation (lead aVR), and ST segment elevation that does not change with repeated ECG evaluations.

BER is a common cause of diffuse, concave ST segment elevation that is often most remarkable in the precordial leads V1–V4. It is most often encountered in the anterior leads alone. It can also be seen simultaneously in the anterior and inferior leads; "isolated" findings limited to the inferior leads are unusual in BER. BER (Figure 25.12) may be identified by an elevated and irregular or notched J point (point at which QRS complex ends and the ST segment begins); the T waves are tall with a symmetric structure. This is a benign variant of normal ECG appearance and is unchanging over time. It is often very difficult to

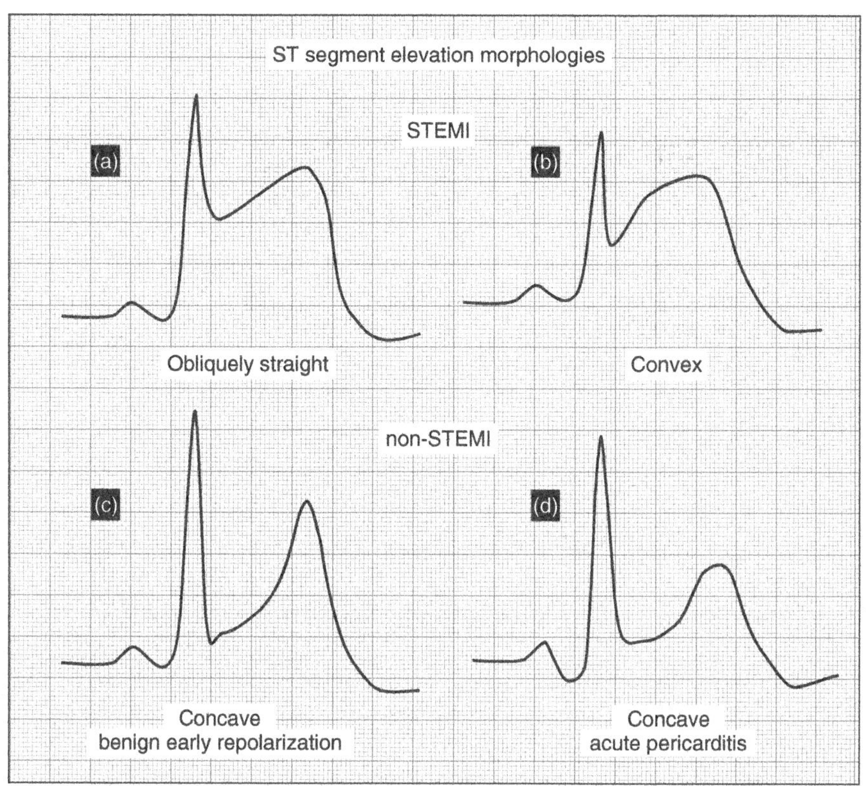

Figure 25.2 ST segment elevation subtypes in STEMI and non-STEMI presentations. (a) STEMI with obliquely straight ST segment elevation; (b) STEMI with convex ST segment elevation; (c) non-STEMI (benign early repolarization, BER) with concave ST segment elevation; (d) non-STEMI (acute pericarditis) with concave ST segment elevation.

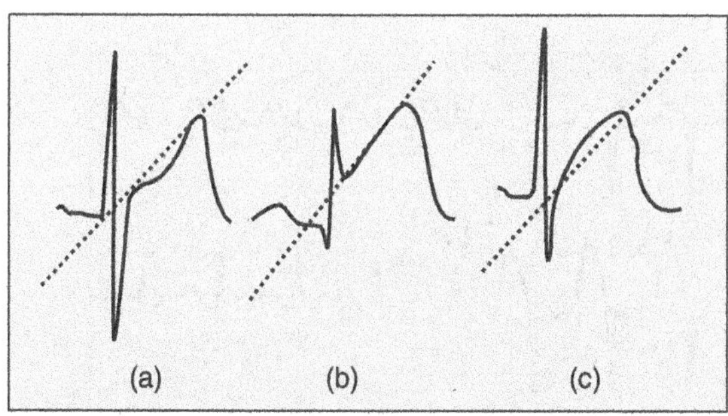

Figure 25.3 Determination of the morphology of the elevated ST segment. (a) Concave – associated with non-STEMI causes of elevation; (b) obliquely straight – associated with STEMI; (c) convex – associated with STEMI.

distinguish from the ST segment elevation seen in acute pericarditis.

Left ventricular aneurysm is a cause of ST segment elevation in patients with past myocardial infarction; in most cases of left ventricular aneurysm, the myocardial infarction has been extensive and has not been interrupted with acute reperfusion therapy. The resulting infarcted segment produces an outpouching, or aneurysm, of the ventricular wall. Most commonly, the left ventricular aneurysm is seen in anterior leads V1–V4 (Figure 25.13). Frequently, significant Q waves are seen, signifying a large, completed myocardial infarction; small, inverted T waves are also found. The magnitude of the ST segment elevation is usually minimal with 1–3 mm encountered in most patients; in the rare patient, ST segment elevation approaching 5 mm is seen. There are often associated non-specific T wave abnormalities, yet reciprocal changes are uncommon; repeated ECG examinations demonstrate an absence of change in the ST segment. Without prior history or old ECGs, this diagnosis may be difficult and is often confused with STEMI.

Brugada syndrome is a genetic syndrome associated with mutations of cardiac sodium ion channels that predispose patients to sudden death from malignant ventricular rhythms, such as polymorphic ventricular tachycardia and ventricular fibrillation. Characteristically, it is seen as an apparent right bundle branch block (RBBB) (rSr′) pattern in leads V1 and/or V2 with associated ST segment elevation. The RBBB can be complete with a QRS complex duration greater than 0.12 seconds in width or incomplete with minimal QRS complex widening. The ST segment elevation can be present in

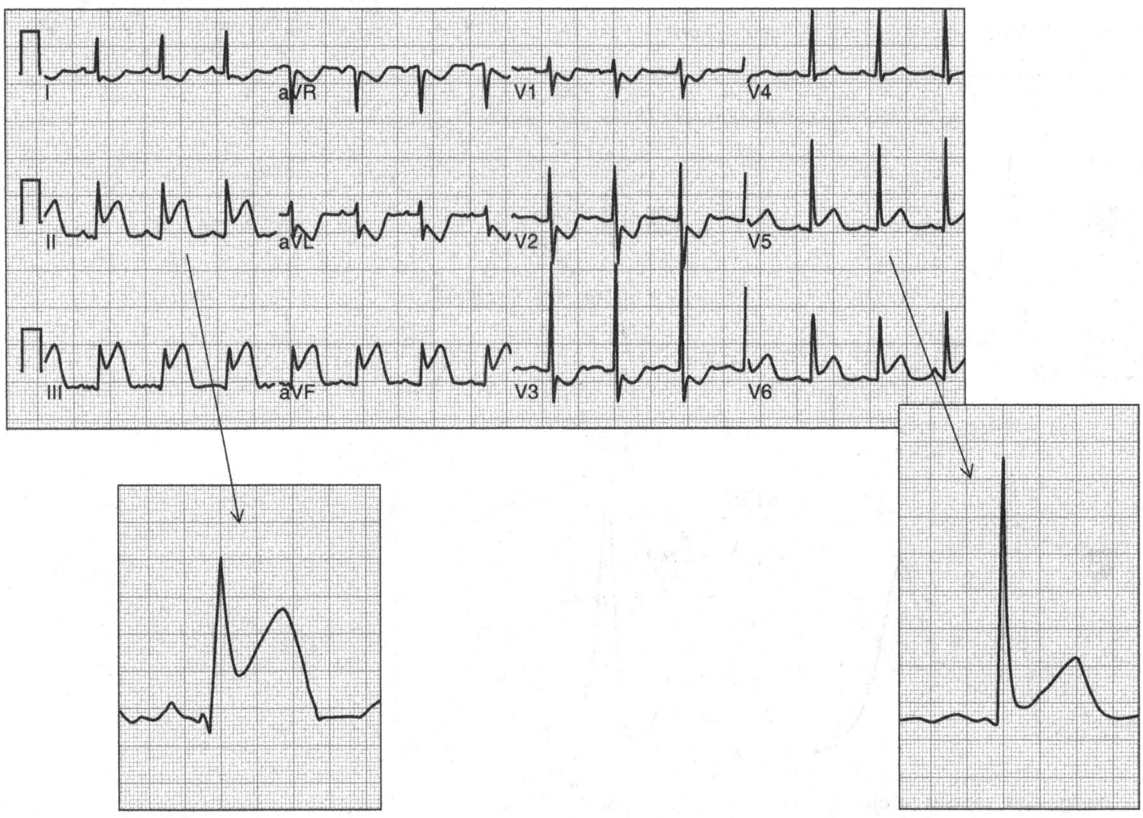

Figure 25.4 Inferolateral STEMI with obvious ST segment elevation in leads II, III, and aVF; less obvious ST segment elevation is seen in leads V5 and V6.

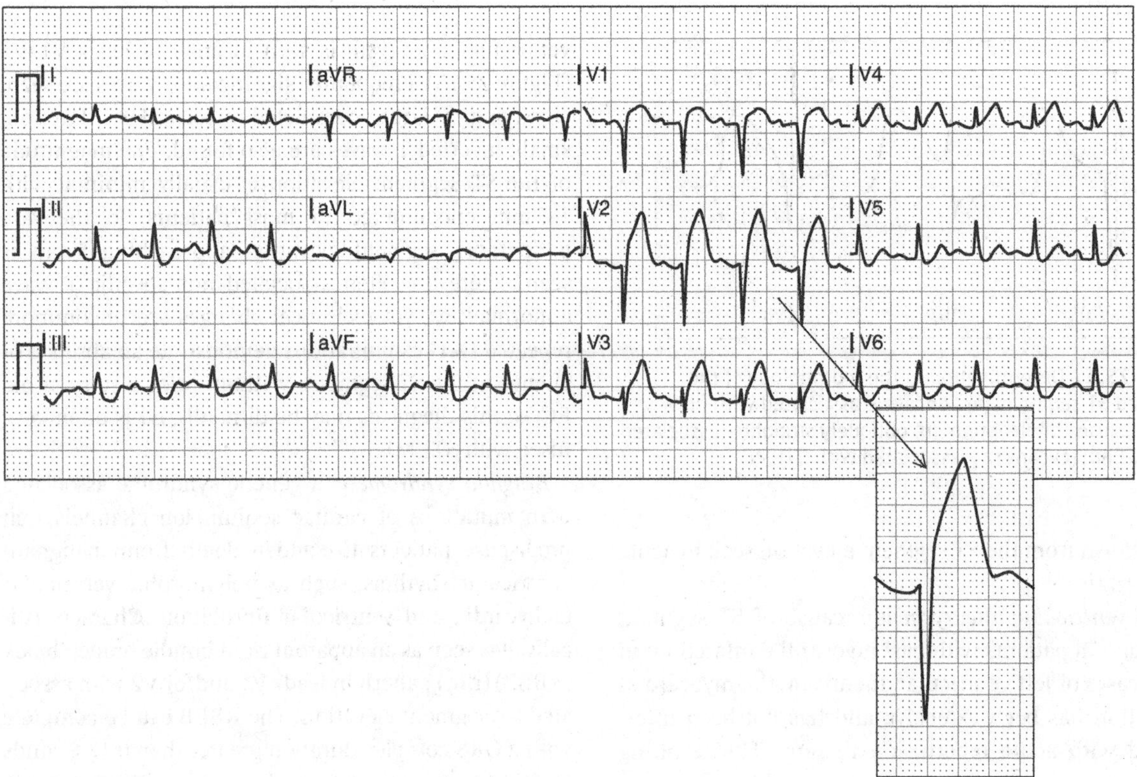

Figure 25.5 Anterior STEMI with ST segment elevation in leads V1–V4.

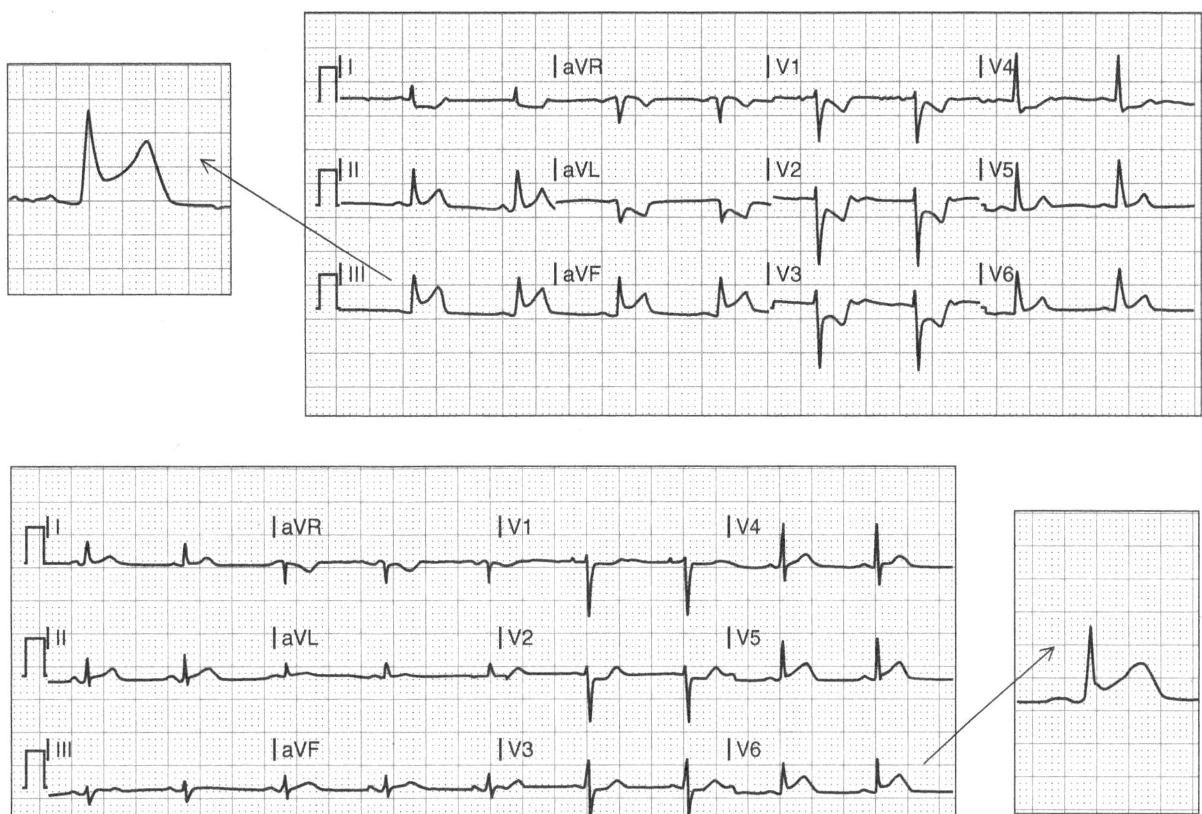

Figure 25.6 STEMI presentations with less obvious ST segment elevation.

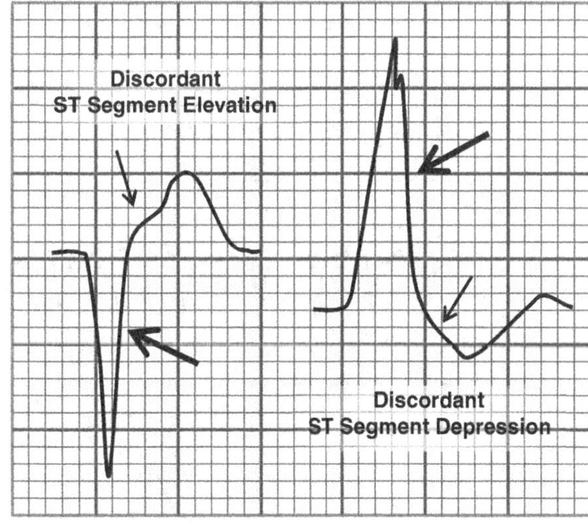

Figure 25.7 Appropriate Discordant Relationship of ST Segment to QRS Complex. This figure demonstrates the anticipated ST segment configuration in LBBB & Right Ventricular Paced patterns. Note that in both cases, the ST segment is directed opposite of the major terminal portion of the QRS complex. The example on the left is discordant ST segment elevation; the ST segment is elevated in a proportional sense on the opposite side of the isoelectric baseline from the QRS complex. The example on the right is discordant ST segment depression; note that the ST segment is depressed and located on the opposite side of the isoelectric baseline from the major terminal portion of the QRS complex. This relationship is found in both left bundle branch block (LBBB) and right ventricular paced (from implanted pacemaker) patterns.

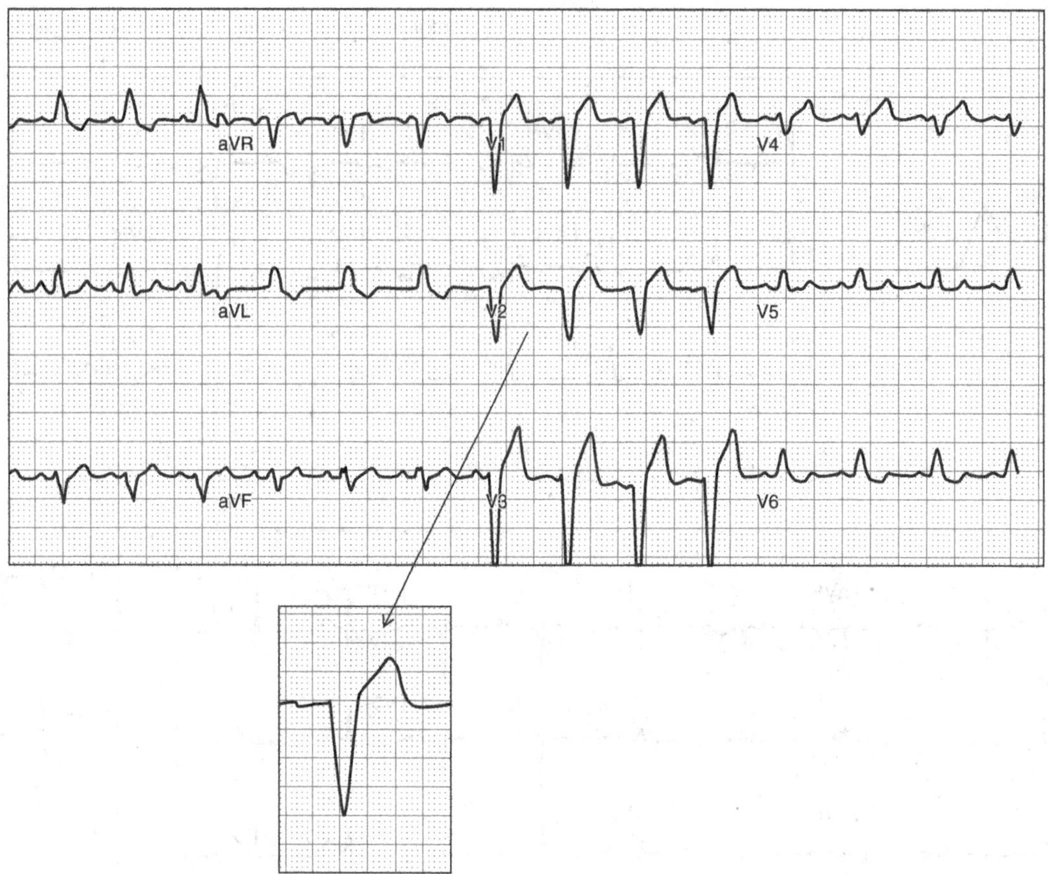

Figure 25.8 ST segment elevation in leads V1–V4, resulting from left bundle branch block (LBBB).

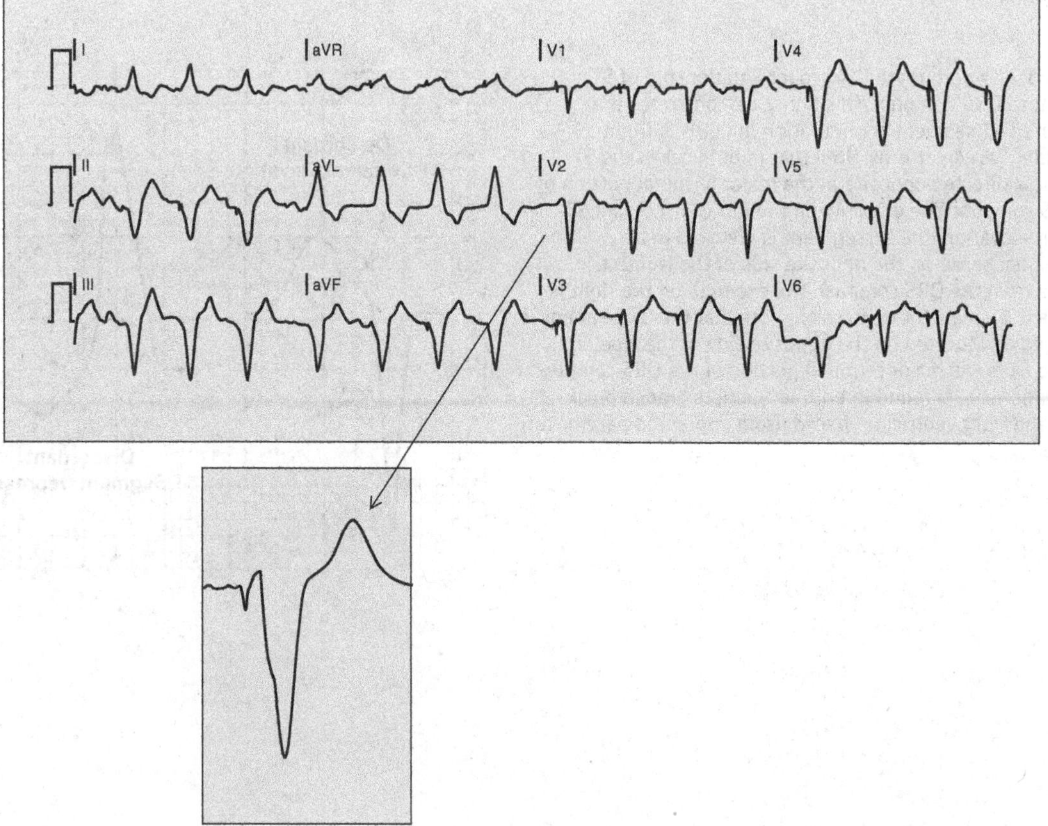

Figure 25.9 ST segment elevation in leads II, III, aVF, and V1–V6, resulting from a ventricular paced pattern.

Clinical Presentation Box 25.1 LBBB is a STEMI Equivalent-Pattern in the Appropriate Clinical Situation

A new LBBB in a patient who previously did not have one, and is experiencing chest pain or an angina equivalent, is considered a STEMI even in the absence of the specific findings discussed above.

one of three morphologies: Type 1 with coved-type ST elevation with at least 2 mm J point elevation and a gradually descending ST segment and a negative T wave; Type II with a saddle-back pattern with at least 2 mm J point elevation and at least 1 mm ST segment elevation with a positive or biphasic T wave; and Type III with a saddle-back pattern with less than 2 mm J point elevation and less than 1 mm ST segment elevation with an upright T wave. These abnormal findings are typically isolated to leads V1 and/or V2.

Other causes of ST segment elevation include *cardiomyopathy, hyperkalemia, intracranial hemorrhage, pulmonary embolism, and aortic dissection.*

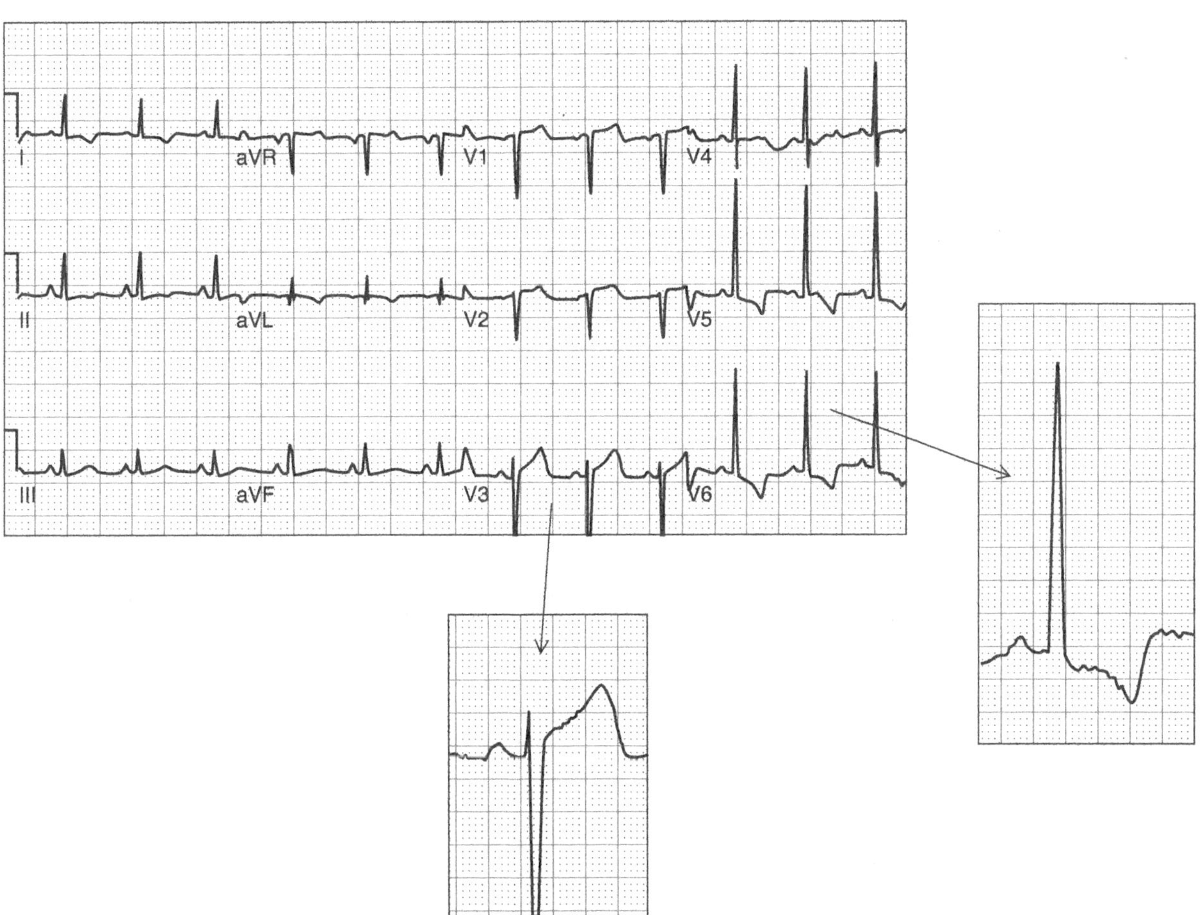

Figure 25.10 Left ventricular hypertrophy by voltage pattern with strain. Note the large QRS complexes in the precordial leads. Also, note the strain pattern, the ST segment, and T wave abnormalities seen in the precordial leads. ST segment elevation is seen in leads V1–V3 along with ST segment depression with T wave inversion in leads V5 and V6.

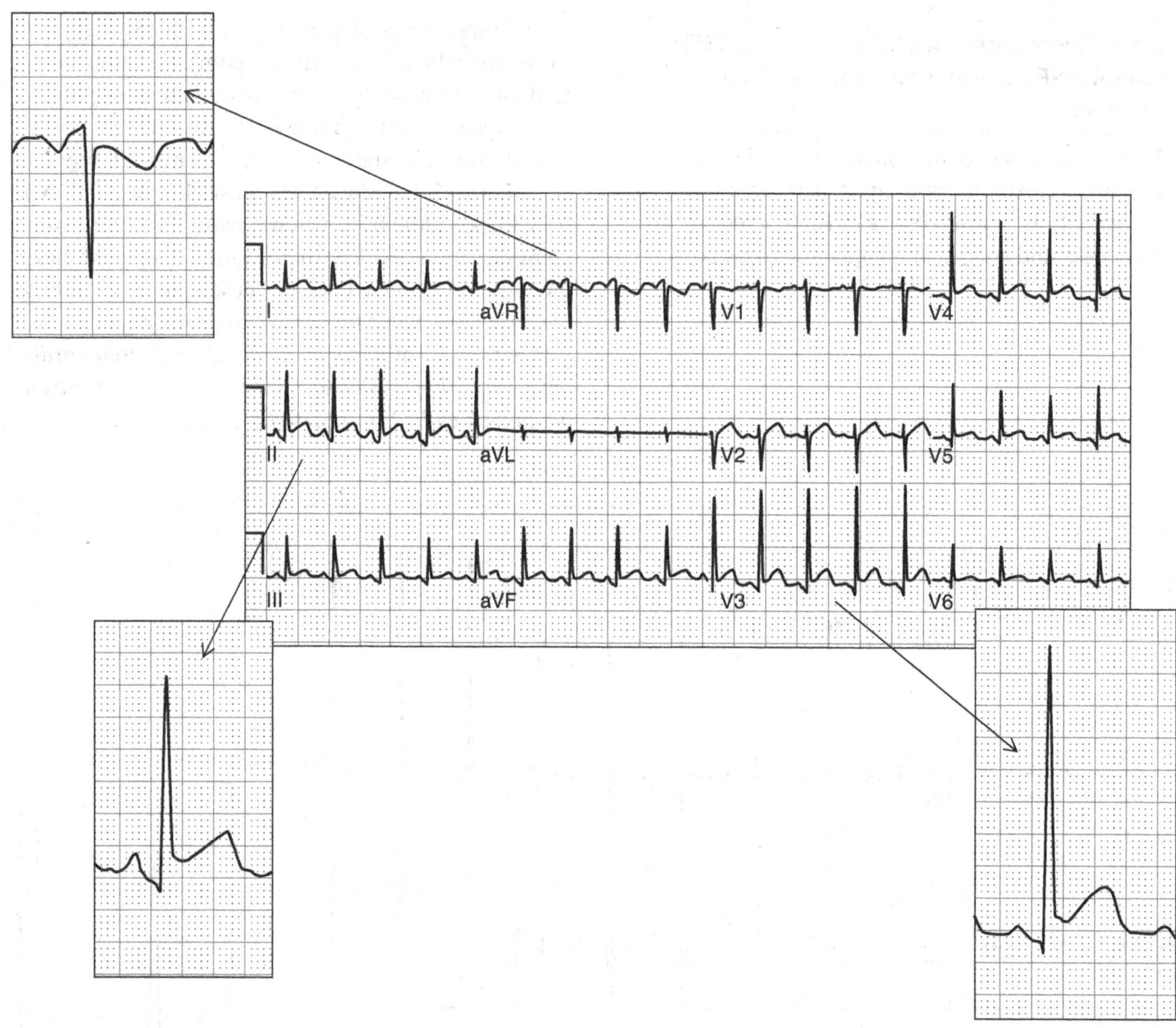

Figure 25.11 Acute myopericarditis, also commonly referred to as *acute pericarditis*, with diffuse ST segment elevation in the anterior and inferior leads. PR segment changes are best seen in the inferior leads (PR segment depression) and lead aVR (PR segment elevation).

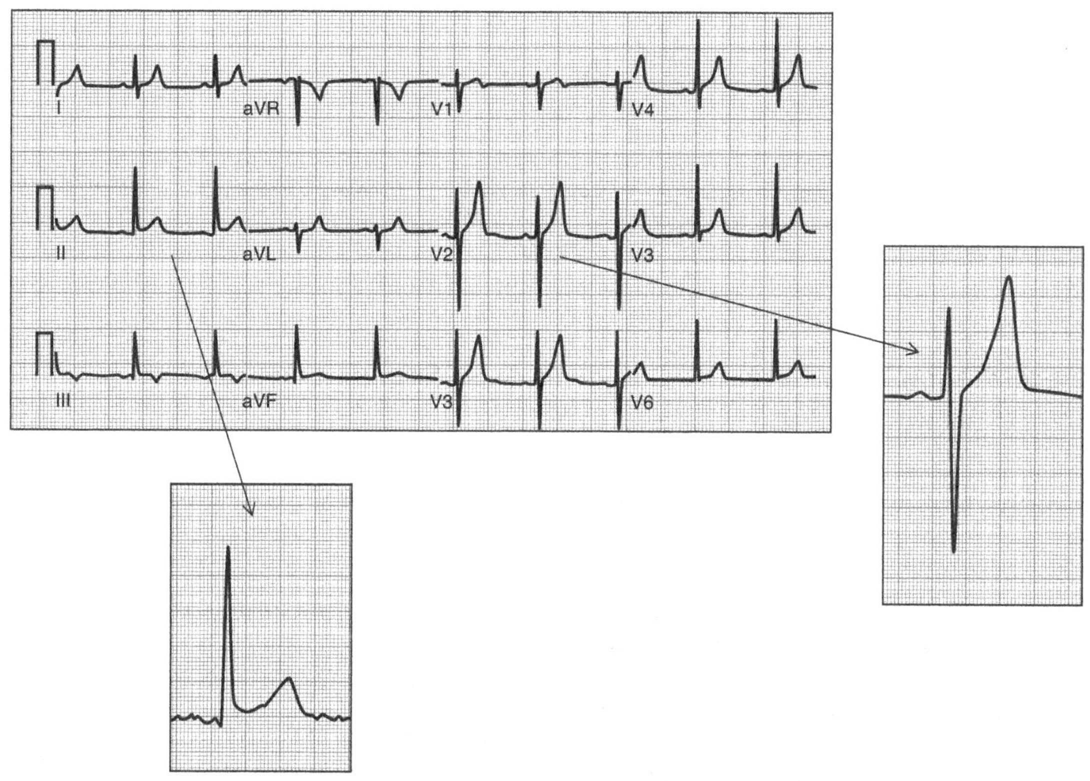

Figure 25.12 Benign early repolarization (BER) with concave ST segment elevation in leads V1–V5 as well as lead II.

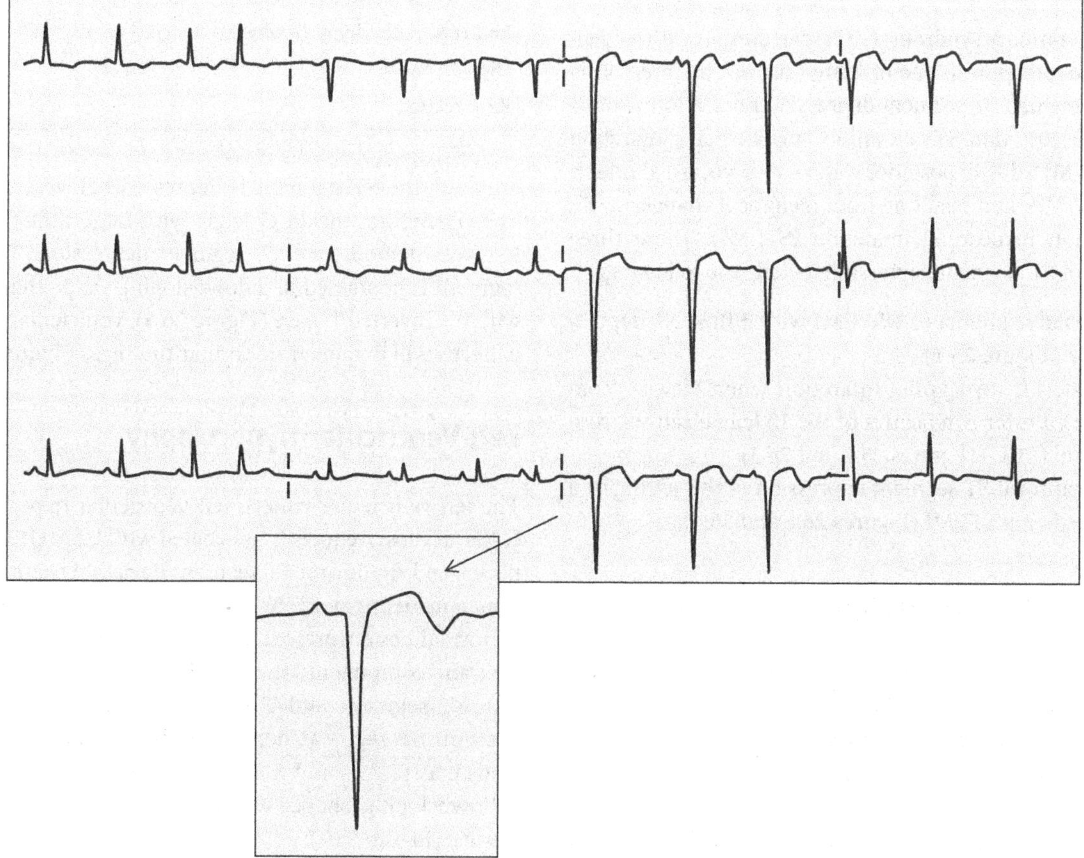

Figure 25.13 Left ventricular aneurysm with ST segment elevation in leads V1–V5; also, note the coexisting Q waves in leads V1–V4 with T wave inversion, indicating past MI.

26

Electrocardiographic Differential Diagnosis of ST Segment Depression

Amita Sudhir[1] *and William J. Brady*[2]

[1] *Department of Emergency Medicine, University of Virginia School of Medicine, Charlottesville, VA, USA*
[2] *Departments of Emergency Medicine and Medicine, University of Virginia School of Medicine, Charlottesville, VA, USA*

ST segment depression is defined as an ST segment that is depressed at least 1 mm or more below the baseline. Although ST segment depression is most commonly clinically associated with ischemia, there are several other possible causes of ST segment depression. Table 26.1 brings out the differential diagnosis of ST segment depression.

Table 26.1 The differential diagnosis of ST segment depression.

Acute coronary syndrome
• Unstable angina/NSTEMI
• Posterior wall myocardial infarction
• Reciprocal change
Left bundle branch block
Ventricular paced pattern
Left ventricular hypertrophy
Digoxin effect
Rate-related

Acute Coronary Syndromes

Acute coronary syndrome (ACS) can present with ST segment depression in one of many forms. The three basic types include ST segment depression related to unstable angina or non-ST elevation myocardial infarction (NSTEMI), due to posterior wall acute myocardial infarction (AMI), and resulting from reciprocal changes in ST elevation myocardial infarction (STEMI). These three types of ST segment depression include the following:

1) Unstable angina or NSTEMI with diffuse ST depression (Figure 26.1).
2) Posterior myocardial infarction when viewed from the anterior perspective of the 12-lead electrocardiogram (ECG) (Figures 26.2 and 26.3).
3) Reciprocal ST segment depression in the setting of a coexisting STEMI (Figures 26.2 and 26.4).

Left Bundle Branch Block

Left bundle branch block (LBBB) pattern is noted when the QRS complex duration is greater than 0.12 seconds with a mainly negatively oriented QRS complex in leads V1 and V2 and mainly positively oriented QRS complexes in leads I, aVL, V5, and V6. In leads where the primary portion of the QRS complex is positively oriented, the ST segment is depressed below the baseline. Therefore, the ECG leads with large monophasic R waves demonstrate ST segment depression. The ST segment is depressed in a downsloping shape that fuses with the inverted T wave (Figure 26.5). Ventricular paced patterns will demonstrate similar findings (Figure 26.6).

Left Ventricular Hypertrophy

The left ventricular pattern left ventricular hypertrophy (LVH) is most frequently associated with large QRS complexes and significant ST segment deviation (both elevation and depression). When ST segment and T wave abnormalities are present, the LVH pattern is said to have a strain component; the "strain" descriptor indicates that ST segment and T wave abnormalities are also present. ST segment depression is seen in the lateral leads I, aVL, V5, and V6. The ST segment is depressed in a downsloping shape, which fuses with the inverted T wave (Figure 26.7).

The Electrocardiogram in Emergency and Acute Care, First Edition.
Edited by Korin B. Hudson, Amita Sudhir, George Glass, and William J. Brady.

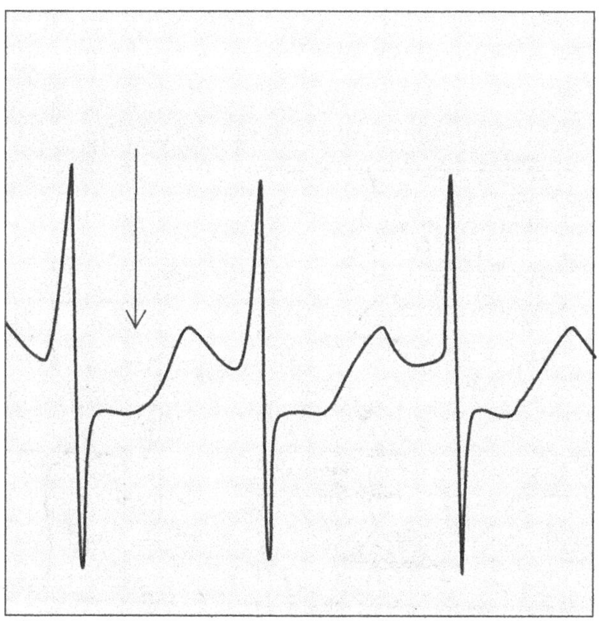

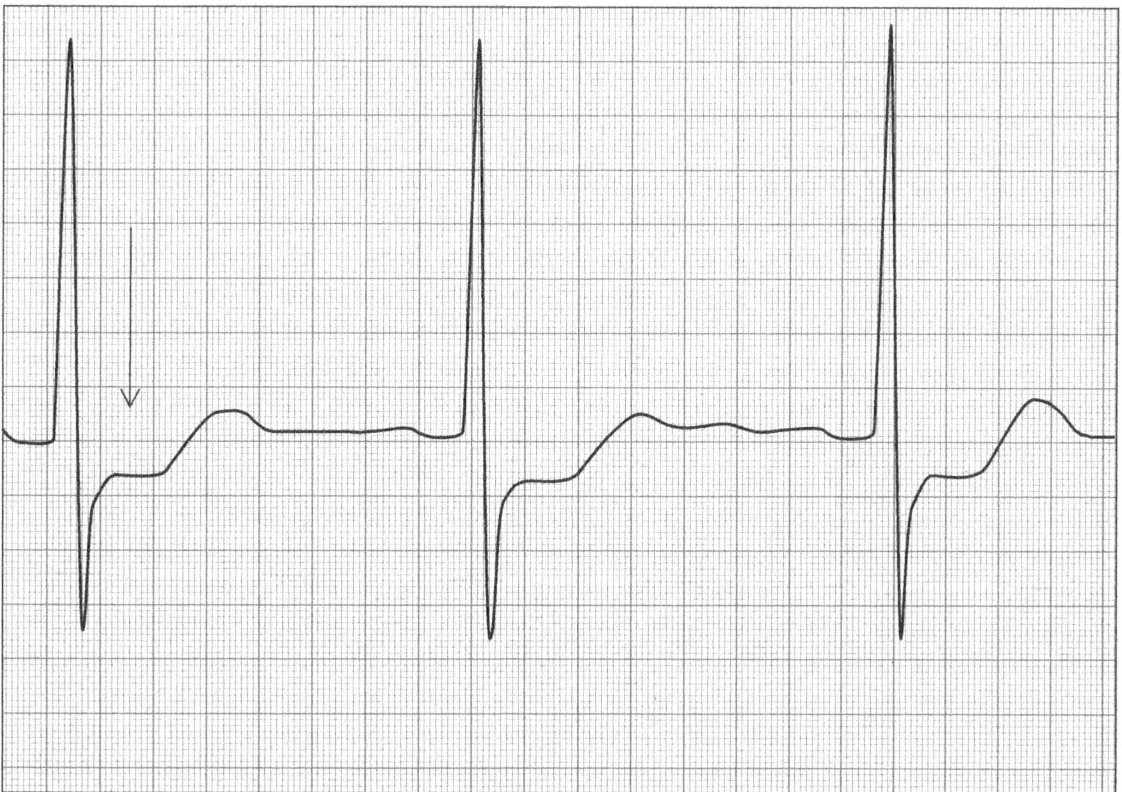

Figure 26.1 ST segment depression (arrows) resulting from ACS. In this situation, either unstable angina with ECG abnormality or non-ST segment elevation AMI could be the final diagnosis in this patient. The primary determinant between these two diagnoses would be an abnormal serum marker, such as an elevated troponin (indicating NSTEMI).

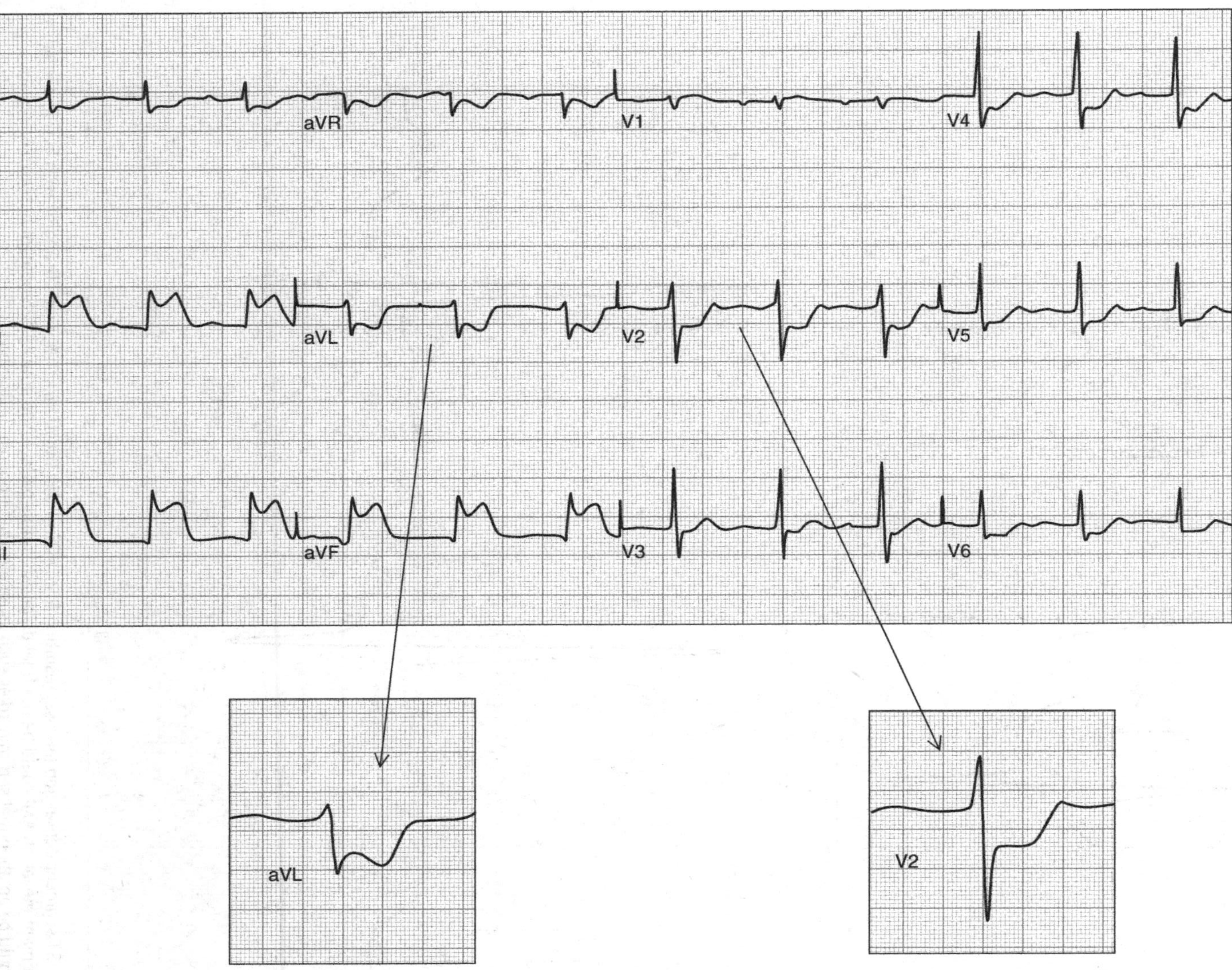

Figure 26.2 Acute inferoposterior STEMI with two forms of ST segment depression – acute posterior wall AMI (lead V2) and reciprocal change (leads I and aVL). ST segment elevation is seen in the inferior leads II, III, and aVF, consistent with inferior STEMI. ST segment depression is seen in lead V2 – this depression is suggestive of posterior wall AMI. ST segment depression is also seen in leads I and aVL – this depression is reciprocal change.

Figure 26.3 ST segment depression in leads V1–V3. This pattern of ST segment depression can suggest either acute posterior wall myocardial infarction or anterior wall ischemia. In this case, posterior wall AMI is suggested by the positive QRS complex (R wave) and upright T waves.

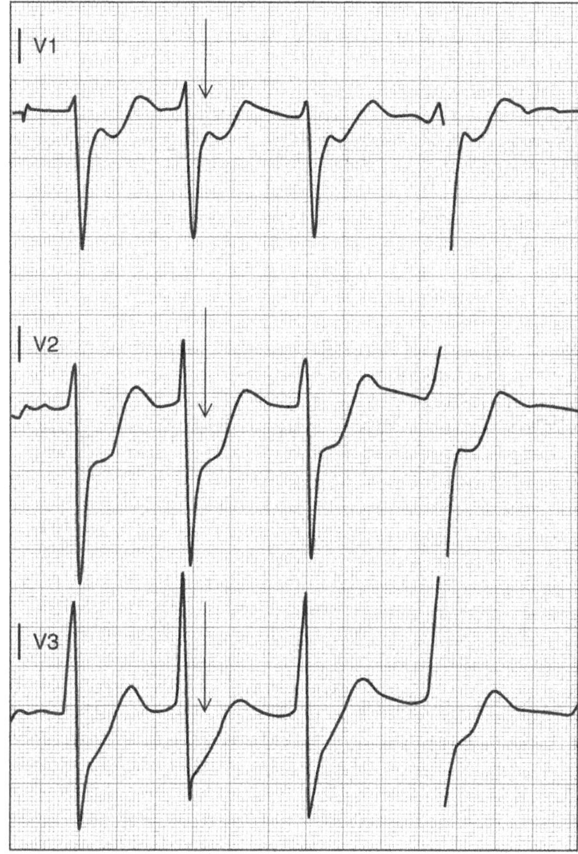

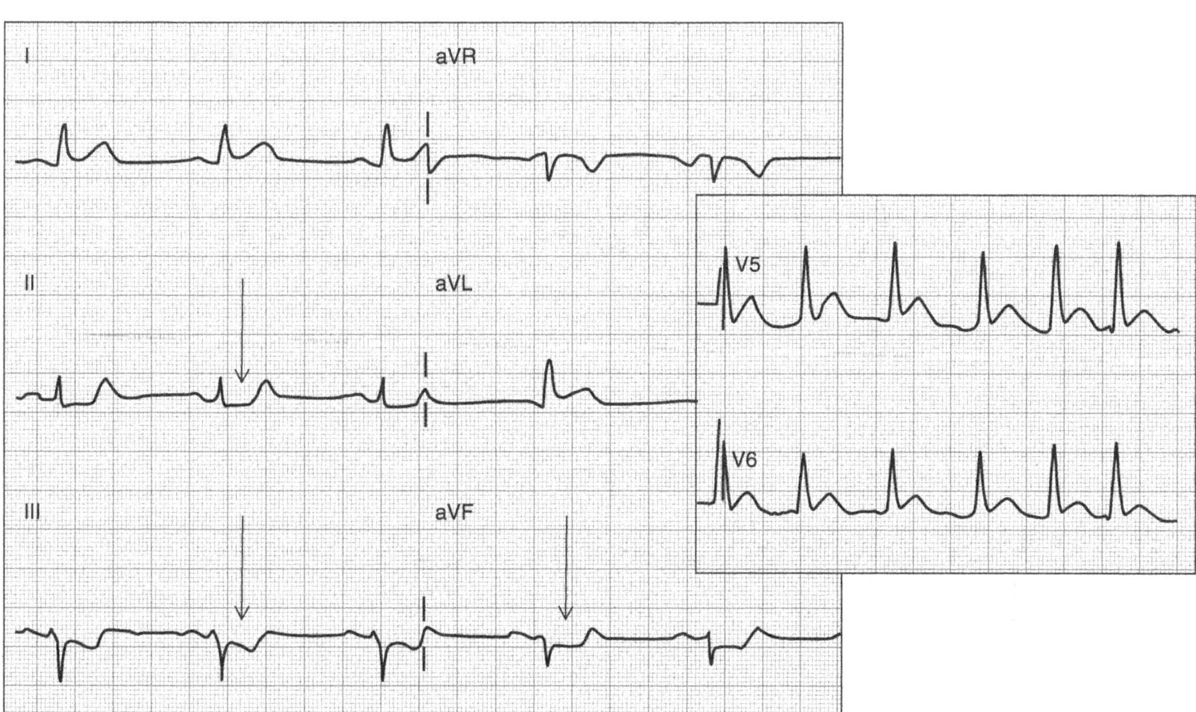

Figure 26.4 ST segment depression (arrows) in leads II, III, and aVF – reciprocal ST segment depression, also known as *reciprocal change*. Note the appearance of subtle ST segment elevation in leads I, aVL, V5, and V6, consistent with lateral wall STEMI. The presence of the reciprocal change in the inferior leads confirms the presence of the lateral STEMI.

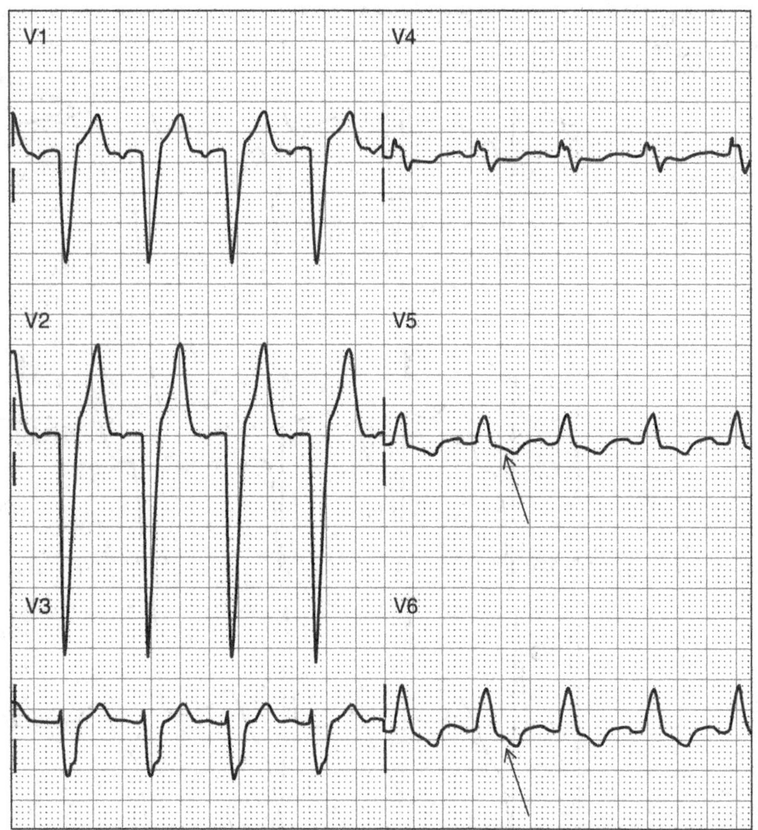

Figure 26.5 Normal appearing left bundle branch block pattern with anticipated – that is, normal for LBBB – ST segment depression (and T wave inversion) in leads V5 and V6 as noted by the arrows.

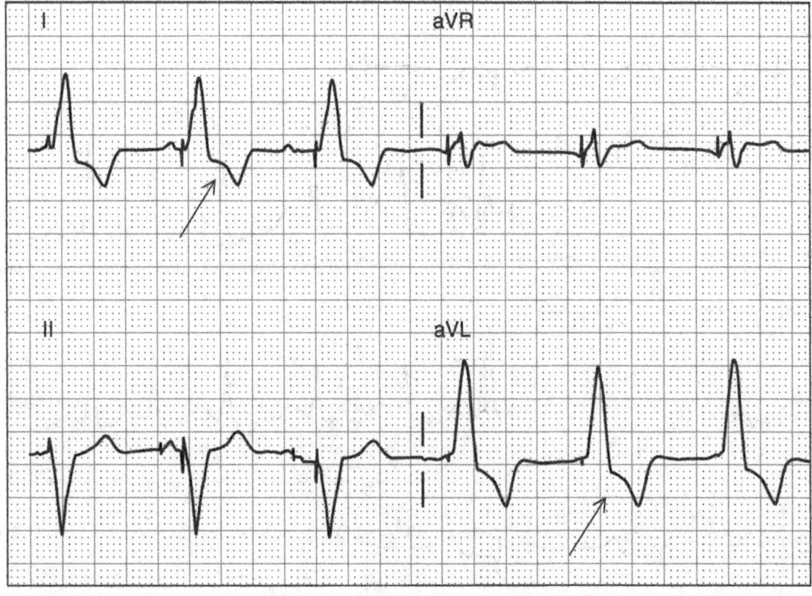

Figure 26.6 ST segment depression (with T wave inversion) indicated by the arrows in leads I and aVL as seen in patients with ventricular paced rhythms.

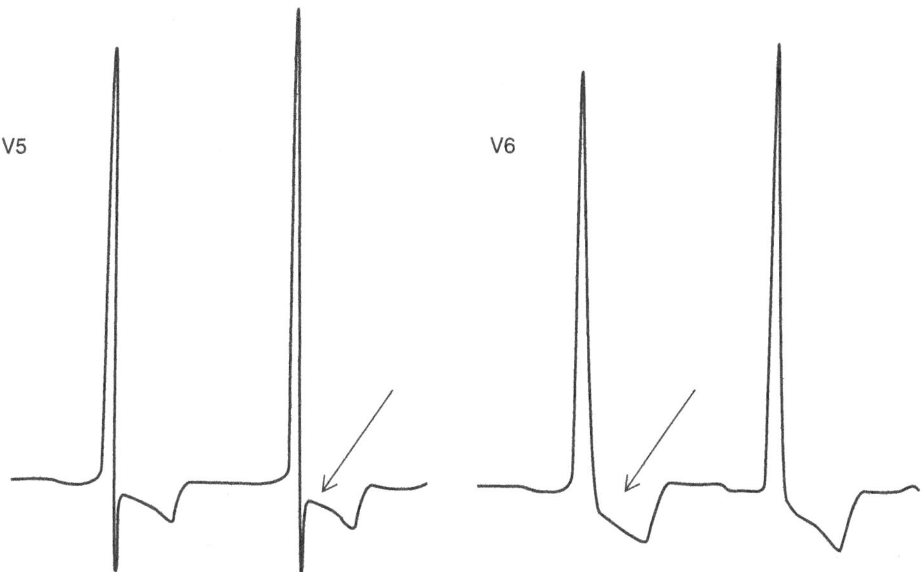

Figure 26.7 ST segment depression (with T wave inversion) as indicated by the arrows in leads V5 and V6 resulting from the left ventricular hypertrophy pattern with strain ("strain" = ST segment abnormality).

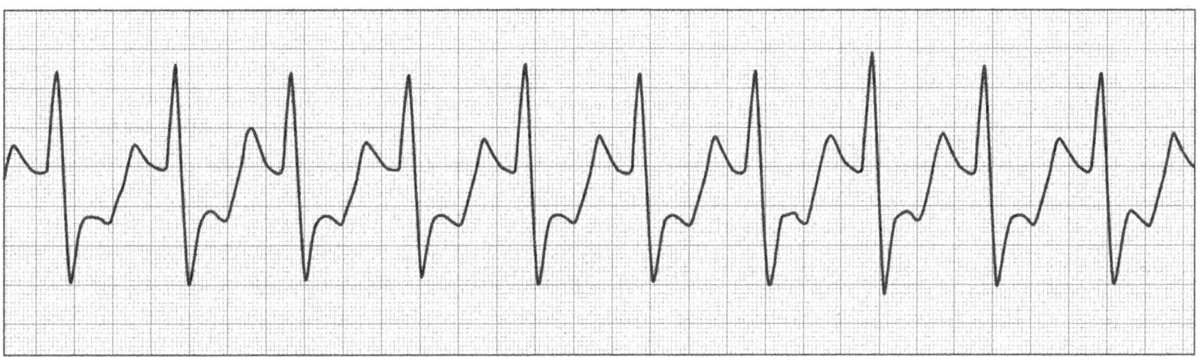

Figure 26.8 Rate-related ST segment depression in a patient with PSVT. This form of ST segment depression is not associated with ACS in most situations unless the clinical scenario suggests active ischemia or infarction.

Rate-Related ST Depression

ST segment depression may also be seen with tachycardia of supraventricular origin, such as paroxysmal supraventricular tachycardia (PSVT) and atrial fibrillation, particularly with rapid ventricular rates. In such a presentation, the ST segment depression does not necessarily indicate ischemia (Figure 26.8).

Other Causes

ST segment depression can also be seen in the following situations: therapeutic digoxin (the digoxin effect; Figure 26.9), hypothermia, hypokalemia, hyperkalemia, and cardiac contusion.

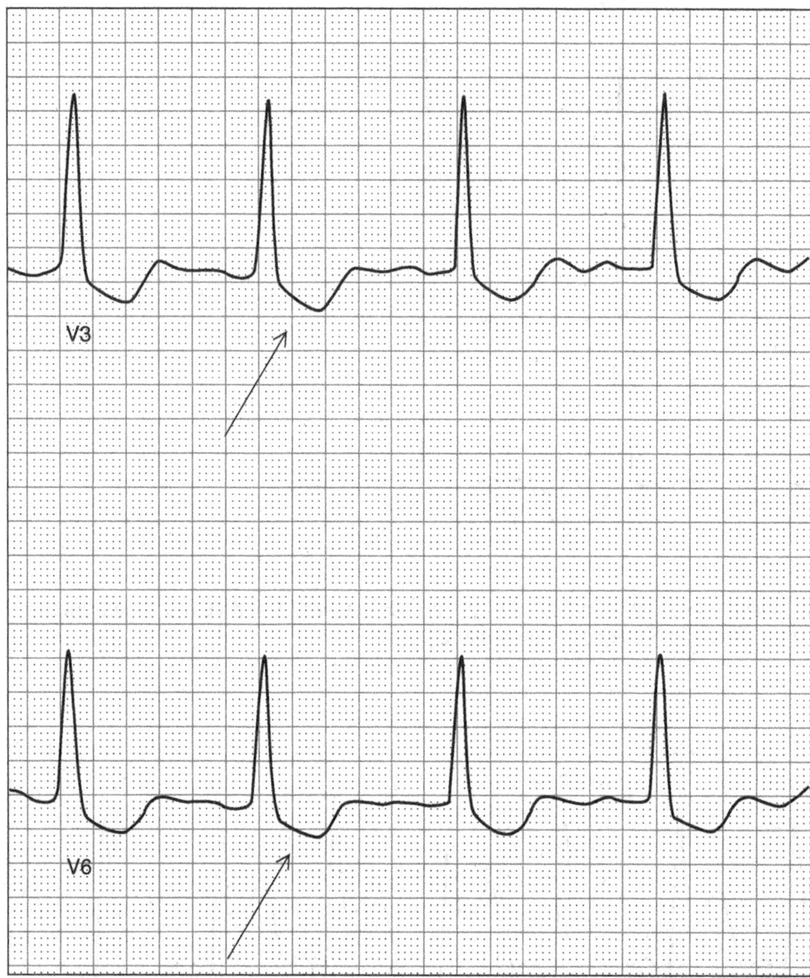

Figure 26.9 ST segment depression (arrows) resulting from the "digoxin effect."

27

Electrocardiographic Differential Diagnosis of T Wave Abnormalities: The Prominent T Wave and T Wave Inversions

Amita Sudhir[1] and William J. Brady[2]

[1] Department of Emergency Medicine, University of Virginia School of Medicine, Charlottesville, VA, USA
[2] Departments of Emergency Medicine and Medicine, University of Virginia School of Medicine, VA, Charlottesville, USA

Prominent T Waves

Hyperacute T waves of early ST segment elevation myocardial infarction: In the setting of an early ST segment elevation myocardial infarction (STEMI), one of the first ECG findings is the prominent, or hyperacute T wave. The hyperacute T wave is seen as early as 5 minutes after the onset of coronary occlusion; it will likely evolve into some form of ST segment elevation by 30 minutes of acute infarction. The T wave is asymmetric in morphology, broad based, and very tall (Figure 27.1). By asymmetric, it is meant that the T wave's upsloping limb is "less steep" compared to the downsloping portion. These T waves are most obvious in the anterior leads V1–V4. As the infarction progresses, the J point (juncture between the QRS complex and ST segment) will elevate along with the ST segment. In essence, the ST segment continues to elevate, producing a prominent form of ST segment elevation, in many cases termed the *giant R wave* or *tombstone ST segment elevation.*

Hyperkalemia: This potentially fatal electrolyte abnormality commonly presents with a number of ECG findings. Abnormalities of T wave are an early finding in this setting with the "peaked" T wave. The T wave of hyperkalemia is quite tall with a symmetric and narrow morphology (Figure 27.2).

Benign early repolarization: Benign early repolarization (BER) is a normal variant pattern that is not associated with any significant underlying cardiac pathology. BER is best known for ST segment elevation, yet also can present with large, prominent T waves. These T waves have a large amplitude and are slightly asymmetric in morphology (Figure 27.3). The T waves may appear "peaked," suggestive of the hyperacute T wave encountered in patients with STEMI. The T waves are concordant with the QRS complex (i.e. on the same side of the major portion of the QRS complex); they are best observed in the precordial leads V1–V4.

Acute pericarditis: In addition to diffuse ST segment elevation and PR segment depression, the ECG in pericarditis may demonstrate prominent T waves (Figure 27.4). These T waves are large in amplitude and broad based with asymmetric structure.

Left bundle branch block: In leads with a predominantly negative QRS, the T waves are likely to be large and upright (Figure 27.5). These T waves, especially in leads V1–V4, have a convex upward shape or a tall, vaulting appearance similar to the hyperacute T wave of early STEMI. The T waves are usually discordant with respect to the primary portion of the QRS complex – that is, the T wave is located on the opposite side of the baseline from the major portion of the QRS complex. Similar findings are noted with ventricular paced rhythms (Figure 27.6).

See Table 27.1.

T Wave Inversion

Normal T wave inversion: Inverted T waves are seen normally in leads III, aVL, aVR, and V1. Inverted T waves are also normal in children and adolescents in the precordial leads; at times, these T wave inversions

The Electrocardiogram in Emergency and Acute Care, First Edition.
Edited by Korin B. Hudson, Amita Sudhir, George Glass, and William J. Brady.

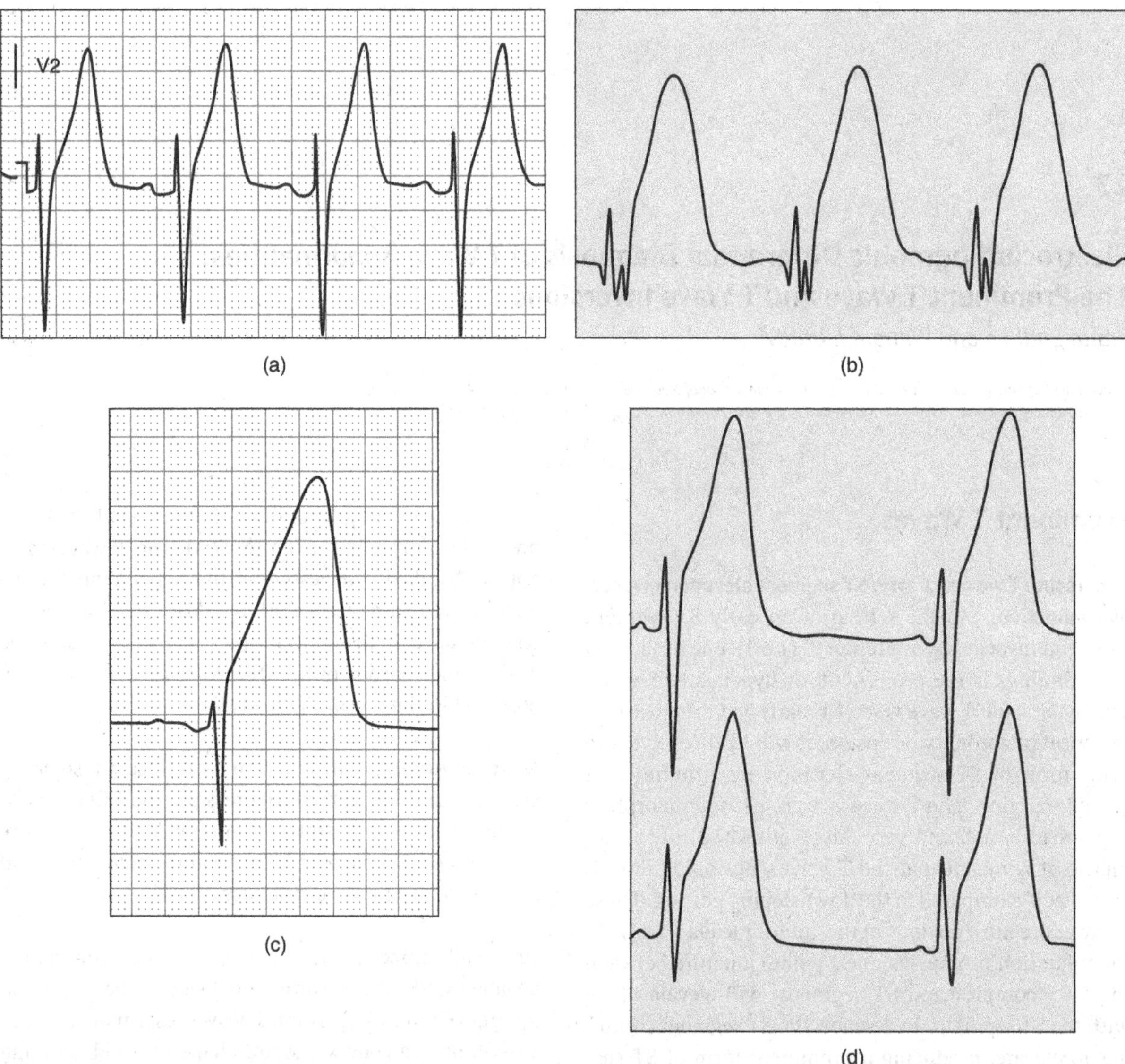

Figure 27.1 Hyperacute T waves of early STEMI. Note the tall appearance with wide base and asymmetric shape.

can persist into early adulthood, demonstrating the persistent juvenile T wave pattern.

Acute coronary syndrome: A concerning cause of T wave inversion is acute coronary syndrome (ACS). T wave inversion can be seen in an anatomic distribution with or without ST segment deviation (elevation or depression; Figures 27.7 and 27.8). T waves related to ACS are usually symmetric in shape with the downsloping and upsloping limbs similar in structure.

Wellen's syndrome: Wellen's syndrome is a constellation of clinical findings associated with critical stenosis of the proximal left anterior descending (LAD) coronary artery; the natural history of Wellen's syndrome is anterior wall myocardial infarction. The T wave abnormalities seen in Wellen's syndrome are quite striking (Figure 27.9). These T waves are present in two ways, including the deeply inverted T wave and the biphasic (both upright and inverted portions) T wave. The deeply inverted T waves are deep and symmetrically inverted. Such T waves are usually seen in the anterior leads V1–V4. Most often, the ST segments are normal. Interestingly, these T wave abnormalities can be seen in patients who are painfree; irrespective of whether the patient is pain free or experiencing discomfort, the risk of anterior wall STEMI remains the same.

Bundle branch block: With a left or right bundle branch block (BBB), any lead that has a positive QRS complex may demonstrate an asymmetric, wide, inverted T wave (Figure 27.10). These T wave inversions fuse with the ST

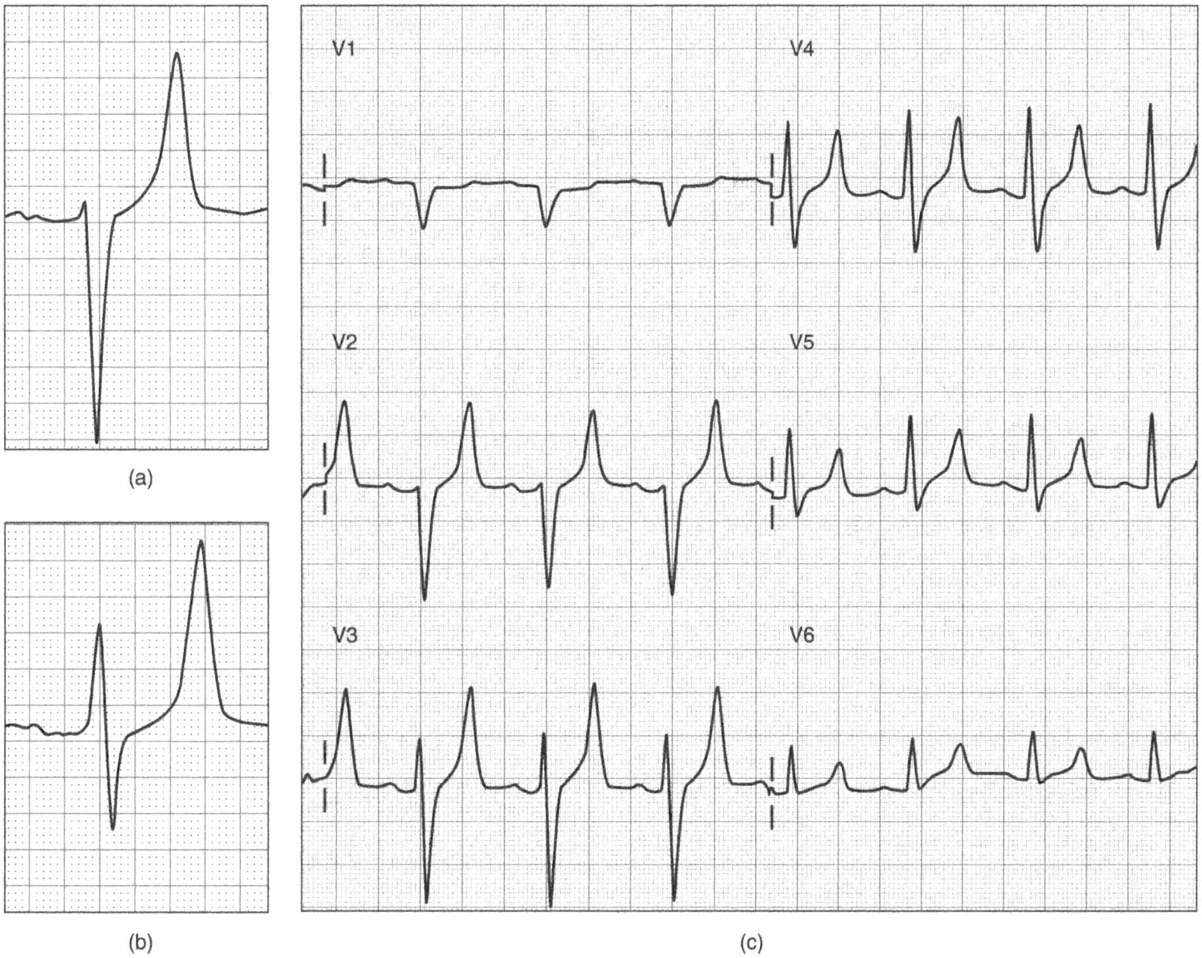

V1
V4
V2
V5
V3
V6

(a)

(b)

(c)

Figure 27.2 Prominent T waves of hyperkalemia. Note the tall appearance with narrow base and symmetric structure.

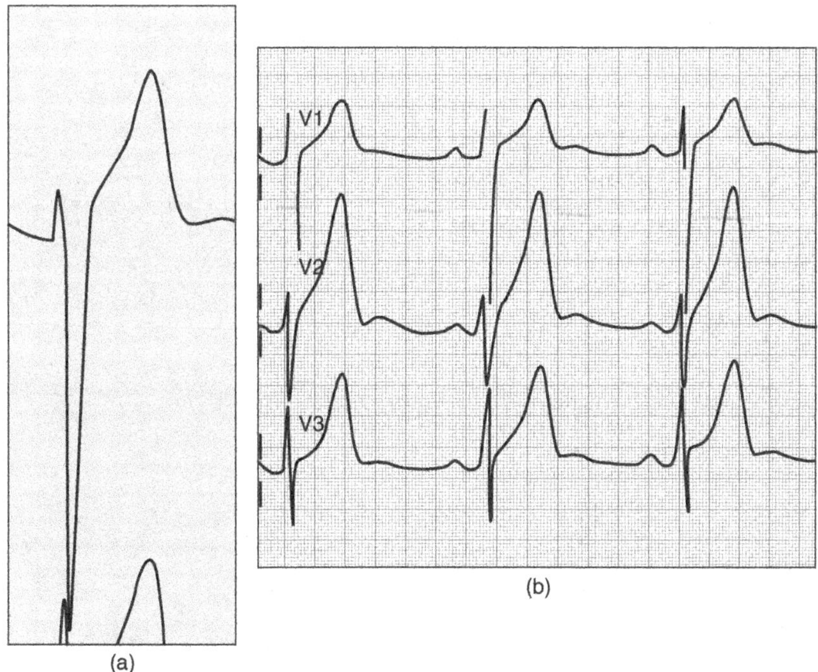

Figure 27.3 Prominent T waves of benign early repolarization.

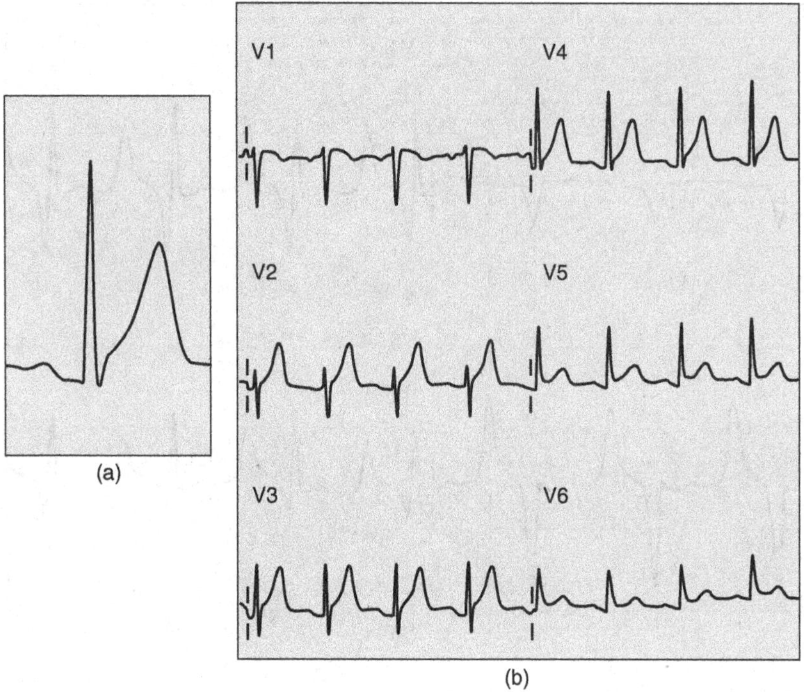

Figure 27.4 Prominent T waves of acute pericarditis.

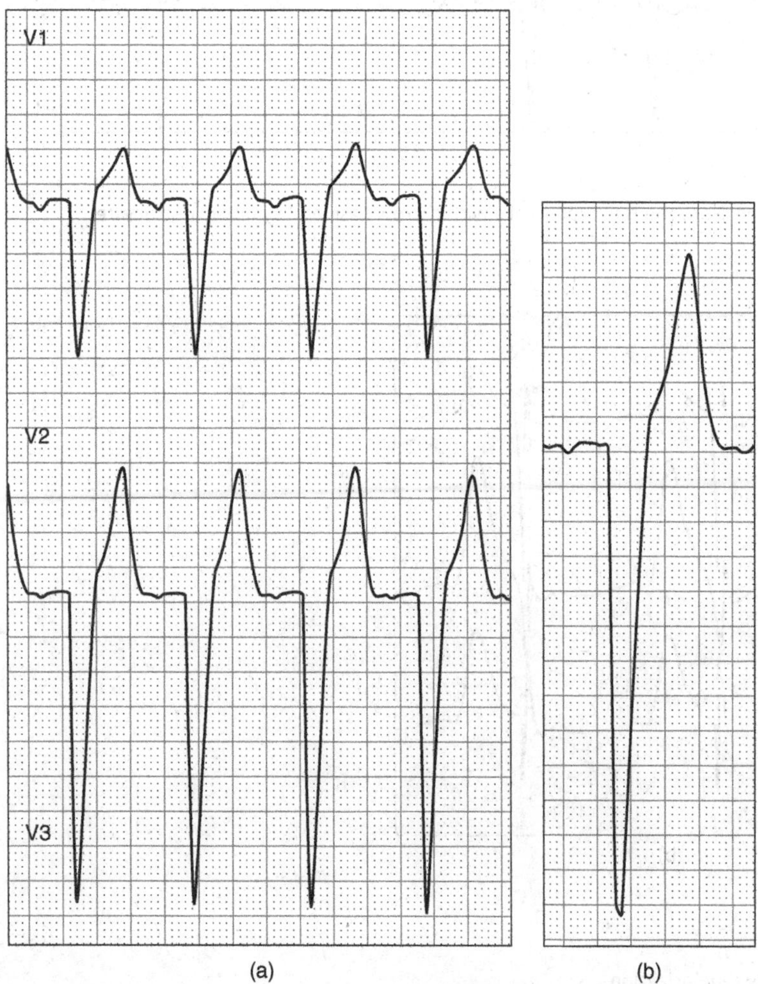

Figure 27.5 Prominent T waves of left bundle branch block.

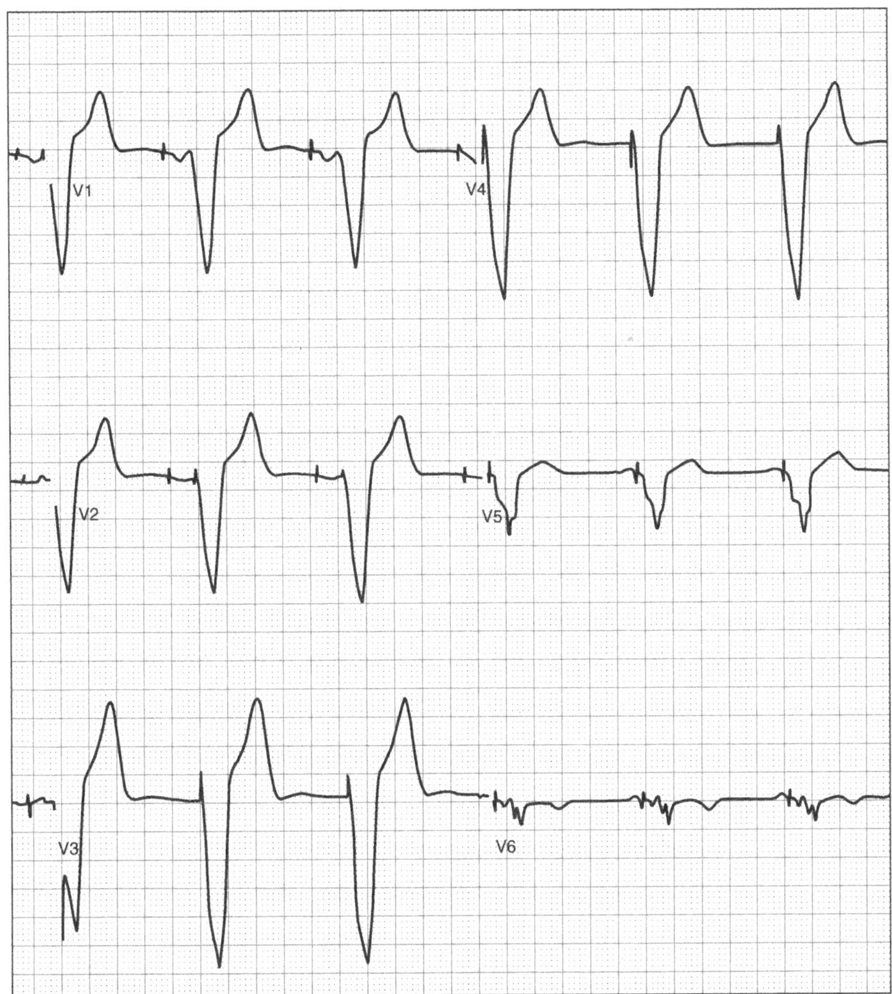

Figure 27.6 Prominent T waves of ventricular paced rhythm in leads V1–V4.

Table 27.1 Differential diagnosis of T wave abnormalities.

Prominent T waves
- Early STEMI
- Hyperkalemia
- Benign early repolarization
- Acute pericarditis
- Left bundle branch block
- Ventricular paced rhythm

Inverted T waves
- Normal T wave inversion
- Persistent juvenile T wave pattern
- Acute coronary syndrome
- Wellen's syndrome
- Bundle branch block
- Ventricular paced rhythm
- Left ventricular hypertrophy
- Digoxin effect
- CNS hemorrhage
- Pericarditis (resolving phase)
- Acute pulmonary embolism
- Wolff-Parkinson–White syndrome

segment, which is often depressed. Similar T wave inversion is seen in the ventricular paced pattern (Figure 27.11).

Left ventricular hypertrophy: The left ventricular pattern (left ventricular hypertrophy [LVH]) is most frequently associated with large QRS complexes and significant ST segment deviation (both elevation and depression). When ST segment and T wave abnormalities are present, the LVH pattern is said to have the strain component; the "strain" descriptor indicates that ST segment and T wave abnormalities are also present. The inverted T waves of the LVH strain pattern are frequently asymmetric in shape. These leads are frequently seen in leads I, aVL, V5, and V6 (Figure 27.12).

Other causes: Other causes of T wave inversion include digoxin therapy, central nervous system (CNS) injury (most often hemorrhage; Figure 27.13), pericarditis (resolving phase), acute pulmonary embolism, ventricular preexcitation syndromes (i.e. Wolff–Parkinson–White [WPW] syndrome), and various metabolic abnormalities.

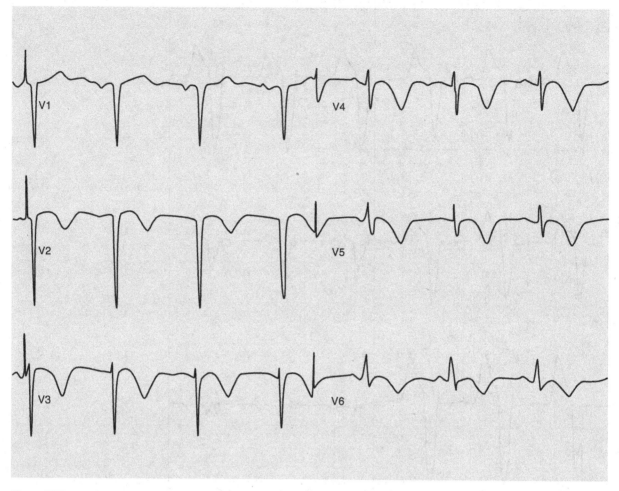

Figure 27.7 Inverted T waves of acute coronary syndrome. Note the symmetric nature of the inverted T waves in leads V2–V6.

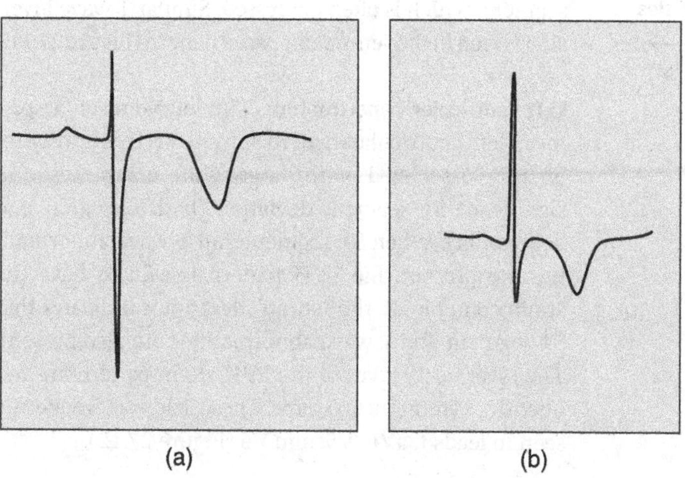

Figure 27.8 Inverted T waves of acute coronary syndrome.

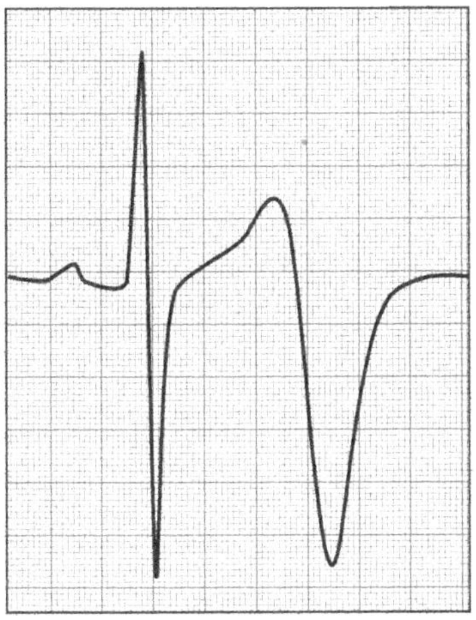

(a)

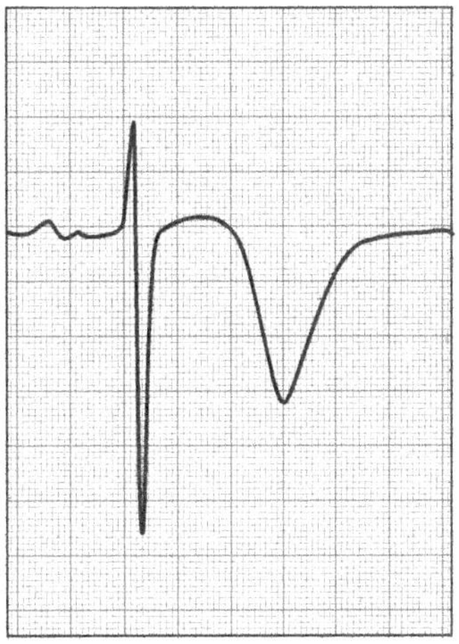

(b)

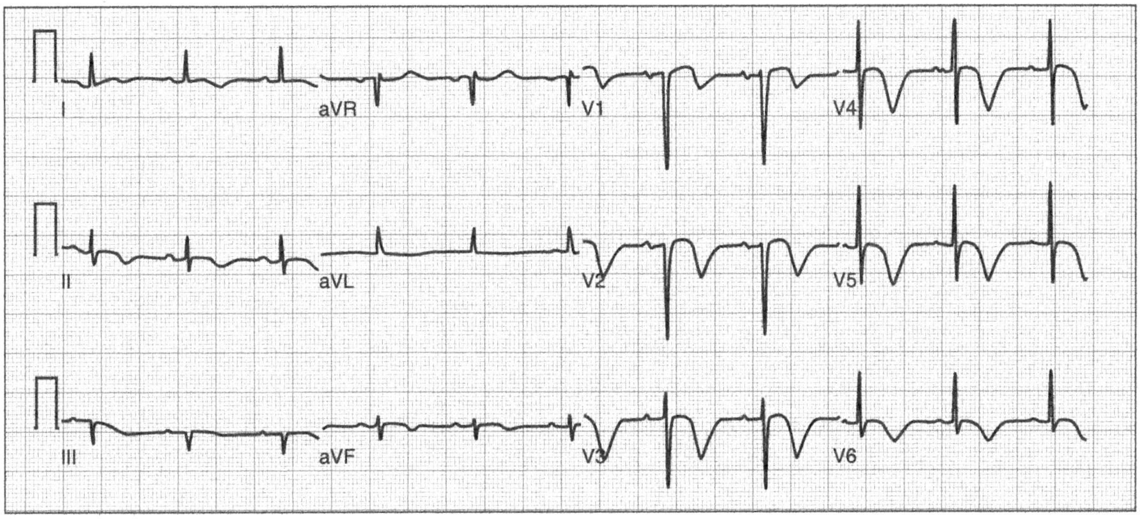

(c)

Figure 27.9 Inverted T waves of Wellen's syndrome. (a) Biphasic T wave (upright and inverted T wave in a single P-QRS-T complex). (b) Deeply inverted T wave. (c) Deeply inverted T waves in leads V1–V6, consistent with Wellen's syndrome.

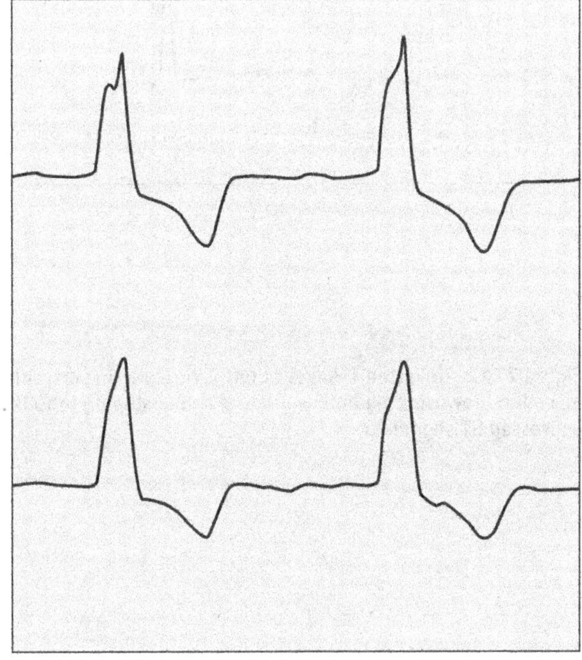

Figure 27.10 Inverted T waves of left bundle branch block pattern. Note the asymmetric nature of the T wave inversion (downsloping limb is gradual and upsloping limb is more abrupt) and blending of the inverted T wave with the depressed ST segment.

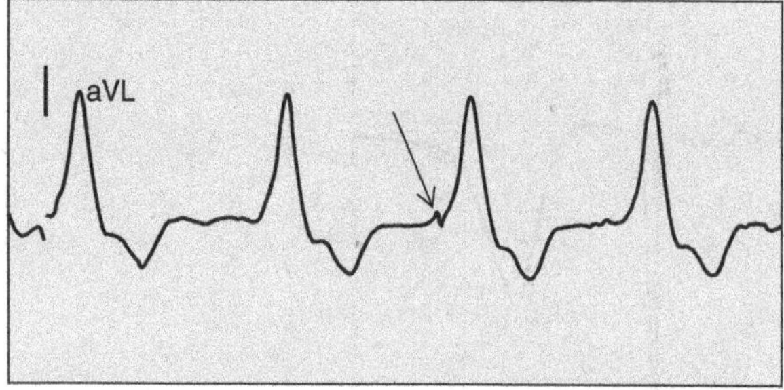

Figure 27.11 Inverted T waves of ventricular paced pattern. A small pacer spike (arrow) is noted preceding the third QRS complex. Note the asymmetric nature of the T wave inversion (downsloping limb is gradual and upsloping limb is more abrupt) and blending of the inverted T wave with the depressed ST segment.

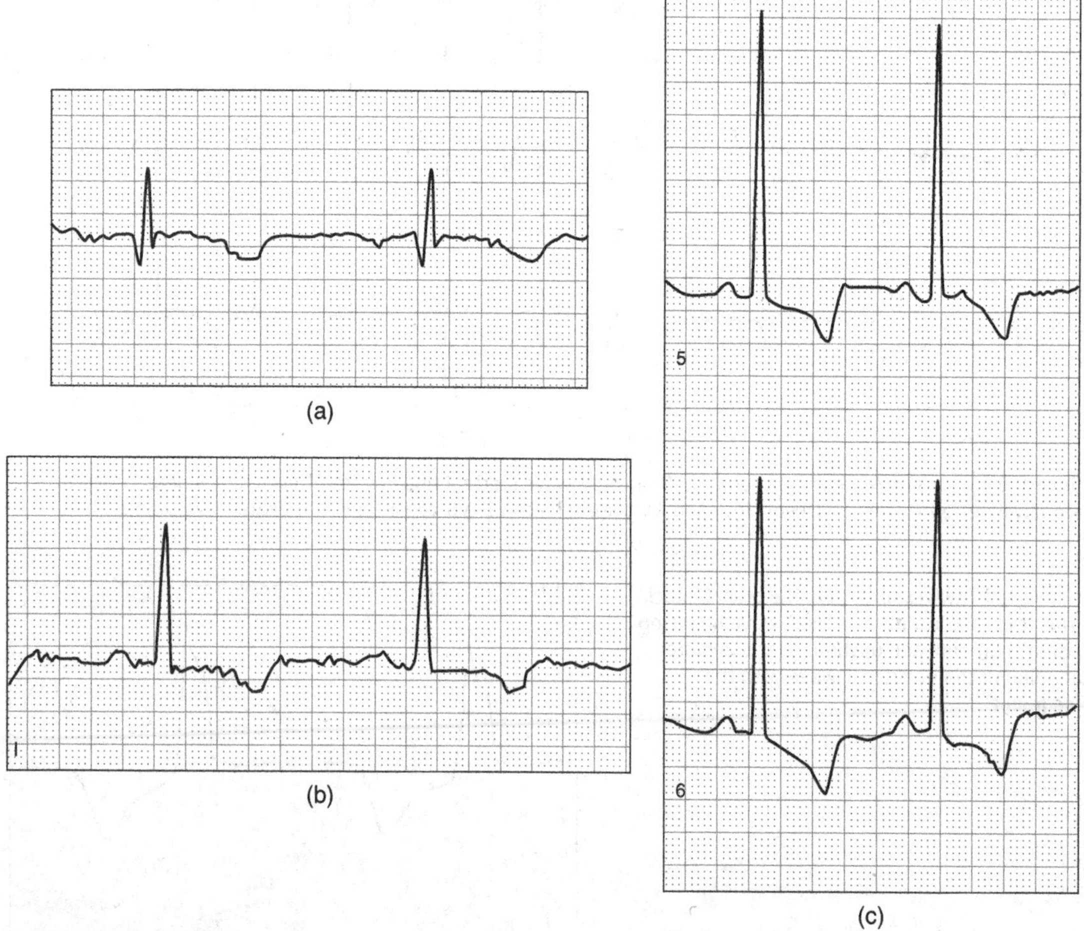

Figure 27.12 Inverted T waves of left ventricular hypertrophy with strain pattern. Note the asymmetric nature of the T wave inversion (downsloping limb is gradual and upsloping limb is more abrupt) and blending of the inverted T wave with the depressed ST segment.

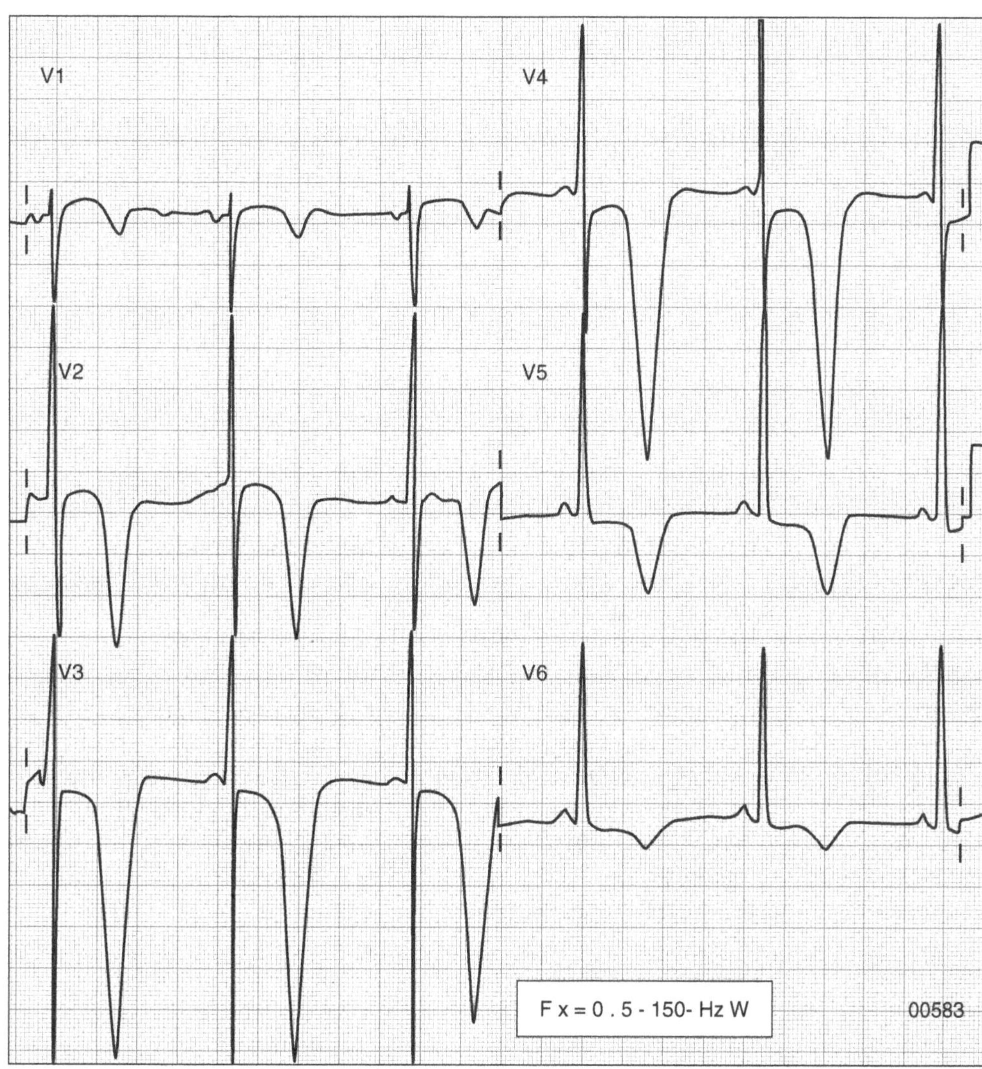

Figure 27.13 Deeply inverted T waves of CNS hemorrhage.

Index

Page locators in **bold** indicate tables. Page locators in *italics* indicate figures. This index uses letter-by-letter alphabetization.

The Electrocardiogram in Emergency and Acute Care, First Edition.
Edited by Korin B. Hudson, Amita Sudhir, George Glass, and William J. Brady.

q